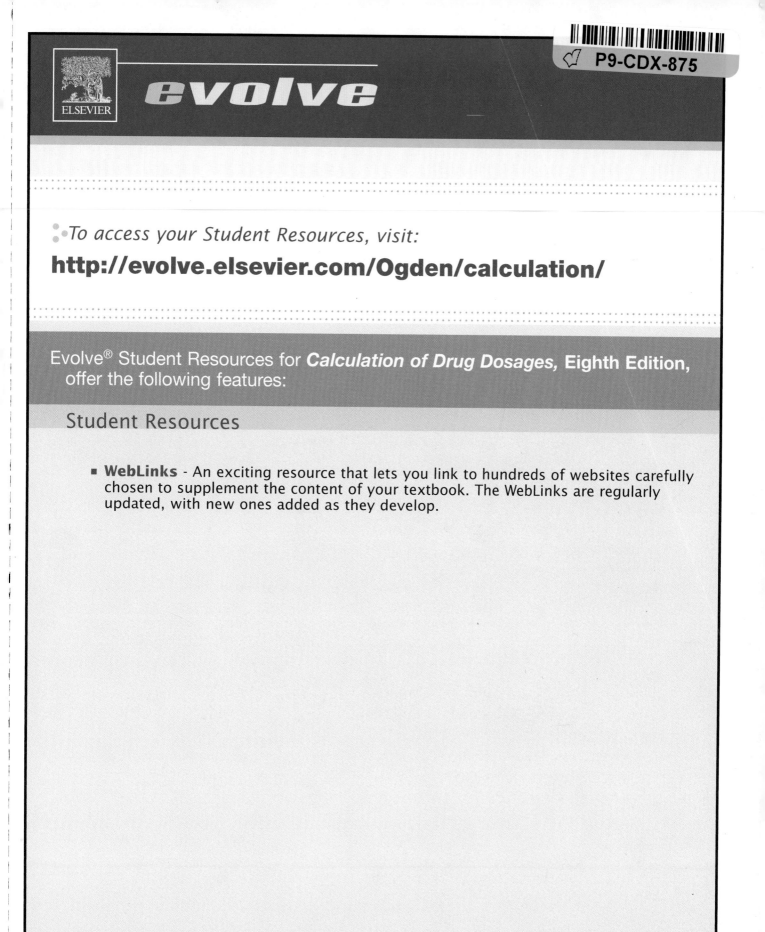

ELSEVIER

evolve

P9-CDX-875

:•*To access your Student Resources, visit:*

http://evolve.elsevier.com/Ogden/calculation/

Evolve® Student Resources for *Calculation of Drug Dosages,* **Eighth Edition,**
offer the following features:

Student Resources

- **WebLinks** - An exciting resource that lets you link to hundreds of websites carefully chosen to supplement the content of your textbook. The WebLinks are regularly updated, with new ones added as they develop.

CALCULATION OF DRUG DOSAGES

EIGHTH EDITION

Sheila J. Ogden, MSN, RN
Director, Orthopaedic Service Line
Clarian Health
Indianapolis, Indiana

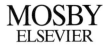

11830 Westline Industrial Drive
St. Louis, Missouri 63146

CALCULATION OF DRUG DOSAGES, EIGHTH EDITION

ISBN: 978-0-323-04588-9

NOTICE

Knowledge and best practice in this field are constantly changing. As new research and experience broaden our knowledge, changes in practice, treatment and drug therapy may become necessary or appropriate. Readers are advised to check the most current information provided (i) on procedures featured or (ii) by the manufacturer of each product to be administered, to verify the recommended dose or formula, the method and duration of administration, and contraindications. It is the responsibility of the practitioner, relying on his or her own experience and knowledge of the patient, to make diagnoses, to determine dosages and the best treatment for each individual patient, and to take all appropriate safety precautions. To the fullest extent of the law, neither the Publisher nor the Author assumes any liability for any injury and/or damage to persons or property arising out of or related to any use of the material contained in this book.

The Publisher

ISBN: 978-0-323-04588-9

Senior Editor: Yvonne Alexopoulos
Senior Developmental Editor: Danielle M. Frazier
Publishing Services Manager: Deborah L. Vogel
Senior Project Manager: Deon Lee
Senior Designer: Jyotika Shroff
Cover Designer: Jyotika Shroff

Printed in Canada

Last digit is the print number: 9 8 7 6 5 4 3 2 1

To
my husband and best friend, David,
for your patience, support, and love

S.J.O.

Contributors

Ruth Anne Burris, MBA, RN
Chief Quality Coordinator
Clarian Health
Indianapolis, Indiana

Linda K. Fluharty, MSN, RN
Associate Professor
ASN Program
Ivy Tech Community College
Indianapolis, Indiana

Mary Ann Reklau, MSN, RN, CPNP
ASN Program
Ivy Tech Community College
Indianapolis, Indiana

Reviewers

Dana Bartlett, RN, MSN, MA, CSPi
Specialist
Philadelphia Poison Control Center
Philadelphia, Pennsylvania

Lou Ann Boose, RN, BSN, MSN
Associate Professor of Nursing
Harrisburg Area Community College
Harrisburg, Pennsylvania

Margaret M. Gingrich, RN, MSN
Associate Professor
Harrisburg Area Community College
Harrisburg, Pennsylvania

April J. Schroer, MSN, RN, CS
Southwest Region Nursing Director
Texas Careers Vocational Nursing Program
Kaplan Higher Education Corporation
San Antonio, Texas

Amy Rine Wake, MSN, RN, BSN
Assistant Professor of Nursing
Jackson State Community College
Jackson, Tennessee

Robert S. Warner, MS, RN
Director of Nursing Program
Assistant Professor
Fulton-Montgomery Community College
Johnstown, NY

Preface to Instructors

This work text is designed for students in professional and vocational schools of nursing and for nurses returning to practice after being away from the clinical setting. It can be used in the classroom or for individual study. The work text contains an extensive review of basic mathematics to assist students who have not mastered the subject in previous educational experiences. It can also be used by those who have not attended school for a number of years and feel a lack of confidence in the area of mathematics computations.

ORGANIZATION OF MATERIAL

A pretest precedes each chapter in Parts I and II and may be used for evaluating present skills. For those students who are comfortable with basic mathematics, a quick assessment for each area will confirm their competency in the subject matter.

Part II begins with the use of the metric system, which is predominant in the medical field; the apothecary system continues to decline in use. However, in remembering that differences in practice exist throughout the United States and the world, it was felt that the content concerning the apothecary system should remain in the text. Still, the number of problems and amount of emphasis have remained reduced in this edition. These chapters remain separate because each system must be learned separately before it can be manipulated in conversions.

Part III helps students prepare for the actual calculation of drug dosages. Chapter 9 is a new chapter that discusses various points concerning patient safety as it relates to medication administration. This chapter also includes safety issues for the nurse in the dispensing of medications. The case scenarios really emphasize the importance of delivering the correct medication to the patient as ordered. Chapter 10 provides an emphasis on the interpretation of the physician's orders, and Chapter 11 explains how to read drug labels. This section ends with Chapter 12, in which dimensional analysis as a method to calculate drug dosages is introduced.

In Part IV, Chapters 13 to 15 introduce the proportion and alternative formula methods for the calculation of drug dosage problems. The actual drug labels have been updated and increased in number in all of the chapters dealing with the calculation of drug dosages. Also, content realted to dosages measured in units has been expanded. Because of the continued increased use of IV fluids in health care, Chapter 16, Intravenous Flow Rates, has again been expanded, as has Chapter 17, Critical Care Intravenous Flow Rates. Chapter 18, Pediatric Dosages, has been expanded and now includes pediatric IV flow rate problems as well.

Part V includes content concerning automated medication-dispensing systems. Chapter 20, on special considerations for the elderly, has been enhanced, as has Chapter 21, which discusses home care considerations. The student needs to remember that the actual calculation of drug dosages does vary based on the setting of the patient. Also, the administration and delivery may be affected by the age and location of the patient in the health care system.

The majority of the calculation problems relating to drug dosages continue to represent actual physicians' orders in various health care settings.

Features in the Eighth Edition

- **Learning objectives** are listed in the beginning of each chapter so that students will know the goals that must be achieved.
- Chapter **work sheets** provide the opportunity to practice solving realistic problems.
- Almost every chapter contains two **posttests** designed to evaluate the student's learning.
- A **comprehensive posttest** at the end of the book will help students assess their total understanding of the process of calculation of drug dosages.
- A **glossary** is included to define important terms.
- Numerous **full-color drug labels** continue to provide a more realistic representation of medication administration.
- NEW! **Chapter 9, Safety in Medication Administration,** has been added to address patient safety in regards to medication administration, as well as nurse safety while administering medications to patients.
- NEW! Eighteen **flash cards** have been included with this edition. They are perforated, which will allow students to divide the cards, perhaps laminate them, and place them on a binder ring and carry them in their pockets for easy access while on the clinical units. The cards contain abbreviations, computer time, temperature, as well as weights and measurements and their equivalents. Cards have also been included for most formulas to show the setup and calculation of drug dosages, IV flow rates, critical care medications, and pediatric drug dosages.

Ancillaries

Instructor's Electronic Resource for Calculation of Drug Dosages, **Eighth Edition.** Designed to enhance student instruction, this CD-ROM corresponds with the chapters of the text and includes the following:

- Suggested class schedules
- Chapter teaching strategies and tips
- Sample transparencies
- Test bank with over 175 questions

This resource is also available on the Evolve site at http://evolve.elsevier.com/Ogden/calculation/.

TEACH CD-ROM for Calculation of Drug Dosages, **Eighth Edition.** This resource is designed to help instructors reduce their lesson preparation time, give them new and creative ideas to promote student learning, and help them to make full use of the rich array of resources in the Ogden teaching package.

TEACH consists of customizable Lesson Plans and Lecture Outlines that are based on the learning objectives from the text. Provided for each book chapter, the lesson plans are divided into 50-minute lessons. These lesson plans include features such as teaching focus summaries, lesson preparation checklists, pretests and background assessment questions, critical thinking questions, and class activities. The lecture outlines are also available for each book chapter and include PowerPoint slides to provide visual presentation and summary of the main chapter points. Lecture notes for each slide highlight key topics and provide thought-provoking questions for discussion to help create an interactive classroom environment.

TEACH is also available online through Evolve at http://evolve.elsevier.com/Ogden/calculation/.

Romans & Daugherty Dosages and Solutions CTB, **Version II.** This generic computerized test bank has been completely updated and is provided as a gratis item to instructors upon adoption of this book. It contains more than 700 questions on general mathematics, converting within systems of measurement, oral dosages, parenteral dosages, flow rates, pediatric dosages, IV calculations, and more. This CTB is available online at the **Evolve** site at http://evolve.elsevier.com/Ogden/calculation/.

ACKNOWLEDGMENTS

I am grateful to the students and instructors who have chosen to use this book; I continue to learn so much from each of you. You have helped me understand the problems that students have with basic mathematics and with the calculation of drug dosages. I appreciate the physicians, nurses, pharmacists, and representatives of various health care agencies who took the time to discuss topics with me. I hope this book will provide readers with a feeling of confidence when working with a variety of mathematical problems.

I want to give special thanks to the reviewers of this text. Your sincere evaluation and critique played an integral part in the revision of this edition, and your attention to detail was most helpful.

I would also like to acknowledge Deon Lee, Danielle Frazier, and Yvonne Alexopoulos for their help and support during the writing of this eighth edition. Deon worked tirelessly to attain accuracy in all areas of the book. Her editing was thorough, helpful, and totally professional. Danielle supplied answers to many questions, pushed to meet deadlines, and offered her services as needed. She also remained calm and offered guidance during the entire revision process. Yvonne has been diligent in providing clarity on the needs of students, faculty, and hospitals as the scope and use of the book continue to grow.

Thank you all so much!

Sheila J. Ogden

Preface to Students

DESCRIPTION AND FEATURES

Calculation of Drug Dosages is an innovative drug calculation work text designed to provide you with a systematic review of mathematics and a simplified method of calculating drug dosages. It affords you the opportunity to move at a comfortable pace to ensure success. It includes information on the ratio and proportion, formula, and dimensional analysis methods of drug calculation, as well as numerous practice problems. Take a look at the following features so that you may familiarize yourself with this text and maximize its value.

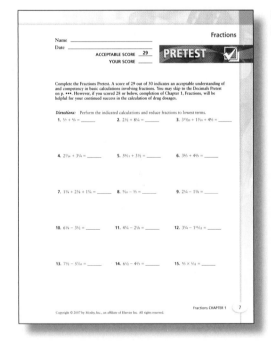

Pretests evaluate your present skills in utilizing mathematics, units, and measurements.

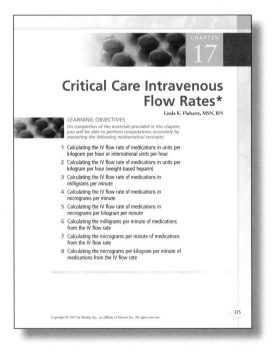

Learning Objectives highlight key content and goals that must be acheived.

Work Sheets provide you with the opportunity to practice solving realistic problems.

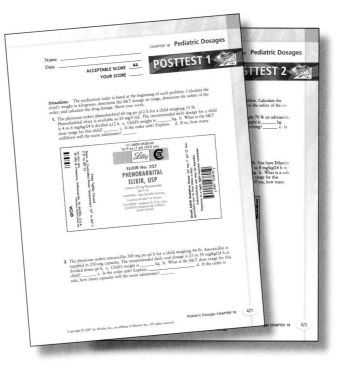

Posttests are designed to assess your learning and identify your strengths and weaknesses.

Drug Calculations Student CD-ROM, Version III. Completely updated, this user-friendly, interactive student tutorial has a brand new organization and design for easier navigation. It includes an extensive menu of various topic areas within drug calculations, such as oral, parenteral, pediatric, and IV calculations, to name a few. It includes animations and interactive exercises where students can fill in syringes to answer problems. Covering the ratio and proportion, formula, and dimensional analysis methods, this CD contains 565 practice problems including a comprehensive posttest. See the sample screen shots below:

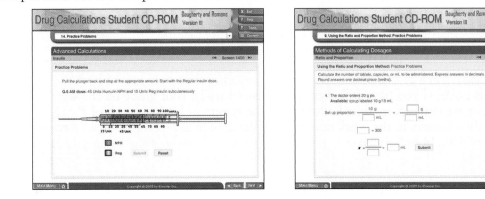

Here is an outline of the table of contents for the *Drug Calculations Student CD-ROM,* Version III:

Look for this icon at the ends of the chapters. It will refer you to the *Drug Calculations Student CD-ROM,* Version III for additional practice problems and content information.

USING THIS WORK TEXT

A pretest precedes each chapter in Parts I and II to assess previous learning. If your grade on the pretest is acceptable (an acceptable score is noted at the top of the test), you may continue to the next pretest. If your score on the pretest indicates a need for further study, read the introduction to the chapter, study the method of solving the problems, and complete the work sheet. If you have difficulty with a problem, refer to the examples in the introduction.

On completion of the work sheet, refer to the answer key in the back of the book to verify that your answers are correct. Rework all the incorrect problems to find your errors. It may be necessary to refer again to the examples in each chapter. Then proceed to the first posttest and grade the test. If your grade is acceptable, as indicated at the top of the test, continue to the next chapter. If your grade is less than acceptable, rework all incorrect problems to find your errors. Review as necessary before completing the second posttest. Again verify that your answers are correct. At this point, if you have followed the system of study, your grade on the second posttest should be more than acceptable. Follow the same system of study in each of the chapters.

When all the chapters in the work text are completed with acceptable scores (between 95% and 100%), you should be proficient in solving problems relating to drug dosages; more importantly, you will have completed the first step toward becoming a safe practitioner of medication administration.

On completion of the material provided in this work text, you will have mastered the following mathematical concepts, to be used for the accurate performance of computations:

1. Solving problems using fractions, decimals, percents, ratios, and proportions
2. Solving problems involving the apothecary, metric, and household systems of measurements
3. Solving problems measured in units and milliequivalents
4. Solving problems related to oral and parenteral dosages
5. Solving problems involving intravenous flow rates and critical care intravenous flow rates
6. Solving problems confirming the correct dosage of pediatric medications
7. Solving problems by using the proportion, formula, or dimensional analysis methods.

You are now ready to begin Chapter 1!

Contents

PART V
Drug Administration Considerations, 431

A solid knowledge base of general mathematics is necessary before you will be able to use these concepts in the more complicated calculations of drug dosages. It is this knowledge that allows for the safe administration of medications to your patients and prevents medication errors.

As you prepare to learn how to calculate drug dosages, an assessment of your current basic mathematics understanding and competency is essential. A general mathematics pretest is provided. Allow 1 to 2 hours in a quiet study area to complete the pretest without the use of a calculator. This is your opportunity to assess your true capability of performing basic math problems. Calculators are very useful tools. In some areas of health care, the use of a calculator is actually required to ensure accuracy in the delivery of medications. Follow the direction of your instructor as to the acceptable use of calculators while using this text on your path to safe administration of medications.

The pretest allows you to assess your need for a more extensive review. After completion of the test, check your answers with the key provided. A score of 95%, or 48 out of 50 problems correct, indicates a firm foundation in basic mathematics. You may then skip to Part II, Units and Measurements for the Calculation of Drug Dosages. However, a score of 47 or below indicates a need to review fraction, decimal, percent, ratio, and/or proportion calculations. Chapters 1 through 5 allow you to work on these basic mathematical skills at your leisure.

The pretest and review chapters are provided to ensure your success in the calculation and administration of your future patients' medications. Begin now, and good luck!

Name _____

Date _____

ACCEPTABLE SCORE ___48___

YOUR SCORE _____

PRETEST ☑

Directions: Perform the indicated computations. Reduce fractions to lowest terms.

1. $\frac{3}{8} + \frac{1}{3} =$ _____

2. $2\frac{3}{7} + 1\frac{2}{3} =$ _____

3. $1\frac{3}{5} + \frac{7}{8} / \frac{1}{3} =$ _____

4. $1.03 + 2.2 + 1.134 =$ _____

5. $1.479 + 28.68 + 4.5 =$ _____

6. $\frac{14}{15} - \frac{1}{6} =$ _____

7. $2\frac{1}{3} - \frac{1}{2} =$ _____

8. $2.04 - 0.987 =$ _____

9. $8.53 - 7.945 =$ _____

10. $3 \times \frac{4}{7} =$ _____

11. $2\frac{1}{2} \times 3\frac{3}{5} =$ _____

12. $0.315 \times 5.8 =$ _____

13. $4.884 \times 6.51 =$ _____

14. $\frac{3}{5} \div \frac{5}{6} =$ _____

15. $\frac{1}{150} \div \frac{1}{20} =$ _____

16. $2\frac{3}{4} \div 6\frac{2}{3} =$ _____

17. $241.73 \div 9.3 =$ _____

18. $128.24 \div 6 =$ _____

19. $22.67 \div 3.5 =$ _____

Directions: Circle the decimal fraction that has the *least* value.

20. 0.3, 0.03, 0.003

21. 0.9, 0.45, 0.66

22. 0.72, 0.721, 0.0072

23. 0.058, 0.1001, 0.07

Directions: Circle the decimal fraction that has the *greatest* value.

24. 0.1, 0.15, 0.155

25. 0.4, 0.8, 0.21

26. 0.249, 0.1587, 0.00633

27. 2.913, 2.99, 2.9

Directions: Change the following fractions to decimals.

28. $\frac{5}{8}$ = _____

29. $\frac{17}{25}$ = _____

Directions: Change the following decimals to fractions reduced to lowest terms.

30. 0.375 = _____

31. 0.05 = _____

Directions: Perform the indicated computations.

32. Express 0.432 as a percent.

33. Express 65% as a proper fraction and reduce to the lowest terms.

34. Express 0.3% as a ratio.

35. What percent of 2.5 is 0.5?

36. What is $\frac{1}{4}$% of 60?

37. What is 65% of 450?

Directions: Change the following fractions and decimals to ratios reduced to lowest terms.

38. $^9/_{42} =$ _____

39. $1\frac{1}{2}/2\frac{2}{3} =$ _____

40. $0.34 =$ _____

Directions: Find the value of x.

41. $7 : ^7/_{100} :: x : 4$

42. $x : 40 :: 7 : 56$

43. $2.5 : 6 :: 10 : x$

44. $x : \frac{1}{4}\% :: 9.6 : \frac{1}{300}$

45. $^1/_{150} : ^1/_{100} :: x : 30$

46. $0.10 : 0.20 :: x : 200$

47. $\frac{1}{200} : \frac{1}{40} :: 100 : x$

48. $x : 85 :: 6 : 10$

49. $^1/_{20}/^1/_5 : 5 :: x : 50$

50. $100 : 5 :: x : 3.4$

Answers on p. 471.

Name _____

Date _____

ACCEPTABLE SCORE ___29___

YOUR SCORE _____

PRETEST ✓

Complete the Fractions Pretest. A score of 29 out of 30 indicates an acceptable understanding of and competency in basic calculations involving fractions. You may skip to the Decimals Pretest on p. 29. However, if you scored 28 or below, completion of Chapter 1, Fractions, will be helpful for your continued success in the calculation of drug dosages.

Directions: Perform the indicated calculations and reduce fractions to lowest terms.

1. $5/7 + 4/9 =$ _____

2. $2\frac{1}{2} + 8\frac{1}{6} =$ _____

3. $3\frac{13}{20} + 1\frac{3}{10} + 4\frac{4}{5} =$ _____

4. $2\frac{5}{16} + 3\frac{1}{4} =$ _____

5. $5\frac{6}{11} + 3\frac{1}{2} =$ _____

6. $3\frac{2}{3} + 4\frac{2}{9} =$ _____

7. $1\frac{3}{4} + 2\frac{3}{8} + 1\frac{5}{6} =$ _____

8. $9/10 - 3/5 =$ _____

9. $2\frac{1}{4} - 1\frac{3}{8} =$ _____

10. $6\frac{1}{8} - 3\frac{1}{2} =$ _____

11. $4\frac{5}{6} - 2\frac{1}{8} =$ _____

12. $3\frac{3}{4} - 1\frac{11}{12} =$ _____

13. $7\frac{1}{2} - 5\frac{7}{10} =$ _____

14. $6\frac{1}{2} - 4\frac{2}{3} =$ _____

15. $4/5 \times 1/12 =$ _____

16. $1\frac{1}{3} \times 3\frac{3}{4} =$ _____

17. $3\frac{2}{7} \times 2\frac{2}{9} =$ _____

18. $\frac{5}{8} \times 1\frac{5}{7} =$ _____

19. $\frac{1}{1000} \times \frac{1}{10} =$ _____

20. $2\frac{4}{9} \times 1\frac{3}{4} =$ _____

21. $4\frac{1}{6} \times 2\frac{9}{10} =$ _____

22. $1\frac{1}{8} \times 2\frac{4}{7} =$ _____

23. $\frac{1}{4} \div \frac{4}{5} =$ _____

24. $2\frac{1}{6} \div 1\frac{5}{8} =$ _____

25. $\frac{1}{3} \div \frac{1}{100} =$ _____

26. $1\frac{3}{4} \div 2 =$ _____

27. $\frac{4}{5} / \frac{3}{5} =$ _____

28. $\frac{1}{3} / \frac{3}{5} =$ _____

29. $2\frac{5}{6} / 1\frac{2}{3} =$ _____

30. $4\frac{1}{2} / 2\frac{1}{4} =$ _____

Answers on p. 471.

CHAPTER 1 Fractions

Fractions

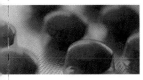

LEARNING OBJECTIVES

On completion of the materials provided in this chapter, you will be able to perform computations accurately by mastering the following mathematical concepts:

1 Changing an improper fraction to a mixed number

2 Changing a mixed number to an improper fraction

3 Changing a fraction to an equivalent fraction with the lowest common denominator

4 Changing a mixed number to an equivalent fraction with the lowest common denominator

5 Adding fractions having the same denominator, having unlike denominators, or involving whole numbers and unlike denominators

6 Subtracting fractions having the same denominator, having unlike denominators, or involving whole numbers and unlike denominators

7 Multiplying fractions and mixed numbers

8 Dividing fractions and mixed numbers

9 Reducing a complex fraction

10 Reducing a complex fraction involving mixed numbers

Study the introductory material for fractions. The processes for the calculation of fraction problems are listed in steps. Memorize the steps for each type of calculation before beginning the work sheet. Complete the work sheet at the end of this chapter, which provides extensive practice in the manipulation of fractions. Check your answers. If you have difficulties, go back and review the steps for that type of calculation. When you feel ready to evaluate your learning, take the first posttest. Check your answers. An acceptable score (number of answers correct) as indicated on the posttest signifies that you are ready for the next chapter. An unacceptable score signifies a need for further study before you take the second posttest.

A **fraction** indicates the number of equal parts of a whole. For example, ¾ means three of four equal parts.

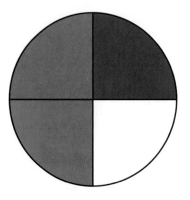

The **denominator** indicates the number of parts into which a whole has been divided. The denominator is the number *below* the fraction line. The **numerator** designates the number of parts that you have of a divided whole. It is the number *above* the fraction line. The line also indicates division to be performed and can be read as "divided by." The example ¾, or three fourths, can therefore be read as "three divided by four." In other words the numerator is "divided by" the denominator. The numerator is the **dividend,** and the denominator is the **divisor.** When numbers are multiplied, the answer is the **product.** When numbers are divided, the answer is the **quotient.**

A fraction can often be expressed in smaller numbers without any change in its real value. This is what is meant by the direction "Reduce to lowest terms." The reduction is accomplished by dividing both numerator and denominator by the same number.

Example 1: ⁶⁄₈

    a. $6 \div 2 = 3$

    b. $8 \div 2 = 4$

    c. $\dfrac{6}{8} = \dfrac{3}{4}$

Example 2: ³⁄₉

    a. $3 \div 3 = 1$

    b. $9 \div 3 = 3$

    c. $\dfrac{3}{9} = \dfrac{1}{3}$

Example 3: ⁴⁄₁₀

    a. $4 \div 2 = 2$

    b. $10 \div 2 = 5$

    c. $\dfrac{4}{10} = \dfrac{2}{5}$

There are several different types of fractions. A **proper fraction** is one in which the numerator is smaller than the denominator. A proper fraction is sometimes called a *common* or *simple fraction.*

Examples: ⅔, ⅛, ⁵⁄₁₂

An **improper fraction** is a fraction in which the numerator is larger than or equal to the denominator.

Examples: ⁸⁄₇, ⁶⁄₆, ⁴⁄₂

A **complex fraction** is one that contains a fraction in its numerator, its denominator, or both.

Examples: 2⅓/3, 2/½, ¾/⅜

Sometimes a fraction is seen in conjunction with a whole number. This combination is called a **mixed number.**

Examples: 2⅜, 4⅓, 6½

IMPROPER FRACTIONS

Changing an Improper Fraction to a Mixed Number

1. Divide the numerator by the denominator.
2. Place any remainder over the denominator and write this proper fraction beside the whole number found in step 1.

Example 1: $5/3$

a. $3\overline{)5} \quad 1 \text{ remainder } 2 = 1\dfrac{2}{3}$
   $\quad\ \underline{3}$
b. $\quad\ \dfrac{3}{2}$

Example 2: $7/2$

a. $2\overline{)7} \quad 3 \text{ remainder } 1 = 3\dfrac{1}{2}$
   $\quad\ \underline{6}$
b. $\quad\ \dfrac{6}{1}$

When an improper fraction is reduced, it will *always* result in a mixed number or a whole number.

Changing a Mixed Number to an Improper Fraction

1. Multiply the denominator of the fraction by the whole number.
2. Add the product to the numerator of the fraction.
3. Place the sum over the denominator.

Example 1: $3\frac{1}{4}$

a. $4 \times 3 = 12$

b. $12 + 1 = 13$

c. $3\dfrac{1}{4} = \dfrac{13}{4}$

Example 2: $1\frac{3}{8}$

a. $8 \times 1 = 8$

b. $8 + 3 = 11$

c. $1\dfrac{3}{8} = \dfrac{11}{8}$

Example 3: $2\frac{7}{10}$

a. $10 \times 2 = 20$

b. $20 + 7 = 27$

c. $2\dfrac{7}{10} = \dfrac{27}{10}$

If fractions are to be added or subtracted, it is necessary for their *denominators to be the same.*

LOWEST COMMON DENOMINATOR

Computations are facilitated when the lowest common denominator is used. The term **lowest common denominator** is defined as the smallest whole number that can be divided evenly by all denominators within the problem.

When trying to determine the lowest common denominator, first observe whether one of the denominators in the problem is evenly divisible by each of the other denominators. If so, this will be the lowest common denominator for the problem.

Example 1: $2/3$ and $5/12$
You find that 12 is evenly divisible by 3; therefore 12 is the lowest common denominator.

Example 2: $1/2$ and $3/8$
You find that 8 is evenly divisible by 2; therefore 8 is the lowest common denominator.

Example 3: $2/7$ and $5/14$ and $1/28$
You find that 28 is evenly divisible by 7 and 14; therefore 28 is the lowest common denominator.

Changing a Fraction to an Equivalent Fraction with the Lowest Common Denominator

1. Divide the lowest common denominator by the denominator of the fraction to be changed.
2. Multiply the quotient by the numerator of the fraction to be changed.
3. Place the product over the lowest common denominator.

Example 1: $2/3 = ?/12$

   a. $12 \div 3 = 4$

   b. $4 \times 2 = 8$

   c. $\dfrac{2}{3} = \dfrac{8}{12}$

Example 2: $1/2 = ?/8$

   a. $8 \div 2 = 4$

   b. $4 \times 1 = 4$

   c. $\dfrac{1}{2} = \dfrac{4}{8}$

Example 3: $2/7 = ?/14$

   a. $14 \div 7 = 2$

   b. $2 \times 2 = 4$

   c. $\dfrac{2}{7} = \dfrac{4}{14}$

Changing a Mixed Number to an Equivalent Fraction with the Lowest Common Denominator

1. Change the mixed number to an improper fraction.
2. Divide the lowest common denominator by the denominator of the fraction.
3. Multiply the quotient by the numerator of the improper fraction.
4. Place the product over the lowest common denominator.

Example 1: $1 3/4$ and $5/12$

   a. $1\dfrac{3}{4} = \dfrac{?}{12}$

      $4 \times 1 = 4$

      $4 + 3 = 7$

   b. $\dfrac{7}{4} = \dfrac{?}{12}$

      $12 \div 4 = 3$

   c. $3 \times 7 = 21$

   d. $1\dfrac{3}{4} = \dfrac{21}{12}$

Example 2: $3 2/3$ and $4/9$

   a. $3\dfrac{2}{3} = \dfrac{?}{9}$

      $3 \times 3 = 9$

      $9 + 2 = 11$

   b. $\dfrac{11}{3} = \dfrac{?}{9}$

      $9 \div 3 = 3$

   c. $3 \times 11 = 33$

   d. $3\dfrac{2}{3} = \dfrac{33}{9}$

    If one of the denominators in the problem is not the lowest common denominator for all, you must look further. One suggestion is to multiply two of the denominators together and if possible use that number as the lowest common denominator.

Example: 3½ and ⅔
Multiply the two denominators: $2 \times 3 = 6$

a. $3\dfrac{1}{2} = \dfrac{?}{6}$

$2 \times 3 = 6$

$6 + 1 = 7$

b. $\dfrac{7}{2} = \dfrac{?}{6}$

c. $6 \div 2 = 3$

d. $3 \times 7 = 21$

e. $3\dfrac{1}{2} = \dfrac{21}{6}$

a. $\dfrac{2}{3} = \dfrac{?}{6}$

b. $6 \div 3 = 2$

c. $2 \times 2 = 4$

d. $\dfrac{2}{3} = \dfrac{4}{6}$

Another method is to multiply one of the denominators by 2, 3, or 4. Determine whether the resulting number can be used as a common denominator.

Example: ¾ and ⅛ and 5⁄12
Multiply the denominator 8 by 3: $8 \times 3 = 24$

a. $\dfrac{3}{4} = \dfrac{?}{24}$

b. $24 \div 4 = 6$

c. $6 \times 3 = 18$

d. $\dfrac{3}{4} = \dfrac{18}{24}$

a. $\dfrac{1}{8} = \dfrac{?}{24}$

b. $24 \div 8 = 3$

c. $3 \times 1 = 3$

d. $\dfrac{1}{8} = \dfrac{3}{24}$

a. $\dfrac{5}{12} = \dfrac{?}{24}$

b. $24 \div 12 = 2$

c. $2 \times 5 = 10$

d. $\dfrac{5}{12} = \dfrac{10}{24}$

ADDITION OF FRACTIONS

Addition of Fractions Having the Same Denominator

1. Add the numerators.
2. Place the sum over the common denominator.
3. Reduce to lowest terms.

Example 1: ⅐ + 2⁄7 = _____

a. $\dfrac{1}{7} + \dfrac{2}{7} =$

b. $\dfrac{1+2}{7} =$

c. $\dfrac{3}{7}$

Example 2: ⅛ + 3⁄8 = _____

a. $\dfrac{1}{8} + \dfrac{3}{8} =$

b. $\dfrac{1+3}{8} =$

c. $\dfrac{4}{8} = \dfrac{1}{2}$

Addition of Fractions with Unlike Denominators

1. Change the fractions to equivalent fractions with the lowest common denominator.
2. Add the numerators.
3. Place the sum over the lowest common denominator.
4. Reduce to lowest terms.

Example 1: $\frac{2}{3} + \frac{1}{5} =$ _____

To find the lowest common denominator, multiply the two denominators together.

$$3 \times 5 = 15$$

Change each fraction to an equivalent fraction with 15 as the denominator.

a. $\dfrac{2}{3} = \dfrac{?}{15}$

$15 \div 3 = 5$

$5 \times 2 = 10$

$\dfrac{2}{3} = \dfrac{10}{15}$

a. $\dfrac{1}{5} = \dfrac{?}{15}$

$15 \div 5 = 3$

$3 \times 1 = 3$

$\dfrac{1}{5} = \dfrac{3}{15}$

b. $\dfrac{10}{15} + \dfrac{3}{15} =$

c. $\dfrac{10+3}{15} = \dfrac{13}{15}$

Example 2: $\frac{1}{6} + \frac{1}{4} + \frac{1}{3} =$ _____

To find a common denominator, try multiplying two of the denominators together and check to see whether that number is divisible by the other denominator.

$$4 \times 3 = 12$$

Is 12 divisible by the other denominator, 6? The answer is YES.

a. $\dfrac{1}{6} = \dfrac{?}{12}$

$12 \div 6 = 2$

$2 \times 1 = 2$

$\dfrac{1}{6} = \dfrac{2}{12}$

a. $\dfrac{1}{4} = \dfrac{?}{12}$

$12 \div 4 = 3$

$3 \times 1 = 3$

$\dfrac{1}{4} = \dfrac{3}{12}$

a. $\dfrac{1}{3} = \dfrac{?}{12}$

$12 \div 3 = 4$

$4 \times 1 = 4$

$\dfrac{1}{3} = \dfrac{4}{12}$

b. $\dfrac{2}{12} + \dfrac{3}{12} + \dfrac{4}{12} =$

c. $\dfrac{2+3+4}{12} = \dfrac{9}{12}$

d. $\dfrac{9}{12} = \dfrac{3}{4}$ (reduced to lowest terms)

Addition of Fractions Involving Whole Numbers and Unlike Denominators

1. Change the fractions to equivalent fractions with the lowest common denominator.
2. Add the numerators.
3. Place the sum over the lowest common denominator.
4. Reduce to lowest terms.
5. Write the reduced fraction next to the sum of the whole numbers.

Example 1: $1\frac{1}{3} + 2\frac{3}{8} =$ _____

To find the lowest common denominator, multiply the two denominators together.

$$3 \times 8 = 24$$

Change the fractions $\frac{1}{3}$ and $\frac{3}{8}$ to equivalent fractions with 24 as their denominators.

a. $\frac{1}{3} = \frac{?}{24}$ 　　　　　　　　　　　a. $\frac{3}{8} = \frac{?}{24}$

$24 \div 3 = 8$ 　　　　　　　　　　　$24 \div 8 = 3$

$8 \times 1 = 8$ 　　　　　　　　　　　$3 \times 3 = 9$

$\frac{1}{3} = \frac{8}{24}$ 　　　　　　　　　　　$\frac{3}{8} = \frac{9}{24}$

b. $1\frac{8}{24} + 2\frac{9}{24} =$

c. $1\frac{8}{24}$

$+2\frac{9}{24}$

d. $3\frac{17}{24}$

Example 2: $5\frac{1}{2} + 3\frac{3}{10} =$ _____

Because 10 is evenly divisible by 2, 10 is the lowest common denominator. Therefore $\frac{1}{2}$ needs to be changed to an equivalent fraction with 10 as the denominator.

a. $\frac{1}{2} = \frac{?}{10}$

$10 \div 2 = 5$

$5 \times 1 = 5$

$\frac{1}{2} = \frac{5}{10}$

b. $5\frac{5}{10} + 3\frac{3}{10} =$

c. $5\frac{5}{10}$

$+3\frac{3}{10}$

d. $8\frac{8}{10} = 8\frac{4}{5}$ (reduced to lowest terms)

SUBTRACTION OF FRACTIONS

Subtraction of Fractions Having the Same Denominator

1. Subtract the numerator of the **subtrahend** (the number being subtracted) from the numerator of the **minuend** (the number from which another number is subtracted).
2. Place the difference over the common denominator.
3. Reduce to lowest terms.

Example 1: $6/8 - 4/8 =$ _____

   a. $\dfrac{6}{8} - \dfrac{4}{8} =$

   b. $\dfrac{6-4}{8} =$

   c. $\dfrac{2}{8} = \dfrac{1}{4}$ (reduced to lowest terms)

Example 2: $7/12 - 1/12 =$ _____

   a. $\dfrac{7}{12} - \dfrac{1}{12} =$

   b. $\dfrac{7-1}{12} =$

   c. $\dfrac{6}{12} = \dfrac{1}{2}$ (reduced to lowest terms)

Subtraction of Fractions with Unlike Denominators

1. Change the fractions to equivalent fractions with the lowest common denominator.
2. Subtract the numerator of the subtrahend from that of the minuend.
3. Place the difference over the lowest common denominator.
4. Reduce to lowest terms.

Example 1: $2/3 - 1/6 =$ _____

The lowest common denominator is 6, because 6 is evenly divisible by 3. Therefore the fraction $2/3$ needs to be changed to an equivalent fraction with 6 as the denominator.

   a. $\dfrac{2}{3} = \dfrac{?}{6}$

      $6 \div 3 = 2$

      $2 \times 2 = 4$

      $\dfrac{2}{3} = \dfrac{4}{6}$

   b. $\dfrac{4}{6} - \dfrac{1}{6} =$

   c. $\dfrac{4-1}{6} =$

   d. $\dfrac{3}{6} = \dfrac{1}{2}$ (reduced to lowest terms)

Example 2: $7/10 - 3/5 =$ _____

The lowest common denominator is 10, because 10 is evenly divisible by 5. Therefore the fraction $3/5$ needs to be changed to an equivalent fraction with 10 as the denominator.

   a. $\dfrac{3}{5} = \dfrac{?}{10}$

      $10 \div 5 = 2$

      $2 \times 3 = 6$

      $\dfrac{3}{5} = \dfrac{6}{10}$

   b. $\dfrac{7}{10} - \dfrac{6}{10} =$

   c. $\dfrac{7-6}{10} = \dfrac{1}{10}$

Subtraction of Fractions Involving Whole Numbers and Unlike Denominators

1. Change the fractions to equivalent fractions with the lowest common denominator.
2. Subtract the numerator of the subtrahend from that of the minuend, borrowing 1 from the whole number if necessary.
3. Place the difference over the lowest common denominator.
4. Reduce to lowest terms.
5. Write the reduced fraction next to the difference of the whole numbers.

Example 1: $3\frac{2}{3} - 1\frac{1}{4} =$ _____

The lowest common denominator is 12 (determined by multiplying 3×4). Each fraction needs to be changed to an equivalent fraction with 12 as the common denominator.

a. $\frac{2}{3} = \frac{?}{12}$

$12 \div 3 = 4$

$4 \times 2 = 8$

$\frac{2}{3} = \frac{8}{12}$

a. $\frac{1}{4} = \frac{?}{12}$

$12 \div 4 = 3$

$3 \times 1 = 3$

$\frac{1}{4} = \frac{3}{12}$

b. $3\frac{8}{12} - 1\frac{3}{12} =$

c. $\quad 3\frac{8}{12}$

$\quad -1\frac{3}{12}$

d. $\quad 2\frac{5}{12}$

Example 2: $8\frac{1}{2} - 3\frac{4}{7} =$ _____

The lowest common denominator is 14 (determined by multiplying 2×7). Each fraction needs to be changed to an equivalent fraction with 14 as the common denominator.

a. $\frac{1}{2} = \frac{?}{14}$

$14 \div 2 = 7$

$7 \times 1 = 7$

$\frac{1}{2} = \frac{7}{14}$

a. $\frac{4}{7} = \frac{?}{14}$

$14 \div 7 = 2$

$2 \times 4 = 8$

$\frac{4}{7} = \frac{8}{14}$

b. $8\frac{7}{14} - 3\frac{8}{14} =$

To perform the subtraction, it is necessary to borrow 1 from the whole number. "One" for this problem can be expressed as $\frac{14}{14}$. Therefore $8\frac{7}{14} = 7\frac{21}{14}$. Now the mathematics may be completed.

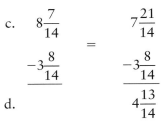

$$
\text{c.} \quad 8\frac{7}{14} \qquad\qquad 7\frac{21}{14}
$$
$$
= \qquad\qquad
$$
$$
-3\frac{8}{14} \qquad\qquad -3\frac{8}{14}
$$
$$
\text{d.} \qquad\qquad\qquad 4\frac{13}{14}
$$

MULTIPLICATION OF FRACTIONS

1. Multiply the numerators.
2. Multiply the denominators.
3. Place the product of the numerators over the product of the denominators.
4. Reduce to lowest terms.

Example 1: $\frac{2}{3} \times \frac{3}{5} = $ _____

$$\frac{2}{3} \times \frac{3}{5} =$$

a.
b. $\dfrac{2\times3}{3\times5} = \dfrac{6}{15}$

c. $\dfrac{6}{15} = \dfrac{2}{5}$ (reduced to lowest terms)

Example 2: $\frac{4}{9} \times \frac{4}{5} = $ _____

$$\frac{4}{9} \times \frac{4}{5} =$$

a.
b. $\dfrac{4\times4}{9\times5} = \dfrac{16}{45}$ (reduced to lowest terms)

The process of multiplying fractions may be shortened by **canceling.** In other words, numbers common to the numerators and denominators may be divided or canceled out.

Example 1: $\frac{2}{3} \times \frac{3}{5} = $ _____

$$\frac{2}{\underset{1}{\cancel{3}}} \times \frac{\overset{1}{\cancel{3}}}{5} = \frac{2\times1}{1\times5} = \frac{2}{5}$$

Example 2: $\frac{7}{20} \times \frac{2}{5} \times \frac{3}{14} = $ _____

$$\frac{\overset{1}{\cancel{7}}}{\underset{10}{\cancel{20}}} \times \frac{\overset{1}{\cancel{2}}}{5} \times \frac{3}{\underset{2}{\cancel{14}}} =$$

$$\frac{1\times1\times3}{10\times5\times2} = \frac{3}{100}$$

Example 3: $\frac{2}{6} \times \frac{3}{4} = $ _____

$$\frac{\overset{1}{\cancel{2}}}{\underset{2}{\cancel{6}}} \times \frac{\overset{1}{\cancel{3}}}{\underset{2}{\cancel{4}}} = \frac{1\times1}{2\times2} = \frac{1}{4}$$

Multiplication of Mixed Numbers

1. Change each mixed number to an improper fraction.
2. Multiply the numerators.
3. Multiply the denominators.
4. Place the product of the numerators over the product of the denominators.
5. Reduce to lowest terms.

18   CHAPTER 1 Fractions

*Remember the denominator of a whole number is *always* 1.

$$6 = \frac{6}{1}$$

$$12 = \frac{12}{1}$$

Example 1: $1\frac{1}{2} \times 2\frac{1}{4} = $ _____

   a.
   b. $\dfrac{3}{2} \times \dfrac{9}{4} = $

   c. $\dfrac{3 \times 9}{2 \times 4} = \dfrac{27}{8} = 3\dfrac{3}{8}$ (reduced to lowest terms)

Example 2: $2 \times 3\frac{5}{6} = $ _____

   a. $\dfrac{2}{1} \times \dfrac{23}{6} = $

   b. $\dfrac{\overset{1}{\cancel{2}}}{1} \times \dfrac{23}{\underset{3}{\cancel{6}}} = $

   c. $\dfrac{1 \times 23}{1 \times 3} = \dfrac{23}{3} = 7\dfrac{2}{3}$ (reduced to lowest terms)

DIVISION OF FRACTIONS

1. Invert (or turn upside down) the divisor.
2. Multiply the two fractions.
3. Reduce to lowest terms.

Example 1: $\frac{2}{3} \div \frac{6}{8} = $ _____

$$\dfrac{2}{3} \div \dfrac{6}{8} = $$

   a. $\dfrac{2}{3} \times \dfrac{8}{6} = $

   b.
   c. $\dfrac{\overset{1}{\cancel{2}}}{3} \times \dfrac{8}{\underset{3}{\cancel{6}}} = \dfrac{1 \times 8}{3 \times 3} = \dfrac{8}{9}$

Example 2: $\frac{3}{4} \div \frac{8}{9} = $ _____

$$\dfrac{3}{4} \div \dfrac{8}{9} = $$

   a. $\dfrac{3}{4} \times \dfrac{9}{8} = $

   b.
   c. $\dfrac{3 \times 9}{4 \times 8} = \dfrac{27}{32}$

Division of Mixed Numbers

1. Change each mixed number to an improper fraction.
2. Invert (or turn upside down) the divisor.
3. Multiply the two fractions.
4. Reduce to lowest terms.

Example 1: $1\frac{3}{4} \div 2\frac{1}{8} = $ _____

   a. $\dfrac{7}{4} \div \dfrac{17}{8} = $

   b.
   c. $\dfrac{7}{\underset{1}{\cancel{4}}} \times \dfrac{\overset{2}{\cancel{8}}}{17} = \dfrac{7 \times 2}{1 \times 17} = \dfrac{14}{17}$

Example 2: $\frac{1}{7} \div 7 = $ _____

   a. $\dfrac{1}{7} \div \dfrac{7}{1} = $

   b.
   c. $\dfrac{1}{7} \times \dfrac{1}{7} = \dfrac{1 \times 1}{7 \times 7} = \dfrac{1}{49}$

REDUCTION OF A COMPLEX FRACTION

1. Rewrite the complex fraction as a division problem.
2. Invert (or turn upside down) the divisor.
3. Multiply the two fractions.
4. Reduce to lowest terms.

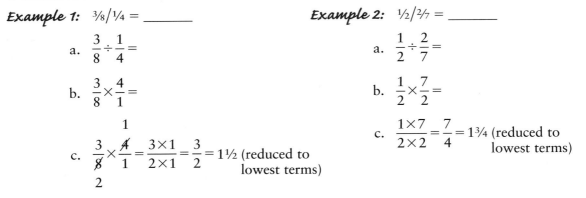

Example 1: ³⁄₈ / ¹⁄₄ = _____

a. $\dfrac{3}{8} \div \dfrac{1}{4} =$

b. $\dfrac{3}{8} \times \dfrac{4}{1} =$

c. $\dfrac{3}{\overset{}{8}} \times \dfrac{\overset{1}{4}}{1} = \dfrac{3 \times 1}{2 \times 1} = \dfrac{3}{2} = 1\frac{1}{2}$ (reduced to lowest terms)

Example 2: ¹⁄₂ / ²⁄₇ = _____

a. $\dfrac{1}{2} \div \dfrac{2}{7} =$

b. $\dfrac{1}{2} \times \dfrac{7}{2} =$

c. $\dfrac{1 \times 7}{2 \times 2} = \dfrac{7}{4} = 1\frac{3}{4}$ (reduced to lowest terms)

Reduction of a Complex Fraction with Mixed Numbers

1. Rewrite the complex fraction as a division problem.
2. Change the mixed numbers to improper fractions.
3. Invert (or turn upside down) the divisor.
4. Multiply the two fractions.
5. Reduce to lowest terms.

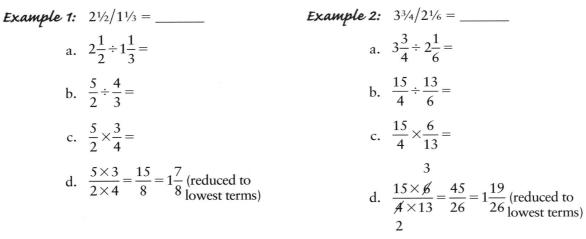

Example 1: 2½ / 1⅓ = _____

a. $2\dfrac{1}{2} \div 1\dfrac{1}{3} =$

b. $\dfrac{5}{2} \div \dfrac{4}{3} =$

c. $\dfrac{5}{2} \times \dfrac{3}{4} =$

d. $\dfrac{5 \times 3}{2 \times 4} = \dfrac{15}{8} = 1\dfrac{7}{8}$ (reduced to lowest terms)

Example 2: 3¾ / 2⅙ = _____

a. $3\dfrac{3}{4} \div 2\dfrac{1}{6} =$

b. $\dfrac{15}{4} \div \dfrac{13}{6} =$

c. $\dfrac{15}{4} \times \dfrac{6}{13} =$

d. $\dfrac{15 \times \overset{3}{6}}{\underset{2}{4} \times 13} = \dfrac{45}{26} = 1\dfrac{19}{26}$ (reduced to lowest terms)

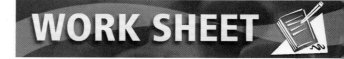

Directions: Change the following improper fractions to mixed numbers.

1. $^4/_3$ = _____   **2.** $^6/_2$ = _____   **3.** $^{16}/_5$ = _____   **4.** $^{13}/_4$ = _____

5. $^{15}/_{10}$ = _____   **6.** $^9/_8$ = _____   **7.** $^{10}/_6$ = _____   **8.** $^{26}/_{12}$ = _____

9. $^{21}/_6$ = _____   **10.** $^{11}/_8$ = _____   **11.** $^7/_2$ = _____   **12.** $^{112}/_{100}$ = _____

Directions: Change the following mixed numbers to improper fractions.

1. $1^1/_2$ = _____   **2.** $3^3/_4$ = _____   **3.** $2^2/_3$ = _____   **4.** $2^5/_6$ = _____

5. $1^3/_5$ = _____   **6.** $3^4/_7$ = _____   **7.** $4^7/_8$ = _____   **8.** $3^7/_{100}$ = _____

9. $2^7/_{10}$ = _____   **10.** $6^5/_8$ = _____   **11.** $1^3/_{25}$ = _____   **12.** $4^1/_4$ = _____

Directions: Add and reduce fractions to lowest terms.

1. $2/3 + 5/6 =$ _____

2. $2/5 + 3/7 =$ _____

3. $3\frac{1}{8} + 2/3 =$ _____

4. $2\frac{1}{2} + 3/4 =$ _____

5. $2\frac{1}{4} + 3\frac{2}{5} =$ _____

6. $1\frac{6}{13} + 1\frac{2}{3} =$ _____

7. $1\frac{1}{2} + 3\frac{3}{4} + 2\frac{3}{8} =$ _____

8. $4\frac{3}{11} + 2\frac{1}{2} =$ _____

9. $2\frac{2}{3} + 3\frac{7}{9} =$ _____

10. $1\frac{3}{10} + 4\frac{2}{5} + 2/3 =$ _____

11. $3\frac{1}{2} + 2\frac{5}{6} + 2\frac{2}{3} =$ _____

12. $5\frac{5}{6} + 2\frac{2}{5} =$ _____

Directions: Subtract and reduce fractions to lowest terms.

1. $2/3 - 3/7 =$ _____

2. $7/8 - 5/16 =$ _____

3. $9/16 - 5/12 =$ _____

4. $1\frac{1}{3} - 5/6 =$ _____

5. $2\frac{17}{20} - 1\frac{3}{4} =$ _____

6. $5\frac{1}{4} - 3\frac{5}{16} =$ _____

7. $5\frac{3}{8} - 4\frac{3}{4} =$ _____

8. $3\frac{1}{4} - 1\frac{11}{12} =$ _____

9. $6\frac{1}{2} - 3\frac{7}{8} =$ _____

10. $4\frac{1}{6} - 2\frac{3}{4} =$ _____

11. $5\frac{2}{3} - 3\frac{7}{8} =$ _____

12. $2\frac{5}{16} - 1\frac{3}{8} =$ _____

Directions: Multiply and reduce fractions to lowest terms.

1. $\frac{1}{3} \times \frac{4}{5} =$ _____

2. $\frac{7}{8} \times \frac{2}{3} =$ _____

3. $6 \times \frac{2}{3} =$ _____

4. $\frac{3}{8} \times 4 =$ _____

5. $2\frac{1}{3} \times 3\frac{3}{4} =$ _____

6. $4\frac{3}{8} \times 2\frac{5}{7} =$ _____

7. $2\frac{5}{12} \times 5\frac{1}{4} =$ _____

8. $\frac{3}{4} \times 2\frac{3}{8} =$ _____

9. $\frac{3}{8} \times \frac{4}{5} \times \frac{2}{3} =$ _____

10. $\frac{1}{10} \times \frac{3}{100} =$ _____

11. $3\frac{1}{2} \times 1\frac{5}{6} =$ _____

12. $2\frac{4}{9} \times 1\frac{3}{11} =$ _____

Fractions **CHAPTER 1**   23

Directions: Divide and reduce fractions to lowest terms.

1. $1\frac{2}{3} \div 3\frac{1}{2} = $ _____

2. $5\frac{1}{2} \div 2\frac{1}{2} = $ _____

3. $3\frac{1}{2} \div 2\frac{1}{4} = $ _____

4. $4\frac{3}{8} \div 1\frac{3}{4} = $ _____

5. $3\frac{1}{2} \div 1\frac{6}{7} = $ _____

6. $\frac{9}{10} \div \frac{2}{3} = $ _____

7. $3 \div 1\frac{5}{6} = $ _____

8. $6\frac{2}{3} \div 1\frac{7}{10} = $ _____

9. $\frac{7}{8} / \frac{1}{4} = $ _____

10. $6\frac{1}{2} / 2\frac{5}{6} = $ _____

11. $5\frac{1}{2} / 2\frac{2}{3} = $ _____

12. $2\frac{2}{3} / 1\frac{7}{9} = $ _____

Answers on p. 472.

Name _____

Date _____

ACCEPTABLE SCORE ___29___

YOUR SCORE _____

POSTTEST 1

Directions: Perform the indicated calculations and reduce fractions to lowest terms.

1. $^2/_3 + ^4/_9 =$ _____

2. $^3/_8 + ^1/_3 =$ _____

3. $2^3/_4 + 2^1/_3 =$ _____

4. $2^2/_3 + ^3/_7 =$ _____

5. $^3/_4 + ^3/_{100} =$ _____

6. $4^2/_5 + 3^3/_4 =$ _____

7. $4^1/_6 + ^2/_3 + 2^3/_4 =$ _____

8. $1^3/_{10} - ^2/_5 =$ _____

9. $2^1/_2 - 1^2/_3 =$ _____

10. $^5/_7 - ^1/_2 =$ _____

11. $3^1/_2 - 1^9/_{16} =$ _____

12. $2^5/_7 - 1^2/_9 =$ _____

13. $9^1/_5 - 3^1/_2 =$ _____

14. $2^1/_4 - ^7/_9 / ^2/_3 =$ _____

15. $^3/_4 \times ^6/_7 =$ _____

16. $3 \times \frac{4}{5} =$ _____

17. $\frac{2}{9} \times 9 =$ _____

18. $2\frac{3}{4} \times 1\frac{1}{6} =$ _____

19. $1\frac{1}{4} \times 2\frac{2}{3} =$ _____

20. $10\frac{1}{2} \times 1\frac{2}{5} =$ _____

21. $5\frac{6}{7} \times \frac{3}{5} =$ _____

22. $\frac{1}{4} \times 3\frac{1}{2} =$ _____

23. $\frac{2}{3} \div \frac{5}{8} =$ _____

24. $\frac{1}{5} \div \frac{1}{50} =$ _____

25. $\frac{1}{3} \div \frac{1}{2} =$ _____

26. $\frac{5}{6} \div \frac{2}{3} =$ _____

27. $\frac{1}{5} / \frac{1}{3} =$ _____

28. $1\frac{1}{5} / \frac{8}{9} =$ _____

29. $\frac{3}{4} / \frac{1}{6} =$ _____

30. $3\frac{1}{8} / 2\frac{3}{4} =$ _____

Answers on p. 472.

Name _____

Date _____

ACCEPTABLE SCORE __29__

YOUR SCORE _____

POSTTEST 2

Directions: Perform the indicated calculations and reduce fractions to lowest terms.

1. $\frac{1}{4} + \frac{5}{6} =$ _____

2. $2\frac{3}{5} + 1\frac{1}{2} =$ _____

3. $\frac{2}{3} + 2\frac{3}{7} =$ _____

4. $1\frac{7}{8} + 3\frac{2}{5} =$ _____

5. $1\frac{3}{4} + \frac{5}{8} + 2\frac{5}{12} =$ _____

6. $10\frac{1}{2} + 1\frac{3}{10} =$ _____

7. $1\frac{5}{14} + 2\frac{3}{21} =$ _____

8. $\frac{4}{9} - \frac{1}{3} =$ _____

9. $2\frac{3}{4} - \frac{7}{8} =$ _____

10. $3\frac{1}{2} - 1\frac{2}{3} =$ _____

11. $3\frac{5}{8} - 1\frac{5}{16} =$ _____

12. $7\frac{1}{3} - 5\frac{5}{6} =$ _____

13. $7\frac{7}{10} - 3\frac{4}{5} =$ _____

14. $3\frac{4}{15} - 2\frac{2}{3} =$ _____

15. $\frac{2}{7} \times \frac{2}{3} =$ _____

16. $3\frac{4}{9} \times 1\frac{4}{5} =$ _____

17. $2 \times \frac{2}{3} =$ _____

18. $\frac{5}{6} \times 2\frac{1}{3} =$ _____

19. $\frac{1}{100} \times \frac{1}{10} = $ _____

20. $6\frac{3}{4} \times 5\frac{1}{3} = $ _____

21. $2\frac{5}{8} \times 1\frac{1}{3} = $ _____

22. $3\frac{1}{2} \times 3\frac{3}{14} = $ _____

23. $\frac{3}{4} \div \frac{8}{9} = $ _____

24. $1\frac{1}{2} \div 1\frac{6}{7} = $ _____

25. $2\frac{1}{3} \div \frac{3}{8} = $ _____

26. $\frac{1}{7} \div 7 = $ _____

27. $\frac{5}{6} / 1\frac{1}{3} = $ _____

28. $1\frac{1}{2} / 2\frac{2}{7} = $ _____

29. $2\frac{1}{4} / 1\frac{1}{3} = $ _____

30. $\frac{3}{8} / \frac{3}{9} = $ _____

Answers on p. 472.

Refer to Review of Mathematics: Fractions on the enclosed CD for additional help and practice problems.

Name _____

Date _____

ACCEPTABLE SCORE ___38___

YOUR SCORE _____

PRETEST ✓

Complete the Decimals Pretest. A score of 38 out of 40 indicates an acceptable understanding of and competency in basic calculations involving decimals. You may skip to the Percents Pretest on p. 51. However, if you score 37 or below, completion of Chapter 2, Decimals, will be helpful for your continued success in the calculation of drug dosages.

Directions: Write the following numbers in words.

1. 0.04 _____

2. 1.6 _____

3. 16.06734 _____

_____

4. 1.015 _____

5. 0.009 _____

Directions: Circle the decimal with the *least value.*

6. 0.2, 0.25, 0.025, 0.02   **7.** 0.4, 0.48, 0.04, 0.004

8. 1.6, 1.64, 1.682, 1.69   **9.** 2.8, 2.82, 2.082, 2.822

10. 0.3, 0.33, 0.003, 0.033

Directions: Perform the indicated calculations.

11. 6.8 + 2.986 + 14.7 + 0.89 = _____

12. 141.71 + 84.98 + 9.98 + 87.63 = _____

13. 1006.48 + 0.008 + 6.2 + 0.179 = _____

14. 47.21 + 48.496 + 0.2976 + 54.67 = _____

15. 5.971 + 63.1 + 8.264 + 7.23 = _____

16. 2.176 − 1.098 = _____

17. $2.006 - 0.998 = $ _____

18. $836.2 - 76.8 = $ _____

19. $100.3 - 98.6 = $ _____

20. $12.6 - 1.654 = $ _____

21. $0.63 \times 0.09 = $ _____

22. $41.545 \times 0.16 = $ _____

23. $5.25 \times 0.37 = $ _____

24. $44.08 \times 0.67 = $ _____

25. $56.7 \times 3.29 = $ _____

26. $0.89 \div 4.32 = $ _____

27. $1.436 \div 0.08 = $ _____

28. $0.689 \div 62.8 = $ _____

29. $12.54 \div 0.02 = $ _____

30. $23 \div 1236 = $ _____

Directions: Change the following decimal fractions to proper fractions.

31. 0.008 = _____   **32.** 0.25 = _____   **33.** 0.322 = _____   **34.** 0.004 = _____

35. 0.34 = _____

Directions: Change the following proper fractions to decimal fractions.

36. $\frac{3}{5}$ = _____   **37.** $\frac{2}{3}$ = _____   **38.** $\frac{3}{500}$ = _____   **39.** $\frac{7}{20}$ = _____

40. $\frac{5}{8}$ = _____

Answers on p. 473.

Decimals

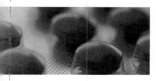

LEARNING OBJECTIVES

On completion of the materials provided in this chapter, you will be able to perform computations accurately by mastering the following mathematical concepts:

1 Reading and writing decimal numbers

2 Determining the value of decimal fractions

3 Adding, subtracting, multiplying, and dividing decimals

4 Rounding decimal fractions to an indicated place value

5 Multiplying and dividing decimals by 10 or a power of 10

6 Multiplying and dividing decimals by 0.1 or a multiple of 0.1

7 Converting a decimal fraction to a proper fraction

8 Converting a proper fraction to a decimal fraction

Study the introductory material for decimals. The processes for the calculation of decimal problems are listed in steps. Memorize the steps for each calculation before beginning the work sheet. Complete the work sheet at the end of this chapter, which provides for extensive practice in the manipulation of decimals. Check your answers. If you have difficulties, go back and review the steps for that type of calculation. When you feel ready to evaluate your learning, take the first posttest. Check your answers. An acceptable score as indicated on the posttest signifies that you are ready for the next chapter. An unacceptable score signifies a need for further study before you take the second posttest.

Decimals are used in the metric system of measurement. **The nurse uses the metric system in the calculation of drug dosages. Therefore it is essential for the nurse to be able to manipulate decimals easily and accurately.**
Each **decimal fraction** consists of a numerator that is expressed in numerals; a decimal point placed so that it designates the value of the denominator; and the denominator, which is understood to be 10 or some power of 10. **In writing a decimal fraction, always place a zero to the left**

of the decimal point so that the decimal point can readily be seen. The omission of the zero may result in a critical medication error. Some examples are as follows:

Fraction	Decimal fraction
$\frac{7}{10}$	0.7
$\frac{13}{100}$	0.13
$\frac{227}{1000}$	0.227

Decimal numbers include an integer (or whole number), a decimal point, and a decimal fraction. The value of the combined integer and decimal fraction is determined by the placement of the decimal point. Whole numbers are written to the *left* of the decimal point, and decimal fractions, to the *right*. Figure 2-1 illustrates the place occupied by the numeral that has the value indicated.

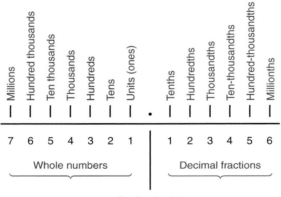

FIGURE 2-1   Decimal place values.

READING DECIMAL NUMBERS

The reading of a decimal number is determined by the place value of the integers and decimal fractions.
1. Read the whole number.
2. Read the decimal point as "and."
3. Read the decimal fraction.

Examples:
0.4	four tenths
0.86	eighty-six hundredths
3.659	three and six hundred fifty-nine thousandths
182.0012	one hundred eighty-two and twelve ten-thousandths
9.47735	nine and forty-seven thousand seven hundred thirty-five hundred-thousandths

DETERMINING THE VALUES OF DECIMAL FRACTIONS

1. Place the numbers in a vertical column with the decimal points in a vertical line.
2. Add zeros on the right in the decimal fractions to make columns even.

3. The largest number in a column to the right of the decimal point has the *greatest* value.
4. If two numbers in a column are of equal value, examine the next column to the right and so on.
5. The smallest number in the column to the right of the decimal point has the *least* value. If two numbers in the first column are of equal value, examine the second column to the right and so on.

Example 1: Of the following fractions (0.623, 0.841, 0.0096, 0.432), which has the greatest value? the least value?

0.6320

0.8410

0.0096

0.4320

0.841 has the greatest value; 0.0096 has the least value.

NOTE: In mixed numbers the values of both the integer and the fraction are considered.

Example 2: Which decimal number (0.4, 0.25, 1.2, 1.002) has the greatest value? the least value?

0.400

0.250

1.200

1.002

1.2 has the greatest value; 0.25 has the least value.

ADDITION AND SUBTRACTION OF DECIMALS

1. Write the numerals in a vertical column with the decimal points in a straight line.
2. Add zeros as needed to complete the columns.
3. Add or subtract each column as indicated by the symbol.
4. Place the decimal point in the sum or difference directly below the decimal points in the column.
5. Place a zero to the left of the decimal point in a decimal fraction.

Example 1: Add: 14.8 + 6.29 + 3.028

$$\begin{array}{r} 14.800 \\ 6.290 \\ +3.028 \\ \hline 24.118 \end{array}$$

Example 2: Subtract: 5.163 − 4.98

$$\begin{array}{r} 5.163 \\ -4.980 \\ \hline 0.183 \end{array}$$

MULTIPLICATION OF DECIMALS

1. Place the shorter group of numbers under the longer group of numbers.
2. Multiply.
3. Add the number of places to the right of the decimal point in the **multiplicand** and the **multiplier** (i.e., the numbers being multiplied). The sum determines the placement of the decimal point within the product.
4. Count from right to left the value of the sum and place the decimal point.

Example 1: 0.19×0.24

$$
\begin{array}{r}
0.19 \quad \text{two place values} \\
\times \quad 0.24 \quad \text{two place values} \\
\hline
076 \\
038 \\
000 \\
\hline
0.0456 \quad \text{four place values}
\end{array}
$$

Example 2: 0.459×0.52

$$
\begin{array}{r}
0.459 \quad \text{three place values} \\
\times \quad 0.52 \quad \text{two place values} \\
\hline
0918 \\
2295 \\
0000 \\
\hline
0.23868 \quad \text{five place values}
\end{array}
$$

Example 3: 8.265×4.36

$$
\begin{array}{r}
8.265 \quad \text{three place values} \\
\times \quad 4.36 \quad \text{two place values} \\
\hline
49590 \\
24795 \\
33060 \\
\hline
36.03540 \quad \text{five place values}
\end{array}
$$

Example 4: 160.41×3.527

$$
\begin{array}{r}
160.41 \quad \text{two place values} \\
\times \quad 3.527 \quad \text{three place values} \\
\hline
112287 \\
32082 \\
80205 \\
48123 \\
\hline
565.76607 \quad \text{five place values}
\end{array}
$$

Multiplying a Decimal by 10 or a Power of 10 (100, 1000, 10,000, 100,000)

1. Move the decimal point to the right the *same number of places as there are zeros in the multiplier.*
2. Zeros may be added as indicated.

Example 1: $0.132 \times 10 = 1.32$

Example 2: $0.053 \times 100 = 5.3$

Example 3: $2.64 \times 1000 = 2640$

Example 4: $49.6 \times 10,000 = 496,000$

Multiplying a Whole Number or Decimal by 0.1 or a Multiple of 0.1 (0.01, 0.001, 0.0001, 0.00001)

1. Move the decimal point to the left the *same number of spaces as there are numbers to the right of the decimal point in the multiplier.*
2. Zeros may be added as indicated.

Example 1: $354.86 \times 0.0001 = 0.035486$

Example 2: $0.729 \times 0.1 = 0.0729$

Example 3: $12.73 \times 0.01 = 0.1273$

Example 4: $5.752 \times 0.001 = 0.005752$

ROUNDING A DECIMAL FRACTION

1. Find the number to the right of the place value desired.
2. If the number is 5, 6, 7, 8, or 9, add 1 to the number in the place value desired and drop the rest of the numbers.
3. If the number is 0, 1, 2, 3, or 4, remove all numbers to the right of the desired place value.

Example 1: Round the following decimal fractions to the nearest tenth.

    a. 0.268

       0.2)68   6 is the number to the right of the tenth place. Therefore 1 should be added to the number 2 and the 68 dropped.

       0.3   correct answer

b. 4.374

4.3)74　　　7 is the number to the right of the tenth place. Therefore 1 should be added to the number 3 and the 74 dropped.

4.4　　　correct answer

c. 5.723

5.7)23　　　2 is the number to the right of the tenth place. Therefore all numbers to the right of the tenth place should be removed.

5.7　　　correct answer

Example 2: Round the following decimal fractions to the nearest hundredth.

a. 0.876

0.87)6　　　6 is the number to the right of the hundredths place. Therefore 1 should be added to the number 7 and the 6 dropped.

0.88　　　correct answer

b. 2.3249

2.32)49　　　4 is the number to the right of the hundredths place. Therefore all numbers to the right of the hundredths place should be removed.

2.32　　　correct answer

Example 3: Round the following decimal fractions to the nearest thousandth.

a. 3.1325

3.132)5　　　5 is the number to the right of the thousandths place. Therefore 1 should be added to the number 2 and the 5 dropped.

3.133　　　correct answer

b. 0.4674

0.467)4　　　4 is the number to the right of the thousandths place. Therefore all numbers to the right of the thousandths place should be removed.

0.467　　　correct answer

Rounding numbers helps to estimate values, compare values, have more realistic and workable numbers, and spot errors. Decimal fractions may be rounded to any designated place value.

DIVISION OF DECIMALS

1. Place a caret ($\wedge$) to the right of the last number in the divisor, signifying the movement of the decimal point that will make the divisor a whole number.
2. Count the number of spaces that the decimal point is moved in the divisor.
3. Count to the right an equal number of spaces in the dividend and place a caret to signify the movement of the decimal.
4. Place a decimal point on the quotient line directly above the caret.
5. Divide, extending the decimal fraction three places to the right of the decimal point.
6. Zeros may be added as indicated to extend the decimal fraction dividend.
7. Round the quotient to the nearest hundredth.

Example 1: 8.326 ÷ 1.062

$$
\begin{array}{r}
7.839 \text{ or } 7.84 \\
1.062_\wedge\overline{)8.326_\wedge000} \\
\underline{7\,434} \\
892\,0 \\
\underline{849\,6} \\
42\,40 \\
\underline{31\,86} \\
10\,540 \\
\underline{9\,558}
\end{array}
$$

Example 2: 386 ÷ 719

$$
\begin{array}{r}
0.536 \text{ or } 0.54 \\
719\overline{)386.000} \\
\underline{359\,5} \\
26\,50 \\
\underline{21\,57} \\
4\,930 \\
\underline{4\,314}
\end{array}
$$

NOTE: The decimal fraction is emphasized by the placement of a zero to the left of the decimal point.

Dividing a Decimal by 10 or a Multiple of 10 (100, 1000, 10,000, 100,000)

1. Move the decimal point to the left the same number of places as there are zeros in the divisor.
2. Zeros may be added as indicated.

Example 1: 6.41 ÷ 10 = 0.641   *Example 2:* 358.0 ÷ 100 = 3.58

Dividing a Whole Number or a Decimal Fraction by 0.1 or a Multiple of 0.1 (0.01, 0.001, 0.0001, 0.00001)

1. Move the decimal point to the right as many places as there are numbers in the divisor.
2. Zeros may be added as indicated.

Example 1: 5.897 ÷ 0.01 = 589.7   *Example 2:* 46.31 ÷ 0.001 = 46,310

CONVERSION

Converting a Decimal Fraction to a Proper Fraction

1. Remove the decimal point and the zero preceding it.
2. The numerals are the numerator.
3. The placement of the decimal point indicates what the denominator will be.
4. Reduce to lowest terms.

Example 1: 0.3

$$\frac{3}{10}$$

Example 2: 0.86

$$\frac{86}{100} = \frac{43}{50}$$

Example 3: 0.375

$$\frac{375}{1000} = \frac{3}{8}$$

Converting a Proper Fraction to a Decimal Fraction

1. Divide the numerator by the denominator.
2. Extend the decimal the desired number of places (often three).
3. Place a zero to the left of the decimal point in a decimal fraction.

Example 1: ⁴/₅

$$
\begin{array}{r}
0.8 \\
5\overline{)4.0} \\
\underline{4\ 0}
\end{array}
$$

⁴/₅ = 0.8

Example 2: ⁷/₈

$$
\begin{array}{r}
0.875 \\
8\overline{)7.000} \\
\underline{6\ 4} \\
60 \\
\underline{56} \\
40 \\
\underline{40}
\end{array}
$$

⁷/₈ = 0.875

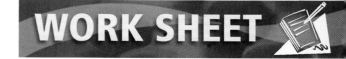

Directions: Write the following numbers in words.

1. 0.2 _____

2. 9.68 _____

3. 0.0003 _____

4. 1968.342 _____

_____

5. 0.02 _____

Directions: Circle the decimal numbers with the *greatest value.*

1. 0.2, 0.15, 0.1, 0.25   **2.** 0.4, 0.45, 0.04, 0.042   **3.** 0.9, 0.09, 0.95, 0.98

4. 0.5, 0.065, 0.58, 0.68   **5.** 1.8, 1.08, 1.18, 1.468   **6.** 7.4, 7.42, 7.423, 7.44

Directions: Circle the decimal numbers with the *least value.*

1. 0.6, 0.66, 0.666, 0.6666   **2.** 0.3, 0.03, 0.003, 0.0003   **3.** 1.2, 1.22, 1.022, 1.0022

4. 0.8, 0.08, 0.868, 0.859   **5.** 0.75, 0.07, 0.007, 0.0075   **6.** 3.015, 3.1, 3.006, 3.02

Directions: Add the following decimal problems.

1. 1.080 + 31.2 +
0.065 + 9.41 = _____

2. 2.2 + 355.6 +
8.125 + 6.75 = _____

3. 24.684 + 5.3697 +
8.025 + 2.9 = _____

4. 18.95 + 1.903 +
8.82 + 9.4 = _____

5. 56.93 + 765.7 +
64.882 + 7.33 = _____

6. 0.3 + 0.874 +
2.763 + 63.2 = _____

7. 13.5 + 1.023 + 8.83 + 3.267 = _____

8. 3.6 + 8.25 + 2.05 + 24 = _____

9. 0.6 + 0.985 + 1.432 + 52.1 = _____

10. 3.75 + 0.718 + 136.95 + 0.8 = _____

Directions: Subtract the following decimal problems.

1. 1321.52 − 63.65 = _____ **2.** 4.745 − 2.896 = _____ **3.** 1.8 − 1.09 = _____

4. 250.7 − 75.896 = _____ **5.** 24.186 − 16.768 = _____ **6.** 6.33 − 2.186 = _____

7. 0.486 − 0.025 = _____ **8.** 1 − 0.012 = _____ **9.** 63 − 0.978 = _____

10. 300 − 12.629 = _____

Directions: Multiply the following decimal problems.

1. $1.3 \times 12.5 =$ _____

2. $127 \times 4.8 =$ _____

3. $1.69 \times 30.8 =$ _____

4. $9.08 \times 6.18 =$ _____

5. $52.4 \times 0.8 =$ _____

6. $420 \times 0.08 =$ _____

7. $2.3 \times 45.21 =$ _____

8. $7.46 \times 54.83 =$ _____

9. $1.19 \times 0.127 =$ _____

10. $7.85 \times 3.006 =$ _____

Directions: Multiply the following numbers by 10 by moving the decimal point.

1. 0.09 _____

2. 0.2 _____

3. 0.18 _____

4. 0.3 _____

5. 0.625 _____

6. 2.33 _____

Directions: Multiply the following numbers by 100 by moving the decimal point.

1. 0.023 _____

2. 1.5 _____

3. 0.004 _____

4. 0.125 _____

5. 8.65 _____

6. 76.4 _____

Directions: Multiply the following numbers by 1000 by moving the decimal point.

1. 0.2 _____

2. 0.005 _____

3. 0.187 _____

4. 9.65 _____

5. 0.46 _____

6. 0.489 _____

Directions: Multiply the following numbers by 0.1 by moving the decimal point.

1. 30.0 _____   **2.** 0.69 _____   **3.** 1.7 _____

4. 0.95 _____   **5.** 0.138 _____   **6.** 5.67 _____

Directions: Multiply the following numbers by 0.01 by moving the decimal point.

1. 0.26 _____   **2.** 90.8 _____   **3.** 5.5 _____

4. 11.2 _____   **5.** 0.875 _____   **6.** 63.3 _____

Directions: Multiply the following numbers by 0.001 by moving the decimal point.

1. 56.0 _____   **2.** 12.55 _____   **3.** 126.5 _____

4. 33.3 _____   **5.** 9.684 _____   **6.** 241 _____

Directions: Round the following decimal fractions to the nearest tenth.

1. 0.33 _____   **2.** 0.913 _____   **3.** 2.359 _____

4. 0.66 _____   **5.** 58.36 _____   **6.** 8.092 _____

Directions: Round the following decimal fractions to the nearest hundredth.

1. 2.555 _____   **2.** 4.275 _____   **3.** 0.284 _____

4. 3.923 _____   **5.** 6.534 _____   **6.** 2.988 _____

Directions: Round the following decimal fractions to the nearest thousandth.

1. 27.86314 _____   **2.** 5.9246 _____   **3.** 2.1574 _____

4. 0.8493 _____   **5.** 321.0869 _____   **6.** 455.7682 _____

Directions: Divide. Round the quotient to the nearest hundredth.

1. $7.02 \div 6 =$ _____   **2.** $124.2 \div 0.03 =$ _____   **3.** $5.46 \div 0.7 =$ _____

4. $24 \div 0.06 =$ _____   **5.** $24 \div 1500 =$ _____   **6.** $4.6 \div 35.362 =$ _____

7. $4.13 \div 0.05 = $ _____   **8.** $9.08 \div 2.006 = $ _____   **9.** $63 \div 132.3 = $ _____

10. $21.25 \div 8.43 = $ _____

Directions: Divide the following numbers by 10 by moving the decimal point.

1. 6.0 _____   **2.** 0.2 _____   **3.** 9.8 _____
4. 0.05 _____   **5.** 0.375 _____   **6.** 0.99 _____

Directions: Divide the following numbers by 100 by moving the decimal point.

1. 0.7 _____   **2.** 8.11 _____   **3.** 700.0 _____
4. 0.19 _____   **5.** 12.0 _____   **6.** 30.2 _____

Directions: Divide the following numbers by 1000 by moving the decimal point.

1. 1.8 _____   **2.** 360.0 _____   **3.** 0.25 _____
4. 54.6 _____   **5.** 7.5 _____   **6.** 7140 _____

Directions: Divide the following numbers by 0.1 by moving the decimal point.

1. 2.8 _____   **2.** 0.1 _____   **3.** 0.65 _____
4. 0.987 _____   **5.** 15.0 _____   **6.** 8.25 _____

Directions: Divide the following numbers by 0.01 by moving the decimal point.

1. 36.0 _____   **2.** 0.16 _____   **3.** 0.48 _____
4. 9.59 _____   **5.** 0.8 _____   **6.** 0.097 _____

Directions: Divide the following numbers by 0.001 by moving the decimal point.

1. 6.2 _____   **2.** 839.0 _____   **3.** 5.0 _____
4. 0.86 _____   **5.** 13.8 _____   **6.** 0.0156 _____

Directions: Change the following decimal fractions to proper fractions.

1. 0.06 _____

2. 0.8 _____

3. 0.68 _____

4. 0.0025 _____

5. 0.625 _____

6. 0.25 _____

7. 0.64 _____

8. 0.005 _____

9. 0.01 _____

10. 0.044 _____

Directions: Change the following proper fractions to decimal fractions.

1. $\frac{1}{8}$ _____

2. $\frac{2}{3}$ _____

3. $\frac{16}{25}$ _____

4. $\frac{3}{5}$ _____

5. $\frac{8}{200}$ _____

6. $\frac{1}{3}$ _____

7. $\frac{4}{5}$ _____

8. $\frac{7}{8}$ _____

9. $\frac{1}{200}$ _____

10. $\frac{5}{6}$ _____

Answers on pp. 473-474.

Name _____

Date _____

ACCEPTABLE SCORE   __33__

YOUR SCORE   _____

POSTTEST 1

Directions: Write the following numbers in words.

1. 634.18 _____

_____

2. 0.9 _____

3. 64.231 _____

_____

Directions: Circle the decimal fractions with the *greatest value*.

4. 0.1, 0.01, 0.15, 0.015

5. 0.666, 0.068, 0.006, 0.66

Directions: Perform the indicated calculations.

6. 1.342 + 0.987 + 8.062 + 44.269 = _____

7. 0.6 + 0.45 + 2.9 + 4.94 = _____

8. 3.004 + 0.848 + 0.9 + 1.6 = _____

9. 2.875 + 0.75 + 0.094 + 2.385 = _____

10. 1981.62 + 4.876 + 146.35 + 19.78 = _____

11. 1 − 0.661 = _____

12. 2.46 − 1.0068 = _____

13. 844.6 − 521.52 = _____

14. 43.69 − 0.0823 = _____

15. 0.9 − 0.689 = _____

16. 72.8 × 9.649 = _____

17. 1.58 × 0.088 = _____

18. $360 \times 0.45 =$ _____   **19.** $26.2 \times 1.69 =$ _____   **20.** $1.5 \times 0.39 =$ _____

21. $268.8 \div 16 =$ _____   **22.** $8.89 \div 0.006 =$ _____   **23.** $12.54 \div 0.02 =$ _____

24. $56.4 \div 40 =$ _____   **25.** $165.9 \div 3.006 =$ _____

Directions: Change the following decimal fractions to proper fractions.

26. 0.09 _____   **27.** 0.0025 _____   **28.** 0.375 _____   **29.** 0.4 _____

30. 0.006 _____

Directions: Change the following proper fractions to decimal fractions.

31. $^5/_7$ _____   **32.** $^1/_{100}$ _____   **33.** $^1/_{250}$ _____   **34.** $^1/_8$ _____

35. $^3/_{32}$ _____

Answers on p. 475.

Name _____

Date _____

ACCEPTABLE SCORE ___33___

YOUR SCORE _____

POSTTEST 2

Directions: Write the following numbers in words.

1. 0.516 _____

_____

2. 4.0002 _____

3. 123.69 _____

_____

Directions: Circle the decimal with the *greatest value*.

4. 0.04, 0.45, 0.8, 0.86   **5.** 1.202, 1.22, 1.2, 1.222

Directions: Perform the indicated calculations.

6. 1.2791 + 327.8 + 123.07 + 4.67 = _____

7. 6.95 + 0.8 + 0.625 + 7.68 = _____

8. 19.29 + 3.5 + 5.869 + 4.55 = _____

9. 1.5 + 6.3 + 10.46 + 29.465 = _____

10. 322 + 0.95 + 6.45 + 9.6 = _____

11. 632.838 − 19.869 = ____

12. 1.572 − 0.985 = _____

13. 6.4 − 3.634 = _____

14. 2.6 − 0.087 = _____

15. 4.819 − 3.734 = _____

16. 57.6 × 2.9 = _____

17. 149.36 × 700 = _____

18. $56.43 \times 0.018 =$ _____   **19.** $12.8 \times 6.5 =$ _____   **20.** $27.5 \times 5.89 =$ _____

21. $5.9 \div 5.3 =$ _____   **22.** $0.295 \div 0.059 =$ _____   **23.** $124 \div 0.008 =$ _____

24. $0.7 \div 2.3 =$ _____   **25.** $5.928 \div 2.4 =$ _____

Directions: Change the following decimal fractions to proper fractions.

26. 0.005 _____   **27.** 0.35 _____   **28.** 0.125 _____   **29.** 0.85 _____

30. 0.6 _____

Directions: Change the following proper fractions to decimal fractions.

31. ⅙ _____   **32.** ¹⁄₄₀₀ _____   **33.** ⅞ _____   **34.** ¹⁄₁₅₀ _____

35. ¹⁄₁₂₅ _____

Answers on p. 475.

 Refer to Review of Mathematics: Decimals on the enclosed CD for additional help and practice problems.

Name _____

Date _____

ACCEPTABLE SCORE __38__

YOUR SCORE _____

PRETEST ✓

Complete the Percents Pretest. A score of 38 out of 40 indicates an acceptable understanding of and competency in basic calculations involving percents. You may skip to the Ratios Pretest on p. 69. However, if you score 37 or below, completion of Chapter 3, Percents, will be helpful for your continued success in the calculation of drug dosages.

Directions: Change the following fractions to percents.

1. $\frac{1}{60}$ _____

2. $\frac{5}{7}$ _____

3. $\frac{1}{8}$ _____

4. $\frac{3}{10}$ _____

5. $\frac{4}{3}$ _____

Directions: Change the following decimals to percents.

6. 0.006 _____

7. 0.35 _____

8. 0.427 _____

9. 3.821 _____

10. 0.7 _____

Directions: Change the following percents to proper fractions.

11. 0.5% _____

12. 75% _____

13. 9½% _____

14. 24.8% _____

15. ⅜% _____

Directions: Change the following percents to decimals.

16. 1⅙% _____

17. 7.5% _____

18. 13³⁄₁₀% _____

19. ⁸⁄₉% _____

20. 63% _____

Directions: What percent of

21. 1.60 is 6 _____

22. ¾ is ⅛ _____

23. 100 is 65 _____

24. 500 is 1 _____

25. 4.5 is 1.5 _____

26. 37.8 is 4.6 _____

27. 1⁴/₉ is ⁵/₈ _____

28. 1000 is 100 _____

29. 3½ is ¼ _____

30. 9.7 is ⅙ _____

Directions:　What is

31. 3% of 60 _____

32. ¼% of 60 _____

33. 4.5% of 57 _____

34. 2⅛% of 32 _____

35. 4% of 77 _____

36. 9.3% of 46 _____

37. ³/₇% of 14 _____

38. 22% of 88 _____

39. 7.6% of 156 _____

40. 5% of 300 _____

Answers on p. 475.

Percents

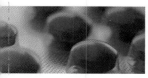

LEARNING OBJECTIVES

On completion of the materials provided in this chapter, you will be able to perform computations accurately by mastering the following mathematical concepts:

1 Changing a fraction or decimal to a percent

2 Changing a percent to a fraction or decimal

3 Changing a percent containing a fraction to a decimal

4 Finding what percent one number is of another

5 Finding the given percent of a number

Study the introductory material on percents. The processes for the calculation of percent problems are listed in steps. Memorize the steps for each calculation before beginning the work sheet. Complete the work sheet at the end of this chapter, which provides for extensive practice in the manipulation of percents. Check your answers. If you have any difficulty, go back and review the steps for that type of calculation. When you feel ready to evaluate your learning, take the first posttest. Check your answers. An acceptable score as indicated on the posttest signifies that you are ready for the next chapter. An unacceptable score signifies a need for further study before taking the second posttest.

A **percent** is a third way of showing a fractional relationship. Fractions, decimals, and percents can all be converted from one form to the others. Conversions of fractions and decimals are discussed in Chapter 2. A percent indicates a value equal to the number of hundredths. Therefore, when a percent is written as a fraction, the denominator is *always* 100. The number beside the percent sign (%) becomes the numerator.

CHANGING A FRACTION TO A PERCENT

1. Multiply by 100.
2. Add the percent sign (%).

Example 1: $^2/_5$

a. $\dfrac{2}{\cancel{5}}\times\dfrac{\cancel{100}^{\,20}}{1}=$

b. $\dfrac{2\times20}{1\times1}=40$

c. 40%

Example 2: $^3/_{10}$

a. $\dfrac{3}{\cancel{10}}\times\dfrac{\cancel{100}^{\,10}}{1}=$

b. $\dfrac{3\times10}{1\times1}=30$

c. 30%

Example 3: $1\frac{1}{4}$

a. $\dfrac{5}{\cancel{4}}\times\dfrac{\cancel{100}^{\,25}}{1}=$

b. $\dfrac{5\times25}{1\times1}=125$

c. 125%

Example 4: $^1/_3$

a. $\dfrac{1}{3}\times\dfrac{100}{1}=$

b. $\dfrac{1\times100}{3\times1}\times\dfrac{100}{3}=33\dfrac{1}{3}$

c. 33⅓%

CHANGING A DECIMAL TO A PERCENT

1. Multiply by 100 (by moving the decimal point two places to the right).
2. Add the percent sign (%).

Example 1: 0.421

a. $0.421\times100=42.1$

b. 42.1%

Example 2: 0.98

a. $0.98\times100=98$

b. 98%

Example 3: 0.2

a. $0.2\times100=20$

b. 20%

Example 4: 1.1212

a. $1.1212\times100=112.12$

b. 112.12%

CHANGING A PERCENT TO A FRACTION

1. Drop the % sign.
2. Write the remaining number as the fraction's numerator.
3. Write 100 as the denominator. (The denominator will *always* be 100.)
4. Reduce to lowest terms.

Example 1: 45%

a. $\dfrac{45}{100}=\dfrac{9}{20}$ (reduced to lowest terms)

Example 2: 0.3%

a. $\dfrac{0.3}{100}=$

b. $\dfrac{\frac{3}{10}}{100}$

c. $\dfrac{3}{10}\div\dfrac{100}{1}=$

d. $\dfrac{3}{10}\times\dfrac{1}{100}=\dfrac{3}{1000}$

Example 3: 3½%

a. $\dfrac{3\frac{1}{2}}{100} = \dfrac{7/2}{100}$

b. $\dfrac{7}{2} \div \dfrac{100}{1} =$

c. $\dfrac{7}{2} \times \dfrac{1}{100} = \dfrac{7}{200}$

CHANGING A PERCENT TO A DECIMAL

1. Drop the % sign.
2. Divide the remaining number by 100 (by moving the decimal point two places to the left).
3. Express the quotient as a decimal. Place a zero before the decimal if there are no whole numbers.

Example 1: 32%

0.32

Example 2: 125%

1.25

CHANGING A PERCENT CONTAINING A FRACTION TO A DECIMAL

1. Drop the % sign.
2. Change the mixed number to an improper fraction.
3. Divide by 100. Remember, the denominator of all whole numbers is 1.
4. Reduce to lowest terms.
5. Divide the numerator by the denominator, expressing the quotient as a decimal.

Example 1: 12½%

a. $\dfrac{25}{2} \div \dfrac{100}{1} =$

b. $\dfrac{\overset{1}{\cancel{25}}}{2} \times \dfrac{1}{\underset{4}{\cancel{100}}} = \dfrac{1}{8}$

c.
```
   0.125
 8)1.000
   8
   20
   16
    40
    40
```

d. 12½% = 0.125

Example 2: 3¾%

a. $\dfrac{15}{4} \div \dfrac{100}{1} =$

b. $\dfrac{\overset{3}{\cancel{15}}}{4} \times \dfrac{1}{\underset{20}{\cancel{100}}} = \dfrac{3}{80}$

c.
```
    0.0375
 80)3.0000
    2 40
    600
    560
     400
     400
```

d. 3¾% = 0.0375

FINDING WHAT PERCENT ONE NUMBER IS OF ANOTHER

1. Write the number following the word *of* as the denominator of a fraction.
2. Write the other number as the numerator of the fraction.
3. Divide the numerator by the denominator, extending the decimal fraction four places to the right of the decimal point.
4. Multiply by 100.
5. Add the % sign.

Example 1: What percent of 24 is 9?

a. $\dfrac{9}{24} = \dfrac{3}{8}$

b.
$$
\begin{array}{r}
0.375 \\
8\overline{)3.000} \\
\underline{2\,4} \\
60 \\
\underline{56} \\
40 \\
\underline{40}
\end{array}
$$

c. $0.375 \times 100 = 37.5$

d. 37.5%

Example 2: What percent of 5.4 is 1.2?

a. $\dfrac{1.2}{5.4} = 5.4\overline{)1.2\,0000}$
$$
\begin{array}{r}
0.2222 \\
\underline{1\,0\,8} \\
1\,20 \\
\underline{1\,08} \\
120 \\
\underline{108} \\
120 \\
\underline{108}
\end{array}
$$

b. $0.2222 \times 100 = 22.22$

c. 22.22%

Example 3: What percent of 2 is ¼?

a. ¼/2

b. $\dfrac{1}{4} \div 2 =$

c. $\dfrac{1}{4} \div \dfrac{2}{1} =$

d. $\dfrac{1}{4} \times \dfrac{1}{2} = \dfrac{1}{8}$

e. $\dfrac{1}{\overset{}{\underset{2}{8}}} \times \dfrac{\overset{25}{\cancel{100}}}{1} = \dfrac{25}{2} = 12.5$

f. 12.5%

Example 4: What percent of 8.7 is 3½?

a. $\dfrac{3½}{8.7} = \dfrac{3.5}{8.7}$

b.
$$
\begin{array}{r}
0.402 \\
8.7\overline{)3.5\,000} \\
\underline{3\,4\,8} \\
20 \\
\underline{00} \\
200 \\
\underline{174}
\end{array}
$$

c. $0.402 \times 100 = 40.2$

d. 40.2%

FINDING THE GIVEN PERCENT OF A NUMBER

1. Write the percent as a decimal number.
2. Multiply by the other number.

Example 1: What is 40% of 180?

a. $\dfrac{40}{100} = 100\overline{)40.0}$ $\begin{array}{r}0.4\\\hline 40.0\\40\,0\\\hline\end{array}$

b. $\begin{array}{r}180\\\times\,0.4\\\hline 72.0\end{array}$

c. 40% of 180 = 72

Example 2: What is ³⁄₁₀% of 52?

a. $\dfrac{\frac{3}{10}}{100} = \dfrac{3}{10} \div \dfrac{100}{1} =$

b. $\dfrac{3}{10} \times \dfrac{1}{100} = \dfrac{3}{1000}$

c. $\dfrac{3}{1000} = 0.003$

d. $\begin{array}{r}0.003\\\times\;\;\;52\\\hline 0\,006\\00\,15\\\hline 00.156\end{array}$

e. ³⁄₁₀% of 52 = 0.156

WORK SHEET

Directions: Change each of the following proper fractions to a percent.

1. $3/4$ _____

2. $3/8$ _____

3. $4/5$ _____

4. $8/25$ _____

5. $3/1000$ _____

6. $7/200$ _____

7. $9/400$ _____

8. $3/20$ _____

9. $9/150$ _____

10. $11/16$ _____

11. $5/6$ _____

12. $75/10,000$ _____

Directions: Change each of the following decimals to a percent.

1. 0.402 _____

2. 0.0367 _____

3. 0.163 _____

4. 0.98 _____

5. 0.3 _____

6. 0.145 _____

7. 0.7 _____

8. 0.42 _____

9. 0.159 _____

10. 0.673 _____

11. 0.3712 _____

12. 2.2 _____

Directions: Change each of the following percents to a mixed number or a proper fraction.

1. 3.5% _____

2. ¾% _____

3. 0.125% _____

4. 10% _____

5. ⅔% _____

6. 20.2% _____

7. 12% _____

8. 0.25% _____

9. 2⅜% _____

10. 6¼% _____

11. 2.1% _____

12. 66⅔% _____

Directions: Change each of the following percents to a decimal.

1. 37.5% _____

2. 3% _____

3. 6¾% _____

4. 0.42% _____

5. ¼% _____

6. 2½% _____

7. 0.23% _____

8. 72.6% _____

9. 16% _____

10. ⁵⁄₁₆% _____

11. ½% _____

12. ⁷⁄₁₂% _____

Directions: What percent of

1. 40 is 22 _____
2. 80 is 6.3 _____
3. 200 is 4 _____
4. 500 is 60 _____

5. 20 is 1 _____
6. 24 is 3.6 _____
7. 275 is 55 _____
8. 1000 is 100 _____

9. 800 is 360 _____
10. 25 is ¼ _____
11. 250 is 5.2 _____
12. 35 is 7 _____

Directions: What is

1. 25% of 478 _____
2. 10% of 34 _____
3. 2.8% of 510 _____

4. ½% of 28 _____
5. 33⅓% of 3000 _____
6. ⅕% of 65 _____

7. 2¼% of 26 _____
8. ⅜% of 32 _____
9. 62% of 871 _____

10. ¼% of 68 _____
11. 41% of 27 _____
12. 8.4% of 128 _____

Answers on p. 476.

Name _____

Date _____

ACCEPTABLE SCORE __29__

YOUR SCORE _____

POSTTEST 1

Directions: Change the following fractions to percents.

1. $^{7}/_{8}$ _____   **2.** $^{11}/_{20}$ _____   **3.** $^{3}/_{1000}$ _____

Directions: Change the following decimals to percents.

4. 0.256 _____   **5.** 0.004 _____   **6.** 0.9 _____

Directions: Change the following percents to proper fractions.

7. 85% _____   **8.** 0.3% _____   **9.** 3½% _____

Directions: Change the following percents to decimals.

10. 86.3% _____   **11.** 4⅝% _____   **12.** 0.36% _____

Directions: What percent of

13. 70 is 7 _____   **14.** 24 is 1.2 _____   **15.** 300 is 1 _____

16. 66⅔ is 8 _____

17. 3.5 is 1.5 _____

18. 2.5 is 0.5 _____

19. ¾ is ⅜ _____

20. 160 is 12 _____

21. 250 is 20 _____

Directions: What is

22. 65% of 800 _____

23. 90% of 40 _____

24. ⅛% of 72 _____

25. 8.5% of 2000 _____

26. 4½% of 940 _____

27. 65% of 450 _____

28. ¼% of 60 _____

29. 4.3% of 56 _____

30. 0.52% of 88 _____

Answers on p. 476.

Name _____

Date _____

ACCEPTABLE SCORE __29__

YOUR SCORE _____

POSTTEST 2

Directions: Change the following fractions to percents.

1. $\frac{1}{8}$ _____   **2.** $\frac{2}{5}$ _____   **3.** $\frac{1}{6}$ _____

Directions: Change the following decimals to percents.

4. 0.065 _____   **5.** 0.005 _____   **6.** 0.2 _____

Directions: Change the following percents to proper fractions.

7. 0.3% _____   **8.** 16½% _____   **9.** 0.25% _____

Directions: Change the following percents to decimals.

10. 3¾% _____   **11.** 7% _____   **12.** 5.55% _____

Directions: What percent of

13. 5.4 is 1.2 _____   **14.** $\frac{1}{4}$ is $\frac{1}{8}$ _____   **15.** 250 is 6 _____

16. 40 is 32 _____

17. 160 is 12 _____

18. 500 is 50 _____

19. 5¾ is 2⅜ _____

20. 120 is 15 _____

21. ⁹⁄₁₆ is ⁵⁄₇ _____

Directions: What is

22. 35% of 650 _____

23. ¼% of 116 _____

24. 4½% of 940 _____

25. 11% of 88 _____

26. 16% of 90 _____

27. 7.5% of 261 _____

28. 45% of 24.27 _____

29. ⅞% of 64 _____

30. 82.4% of 118 _____

Answers on p. 477.

 Refer to Review of Mathematics: Percents on the enclosed CD for additional help and practice problems.

Name _____

Date _____

ACCEPTABLE SCORE __29__

YOUR SCORE _____

PRETEST ✓

Complete the Ratios Pretest. A score of 29 out of 30 indicates an acceptable understanding of and competency in basic calculations involving ratios. You may skip to the Proportions Pretest on p. 83. However, if you score 28 or below, completion of Chapter 4, Ratios, will be helpful for your continued success in the calculation of drug dosages.

Directions: Convert to equivalents.

	Ratio	Fraction	Decimal	Percent
1.	17 : 51			
2.			0.715	
3.		$^8/_{20}$		
4.				12½%
5.	21 : 420			
6.		$^5/_{32}$		
7.			0.286	
8.				71³/₇%
9.				16¼%
10.			0.462	

Answers on p. 477.

Ratios

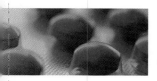

LEARNING OBJECTIVES

On completion of the materials provided in this chapter, you will be able to perform computations accurately by mastering the following mathematical concepts:

1 Changing a proper fraction, decimal fraction, and percent to a ratio reduced to lowest terms

2 Changing a ratio to a proper fraction, a decimal fraction, and a percent

Study the introductory material on ratios. The processes for the calculation of ratio problems are listed in steps. Memorize the steps for each calculation before beginning the work sheet. Review previous chapters on fractions, decimals, and percents as necessary. Complete the work sheet at the end of this chapter, which provides for extensive practice in the manipulation of ratios. Check your answers. If you have difficulties, go back and review the steps for that type of calculation. When you feel ready to evaluate your learning, take the first posttest. Check your answers. An acceptable score as indicated on the posttest signifies that you are ready for the next chapter. An unacceptable score signifies a need for further study before taking the second posttest.

A **ratio** is another way of indicating a relationship between two numbers. In other words, it is another way to express a fraction. A ratio indicates *division*.

Example 1: ¾ written as a ratio is 3 : 4

In reading a ratio, one reads the colon as "is to." The example would then be read as "three is to four."

Example 2: 7 written as a ratio is 7 : 1

To express any whole number as a ratio, the number following the colon is *always* 1. The example would be read as "seven is to one."

CHANGING A PROPER FRACTION TO A RATIO REDUCED TO LOWEST TERMS

1. Reduce the fraction to lowest terms.
2. Write the numerator of the fraction as the first number of the ratio.
3. Place a colon after the first number.
4. Write the denominator of the fraction as the second number of the ratio.

Example 1: $^4/_{12}$
  a. $^4/_{12}$ reduced to lowest terms equals $^1/_3$
  b. $^1/_3$ written as a ratio is $1 : 3$

Example 2: $^1/_{1000}/^1/_{10}$

  a. $\dfrac{1}{1000} \div \dfrac{1}{10} =$ c. $^1/_{1000}/^1/_{10}$ reduced to lowest terms equals $^1/_{100}$

  b. $\dfrac{1}{\overset{}{\underset{100}{\cancel{1000}}}} \times \dfrac{\overset{1}{\cancel{10}}}{1} = \dfrac{1}{100}$ d. $^1/_{100}$ written as a ratio is $1 : 100$

CHANGING A DECIMAL FRACTION TO A RATIO REDUCED TO LOWEST TERMS

1. Express the decimal fraction as a proper fraction reduced to lowest terms.
2. Write the numerator of the fraction as the first number of the ratio.
3. Place a colon after the first number.
4. Write the denominator of the fraction as the second number of the ratio.

Example 1: 0.85

  a. $\dfrac{85}{100} = \dfrac{17}{20}$ (reduced to lowest terms)

  b. $\dfrac{17}{20}$ written as a ratio is $17 : 20$

Example 2: 0.125

  a. $\dfrac{125}{1000} = \dfrac{1}{8}$ (reduced to lowest terms)

  b. $\dfrac{1}{8}$ written as a ratio is $1 : 8$

CHANGING A PERCENT TO A RATIO REDUCED TO LOWEST TERMS

1. Express the percent as a proper fraction reduced to lowest terms.
2. Write the numerator of the fraction as the first number of the ratio.
3. Place a colon after the first number.
4. Write the denominator of the fraction as the second number of the ratio.

Example 1: 30%

  a. $\dfrac{30}{100} = \dfrac{3}{10}$ (reduced to lowest terms)

  b. $\dfrac{3}{10}$ written as a ratio is $3 : 10$

Example 2: ½%

a. $\dfrac{\dfrac{1}{2}}{100} =$

b. $\dfrac{1}{2} \div \dfrac{100}{1} =$

c. $\dfrac{1}{2} \times \dfrac{1}{100} = \dfrac{1}{200}$

d. $\dfrac{1}{200}$ written as a ratio is 1 : 200

Example 3: 3⁹⁄₁₀%

a. $\dfrac{3\dfrac{9}{10}}{100} =$

b. $\dfrac{39}{10} \div \dfrac{100}{1} =$

c. $\dfrac{39}{10} \times \dfrac{1}{100} = \dfrac{39}{1000}$

d. $\dfrac{39}{1000}$ written as a ratio is 39 : 1000

CHANGING A RATIO TO A PROPER FRACTION REDUCED TO LOWEST TERMS

1. Write the first number of the ratio as a numerator.
2. Write the second number of the ratio as the denominator.
3. Reduce to lowest terms.

Example 1: 9 : 15

$\dfrac{9}{15} = \dfrac{3}{5}$ (reduced to lowest terms)

Example 2: 11 : 22

$\dfrac{11}{22} = \dfrac{1}{2}$ (reduced to lowest terms)

CHANGING A RATIO TO A DECIMAL FRACTION

Divide the first number of the ratio by the second number of the ratio, using long division.

Example 1: 4 : 5

a. $5\overline{)4.0}$ with quotient 0.8, $4\,0$

b. 4 : 5 written as a decimal is 0.8

Example 2: $3\frac{1}{2} : 2\frac{1}{4}$

  a. $3.5 : 2.25$

  b.
$$
2.25 \overline{\smash{\big)}\,3.50 \land 000} \quad 1.555
$$

```
              1 . 5 5 5
2.25 ⋏)3.50⋏000
      2 25
      1 25   0
      1 12   5
         12  50
         11  25
          1  250
          1  125
```

  c. $3\frac{1}{2} : 2\frac{1}{4}$ written as a decimal is 1.555

CHANGING A RATIO TO A PERCENT

1. Express the ratio as a proper fraction or a decimal fraction, whichever you prefer to work with.
2. Multiply by 100.
3. Add the percent sign (%).

Example 1: $3 : 5$

Changing to a proper fraction:

  a. $\dfrac{3}{\cancel{5}_{1}} \times \dfrac{\cancel{100}^{20}}{1} = \dfrac{60}{1}$

  b. 60%

Changing to a decimal fraction:

  a.
```
      0.6
  5)3.0
    3 0
```

  b. $0.6 \times 100 = 60$

  c. 60%

Example 2: $60 : 180$

Changing to a proper fraction:

  a. $\dfrac{60}{180} = \dfrac{1}{3}$

  b. $\dfrac{1}{3} \times \dfrac{100}{1} = \dfrac{100}{3} = 33\frac{1}{3}$

  c. $33\frac{1}{3}\%$

Changing to a decimal fraction:

  a.
```
      0.333
  180)60.000
      54 0
       6 00
       5 40
         600
         540
          600
          540
           60
```

  b. $0.333 \times 100 = 33.3$

  c. 33.3%

WORK SHEET

Directions: Change the following fractions to ratios reduced to lowest terms.

1. $^9/_{12}$ _____

2. $^4/_6$ _____

3. $^{11}/_{22}$ _____

4. $^{56}/_{100}$ _____

5. $^{20}/_{50}$ _____

6. $^{310}/_{1000}$ _____

7. $^{10}/_{16}$ _____

8. $^5/_6 / 3^1/_3$ _____

9. $1^3/_5 / 2^7/_{10}$ _____

10. $^1/_{10} / ^1/_{100}$ _____

11. $^{14}/_{30} / 2$ _____

12. $3^1/_3 / 3^1/_3$ _____

Directions: Change the following decimal fractions to ratios reduced to lowest terms.

1. 0.896 _____

2. 0.96 _____

3. 0.06 _____

4. 0.6 _____

5. 0.4032 _____

6. 0.74 _____

7. 0.166 _____

8. 0.26 _____

9. 0.492 _____

10. 0.95 _____

11. 0.235 _____

12. 0.172 _____

Directions: Change the following percents to ratios reduced to lowest terms.

1. 10% _____

2. 33⅓% _____

3. ⅜% _____

4. 2⁷⁄₁₀% _____

5. 44% _____

6. 15.7% _____

7. 7¾% _____

8. 0.44% _____

9. 7.8% _____

10. 1% _____

11. ⅗% _____

12. 3³⁄₇% _____

Directions: Change the following ratios to fractions reduced to lowest terms.

1. 4 : 64 _____

2. 4 : 800 _____

3. 3 : 150 _____

4. ³⁄₈ : ¹⁄₄ _____

5. ⁸⁄₁₂ : ²⁄₃ _____

6. 2¹⁄₂ : 7¹⁄₂ _____

7. ⁴⁄₅ : ¹⁄₄ _____

8. ¹⁄₁₀ : ⁴⁄₂₀ _____

9. ⁴⁄₇₅ : ³⁄₁₀ _____

10. 0.68 : 0.44 _____

11. 1.85 : 3.35 _____

12. 1.64 : 2.54 _____

Directions: Change the following ratios to decimal numbers.

1. 7 : 14 _____

2. 5 : 20 _____

3. 3 : 8 _____

4. 11 : 33 _____

5. ⁵⁄₈ : ¹⁄₁₀ _____

6. ¹⁄₁₀₀₀ : ¹⁄₅₀₀ _____

7. ¾ : ½ _____

8. ³⁄₁₀₀₀ : ³⁄₁₀₀ _____

9. 2 : 5 _____

10. ½ : ⁵⁄₉ _____

11. 7 : 259 _____

12. 1²⁄₅ : ¹²⁄₃₀ _____

Directions: Change the following ratios to percents.

1. 2 : 4 _____

2. 7 : 231 _____

3. 25 : 250 _____

4. 30 : 150 _____

5. 1¼ : 3⅜ _____

6. 1 : 1000 _____

7. 0.15 : 0.6 _____

8. ⁵⁄₁₆ : ⅗ _____

9. 1 : 500 _____

10. 1⁸⁄₁₂ : 2³⁄₆ _____

11. 2.5 : 4.5 _____

12. 4 : ³⁄₁₆ _____

Answers on pp. 477-478.

Name _____

Date _____

ACCEPTABLE SCORE __29__

YOUR SCORE _____

POSTTEST 1

Directions: Convert to equivalents.

	Ratio	Fraction	Decimal	Percent
1.	42 : 48			
2.			0.004	
3.		$^{13}/_{20}$		
4.				2¼%
5.			0.35	
6.		$^{6}/_{25}$		
7.	$^{3}/_{8} : ^{5}/_{9}$			
8.				0.3%
9.			0.205	
10.		$^{4}/_{11}$		

Answers on p. 478.

Name _____

Date _____

ACCEPTABLE SCORE ___29___

YOUR SCORE _____

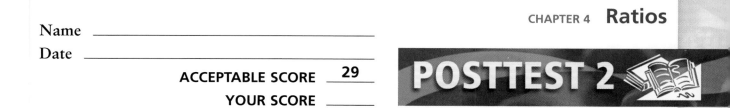

POSTTEST 2

Directions: Convert to equivalents.

	Ratio	Fraction	Decimal	Percent
1.	7 : 10			
2.		⁵/₁₆		
3.			0.075	
4.				6%
5.				⅜%
6.		¹/₁₅₀		
7.			0.007	
8.	6 : 21			
9.			0.322	
10.				18.2%

Answers on p. 478.

Refer to Review of Mathematics: Ratios on the enclosed CD for additional help and practice problems.

Name _____

Date _____

ACCEPTABLE SCORE ___19___

YOUR SCORE _____

PRETEST ✓

Complete the Proportions Pretest. A score of 19 out of 20 indicates an acceptable understanding of and competency in basic calculations involving proportions. You may skip to the Review of Mathematics Posttest on p. 97. However, if you score 18 or below, completion of Chapter 5, Proportions, will be helpful for your continued success in the calculation of drug dosages.

Directions: Find the value of x. Show your work.

1. $25 : 75 :: x : 300$ _____

2. $450 : 15 :: 225 : x$ _____

3. $x : \frac{1}{4}\% :: 8 : 12$ _____

4. $12 : 3 :: x : 0.8$ _____

5. $0.6 : 2.4 :: 32 : x$ _____

6. $150 : x :: 75 : 2$ _____

7. $\frac{1}{8} : \frac{2}{3} :: 75 : x$ _____

8. $\frac{1}{200} : 8 :: x : 800$ _____

9. $x : \frac{1}{2} :: \frac{3}{4} : \frac{7}{8}$ _____

10. $16 : x :: 24 : 12$ _____

11. $\frac{2}{3} : \frac{1}{5} :: x : 24$ _____

12. $x : 9 :: \frac{2}{3} : 36$ _____

13. $\frac{1}{7} : x :: \frac{1}{2} : 49$ _____

14. $0.8 : 4 :: 9.6 : x$ _____

15. $\frac{4}{5} : x :: \frac{2}{3} : \frac{1}{4}$ _____

16. $40 : 80 :: x : 160$ _____   **17.** $2.5 : x :: 4 : 16$ _____   **18.** $8 : 72 :: 14 : x$ _____

19. $x : \frac{1}{15} :: 50 : 500$ _____   **20.** $5 : 100 :: x : 325$ _____

Answers on p. 478.

Proportions

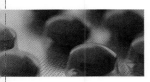

LEARNING OBJECTIVES

On completion of the materials provided in this chapter, you will be able to perform computations accurately by mastering the following mathematical concepts:

1 Solving simple proportion problems

2 Solving proportion problems involving fractions, decimals, and percents

Most problems concerning drug dosage can be solved by a proportion problem, whether it involves fractions, decimals, or percents. If a proportion problem contains any combination of fractions, decimals, or percents, all forms within the problem must be converted to either fractions or decimals.

Study the introductory material on proportions. The process for the calculation of proportion problems is listed in steps. Memorize the steps before beginning the work sheet. Complete the work sheet at the end of this chapter, which provides for extensive practice in the manipulation of proportions. Check your answers. If you have difficulties, go back and review the necessary steps. When you feel ready to evaluate your learning, take the first posttest. Check your answers. An acceptable score as indicated on the posttest signifies that you are ready for the next chapter. An unacceptable score signifies a need for further study before taking the second posttest.

A **proportion** consists of two ratios of equal value. The ratios are connected by a double colon ($::$), which symbolizes the word *as.*

$$2 : 3 :: 4 : 6$$

Read the above proportion: "Two is to three as four is to six."

The first and fourth terms of the proportion are the **extremes.** The second and third terms are the **means.**

$$2 : 3 :: 4 : 6$$

2 and 6 are the extremes
3 and 4 are the means

A helpful way to remember the correct location of the extremes and means is

E = The *end* of the problem
M = The *middle* of the problem

In a proportion the product of the means equals the product of the extremes because the ratios are of equal value. This principle may be used to verify your answer in a proportion problem.

$3 \times 4 = 12$, product of the means
$2 \times 6 = 12$, product of the extremes

If three terms in the proportions are known and one term is unknown, an x is inserted in the space for the unknown term.

$$2 : 3 :: 4 : x$$

SOLVING A SIMPLE PROPORTION PROBLEM

1. Multiply the means.
2. Multiply the extremes.
3. Place the product that includes the x on the *left* of the equal sign and the product of the known terms on the *right* of the equal sign.
4. Divide the product of the known terms by the number next to x. The quotient will be the value of x.

Proportion Problem Involving Whole Numbers

Example: $2 : 3 :: 4 : x$

    a. $2x = 3 \times 4$

    b. $2x = 12$

    c. $x = 12 \div 2$

    d. $x = \dfrac{12}{2}$

    e. $x = 6$

Proportion Problem Involving Fractions

Example: $\dfrac{1}{150} : \dfrac{1}{100} :: x : 60$

    a. $\dfrac{1}{100}x = \dfrac{1}{150} \times 60$

    b. $\dfrac{1}{100}x = \dfrac{2}{5}$

    c. $x = \dfrac{2}{5} \div \dfrac{1}{100}$

    d. $x = \dfrac{2}{\cancel{5}_{1}} \times \dfrac{\cancel{100}^{20}}{1}$

    e. $x = 40$

Proportion Problem Involving Decimals

Example: $0.4 : 0.8 :: 0.25 : x$

a. $0.4x = 0.8 \times 0.25$

b. $0.4x = 0.2$

c. $x = 0.2 \div 0.4$

d. $x = 0.5$

Proportion Problem Involving Fractions and Percents

Example: $x : \frac{1}{4}\% :: 9\frac{3}{5} : \frac{1}{200}$

Convert ¼% to a proper fraction and 9⅗ to an improper fraction. Then rewrite the proportion using these fractions.

a. $x : \dfrac{1}{400} :: \dfrac{48}{5} : \dfrac{1}{200}$

b. $\dfrac{1}{200}x = \dfrac{1}{400} \times \dfrac{48}{5}$

c. $\dfrac{1}{200}x = \dfrac{1}{\underset{25}{\cancel{400}}} \times \dfrac{\overset{3}{\cancel{48}}}{5}$

d. $\dfrac{1}{200}x = \dfrac{3}{125}$

e. $x = \dfrac{3}{125} \div \dfrac{1}{200}$

f. $x = \dfrac{3}{\underset{5}{\cancel{125}}} \times \dfrac{\overset{8}{\cancel{200}}}{1}$

g. $x = \dfrac{24}{5}$

h. $x = 4\frac{4}{5}$

Proportion Problem Involving Decimals and Percents

Example: $0.3\% : 1.8 :: x : 14.4$

Convert 0.3% to a decimal.

a. $0.003 : 1.8 = x : 14.4$

b. $1.8x = 0.003 \times 14.4$

c. $1.8x = 0.0432$

d. $x = 0.0432 \div 1.8$

e. $x = 0.024$

Proportion Problem Involving Numerous Zeros

Example: $250{,}000 : x :: 500{,}000 : 4$

     a. $500{,}000x = 250{,}000 \times 4$

     b. $500{,}000x = 1{,}000{,}000$

     c. $x = 1{,}000{,}000 \div 500{,}000$

     d. $x = \dfrac{1{,}000{,}000}{500{,}000}$

     e. $x = 2$

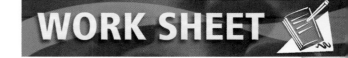

Directions: Find the value of x. Show your work.

1. $20 : 400 :: x : 1680$ _____

2. $0.9 : 2.4 :: x : 75$ _____

3. $\frac{5}{6} : x :: \frac{5}{9} : \frac{4}{5}$ _____

4. $3 : 90 :: 1\frac{3}{4} : x$ _____

5. $75 : x :: 100 : 2$ _____

6. $\frac{1}{6} : 1 :: \frac{1}{8} : x$ _____

7. $200,000 : x :: 1,000,000 : 5$ _____

8. $x : \frac{3}{4}\% :: 3\frac{1}{5} : \frac{1}{200}$ _____

9. $\frac{1}{150} : 1 :: \frac{1}{100} : x$ _____

10. $3 : 150 :: 40 : x$ _____

11. $\frac{1}{8} : x :: 7 : 56$ _____

12. $\frac{1}{200} : 40 :: \frac{1}{100} : x$ _____

13. $12\frac{1}{2} : x :: 50 : 2400$ _____

14. $\frac{1}{2}\% : \frac{1}{100} :: x : 80$ _____

15. $x : 6.4 :: 0.03 : 6$ _____

16. $0.25 : 1 :: 0.05 : x$ _____

17. $\frac{1}{120} : 2 :: 4 : x$ _____

18. $x : \frac{1}{1000} :: 5 : \frac{1}{5000}$ _____

19. $6 : 15 :: 8 : x$ _____

20. $x : 3 :: 9 : 54$ _____

21. $1.4 : 0.4 :: 4.2 : x$ _____

22. $x : 0.65 :: 9 : 5$ _____

23. $12\frac{1}{2}\% : 5 :: x : 120$ _____

24. $\frac{1}{300} : 6 :: \frac{1}{120} : x$ _____

25. $25 : 75 :: 16 : x$ _____

26. $0.3 : x :: 7 : 21$ _____

27. $4 : x :: 12 : 48$ _____

28. $x : 12 :: 2 : 4$ _____

29. $\frac{4}{5} : x :: \frac{1}{3} : \frac{5}{9}$ _____

30. $0.6 : x :: 7 : 42$ _____

31. $15 : x :: 20 : 600$ _____

32. $9\% : x :: 11 : 73$ _____

33. $500{,}000 : 1 :: 300{,}000 : x$ _____

34. $\frac{1}{6} : \frac{9}{10} :: \frac{1}{2} : x$ _____

35. $2.8 : 12 :: 40 : x$ _____

36. $8 : \frac{8}{100} :: x : 5$ _____

37. $\frac{1}{8}\% : \frac{1}{200} :: x : 40$ _____

38. $x : 25 :: 18 : 36$ _____

39. $0.15 : 0.25 :: x : 400$ _____

40. $\frac{1}{20} : \frac{1}{15} :: x : 25$ _____

41. $800,000 : 5 :: 960,000 : x$ _____

42. $27 : x :: 9 : 60$ _____

43. $\frac{1}{20} : \frac{1}{5} :: x : 50$ _____

44. $\frac{1}{150} : \frac{1}{200} :: x : 60$ _____

45. $\frac{1}{2}\% : 4 :: x : 25$ _____

46. $500 : 2.5 :: x : 8.1$ _____

Answers on p. 478.

Name _____

Date _____

ACCEPTABLE SCORE ___19___

YOUR SCORE _____

POSTTEST 1

Directions: Find the value of x. Show your work.

1. $x : 2.5 :: 4 : 5$ _____

2. $\frac{7}{8} : x :: \frac{4}{5} : \frac{2}{3}$ _____

3. $30 : 90 :: 2 : x$ _____

4. $x : 3.5 :: 25 : 14$ _____

5. $\frac{2}{7} : \frac{1}{2} :: x : 56$ _____

6. $\frac{1}{4} : x :: 160 : 320$ _____

7. $x : 7 :: 5 : 14$ _____

8. $3 : x :: 18 : 12$ _____

9. $\frac{1}{5} : 90 :: x : 250$ _____

10. $1.8 : 4.8 :: x : 96$ _____

11. $x : 8 :: 10 : 20$ _____

12. $\frac{2}{3} : x :: 4.5 : 27$ _____

13. $\frac{1}{150} : x :: \frac{1}{200} : 6$ _____

14. $\frac{2}{3}\% : \frac{1}{5} :: 50 : x$ _____

15. $14 : x :: 6 : 18$ _____

16. $x : \frac{2}{3} :: 12 : 18$ _____   **17.** $50 : 250 :: \frac{4}{5} : x$ _____   **18.** $50 : 3 :: x : 6$ _____

19. $\frac{1}{2} : x :: 40 : 80$ _____   **20.** $0.8 : 10 :: x : 40$ _____

Answers on p. 478.

Name _____

Date _____

ACCEPTABLE SCORE ___19___

YOUR SCORE _____

POSTTEST 2

Directions: Find the value of x. Show your work.

1. $x : 300 :: 9 : 12$ _____

2. $4 : 32\% :: 16 : x$ _____

3. $18 : x :: 6 : 40$ _____

4. $1.8 : 2.5 :: x : 9.5$ _____

5. $x : 30 :: \frac{1}{3} : \frac{3}{4}$ _____

6. $\frac{7}{8} : x :: \frac{5}{8} : 40$ _____

7. $400 : 500 :: \frac{4}{5} : x$ _____

8. $x : 7.6 :: 3 : 6$ _____

9. $\frac{1}{4} : x :: \frac{2}{3} : \frac{2}{5}$ _____

10. $\frac{1}{150} : \frac{1}{100} :: x : 60$ _____

11. $0.6 : x :: 15 : 90$ _____

12. $3.5 : 12 :: x : 360$ _____

13. $\frac{2}{9} : \frac{4}{5} :: \frac{3}{4} : x$ _____

14. $\frac{1}{8} : x :: \frac{1}{7} : \frac{5}{9}$ _____

15. $x : 2.5 :: 16 : 4$ _____

16. $0.6 : 3 :: 72 : x$ _____

17. $20 : x :: 6 : 4.5$ _____

18. $x : ¼ :: 96 : ⅓$ _____

19. $300 : 5000 :: x : 18$ _____

20. $⅓ : x :: ⅕ : 90$ _____

Answers on p. 479.

Refer to Review of Mathematics: Proportions on the enclosed CD for additional help and practice problems.

Name _____

Date _____

ACCEPTABLE SCORE ___95___

YOUR SCORE _____

POSTTEST

After your successful completion of Chapters 1 through 5, complete the Review of Mathematics Posttest. A score of 95 out of 100 indicates an acceptable understanding of and competency in basic mathematics. You are now ready to begin Part II, Units and Measurements for the Calculation of Drug Dosages. However, if you score 94 or below, an additional review of previous chapter content may be helpful before beginning Part II.

Directions: Complete the following definitions and exercises.

1. *Improper fractions* can be reduced to a _____ number or a _____ number.

2. In the following fractions, circle only those that are *improper fractions*.

   $\frac{4}{12}$ $\frac{7}{6}$ $\frac{6}{3}$ $\frac{4}{7}$ $\frac{9}{9}$ $\frac{14}{21}$

3. A *complex fraction* contains a _____ in its numerator, its denominator, or both.

4. In the following examples, circle only the *complex fractions*.

   $1\frac{2}{3}$ $\frac{1/2}{4}$ $\frac{12}{4}$ $\frac{3/7}{4/2}$ $21\frac{5}{6}$ $\frac{21}{2/3}$

5-6. A *ratio* is the _____ between _____ numbers.

Write each of the following numbers as a *ratio*.

7. $\frac{4}{12}$ _____

8. 24% _____

9. 0.03 _____

10. $1\frac{3}{8}$ _____

11. 2.2% _____

12. 1.24 _____

13. The *divisor* of a fraction is known as the _____.

Division problems can be expressed in different ways. Circle the *divisor* in each of the following examples.

14. $\frac{2}{3}$ 15. $4 \div 8$ 16. $10 : 5$ 17. $4\overline{)12}$ 18. $\frac{14}{8}$ 19. $6 \div 24$ 20. $42\overline{)7}$ 21. $7 : 10$

22-24. The number shown in a decimal is the _____ of a fraction. The denominator of this fraction is implied by the number of decimal places shown and is _____ or some power of _____.

Write the fraction values for the following *decimal fraction* numbers.

25. 0.436 _____

26. 0.051 _____

27. 1.0042 _____

28. 0.9684 _____

29. 0.0019 _____

30. 1.02064 _____

Directions: Add and reduce fractions to lowest terms.

31. $5/9 + 2/5 + 2/3 =$ _____

32. $4\frac{1}{4} + 2\frac{5}{6} =$ _____

33. $5\frac{1}{2} + 3/9 =$ _____

34. $3/4 / 5/6 + 4\frac{3}{5} =$ _____

Directions: Add and round answers to hundredths.

35. $4.02 + 3.4 + 1.099 =$ _____

36. $45.009 + 0.076 + 1.2 =$ _____

37. $0.0082 + 0.923 + 234 =$ _____

38. $456 + 3.56 + 0.0029 =$ _____

Directions: Subtract and reduce fractions to lowest terms.

39. $2/4 - 3/9 =$ _____

40. $4/7 / 2/8 - 2/3 =$ _____

41. $3\frac{4}{5} - 2\frac{8}{9} =$ _____

42. $6\frac{1}{2} - 8/9 =$ _____

Directions: Subtract and round answers to tenths.

43. $23.98 - 0.0987 =$ _____

44. $23.191 - 23.099 =$ _____

45. $9.002 - 4.9089 =$ _____

46. $2.009 - 0.9834 =$ _____

Directions: Multiply and reduce fractions to lowest terms.

47. $9 \times \frac{5}{8} =$ _____

48. $\frac{3}{4} \times \frac{8}{9} =$ _____

49. $4\frac{8}{9} \times 1\frac{5}{6} =$ _____

50. $3\frac{4}{5} \times 7 =$ _____

Directions: Multiply and round answers to hundredths.

51. $3.45 \times 0.56 =$ _____

52. $21.4 \times 0.092 =$ _____

53. $0.0452 \times 99.1 =$ _____

54. $739 \times 0.246 =$ _____

Directions: Divide and reduce fractions to lowest terms.

55. $\frac{7}{8} \div \frac{4}{9} =$ _____

56. $\frac{2}{5} \div \frac{7}{9} =$ _____

57. $\frac{1}{300} \div \frac{3}{4} =$ _____

58. $4\frac{7}{9} \div 5\frac{9}{11} =$ _____

Directions: Divide and round answers to thousandths.

59. $52.014 \div 9.2 =$ _____

60. $0.0982 \div 75 =$ _____

61. $3200 \div 0.04 =$ _____

62. $78.09 \div 4.501 =$ _____

Directions: Number the following decimal numbers in order from *lesser to greater value.*

63. 0.45 _____ 1.46 _____ 0.407 _____ 2.401 _____ 0.048 _____ 0.014 _____

64. 0.15 _____ 0.015 _____ 1.015 _____ 1.15 _____ 0.155 _____ 1.0015 _____

65. 9.09 _____ 0.99 _____ 0.090 _____ 0.90 _____ 90.90 _____ 9.009 _____

66. 0.6 _____ 0.4 _____ 0.7 _____ 0.52 _____ 0.44 _____ 0.24 _____

67. 0.21 _____ 0.191 _____ 0.021 _____ 0.1091 _____ 0.201 _____ 0.2 _____

Directions: Change the following fractions to decimals and round the answers to hundredths.

68. $5/6$ _____   **69.** $5/9$ _____

70. $9/16$ _____   **71.** $1/150$ _____

Directions: Change the following decimals to fractions and reduce to lowest terms.

72. 0.225 _____   **73.** 0.465 _____

74. 0.06 _____   **75.** 0.372 _____

Directions: Make the following calculations.

76. Express 0.275 as a percent. _____   **77.** Express $3/8$ as a percent. _____

78. Express 42% as a proper fraction and reduce to lowest terms. _____

79. Express 0.62% as a ratio. _____   **80.** What percent of 3.2 is 0.4? _____

81. What percent of $5/7$ is $5/28$? _____   **82.** What percent of 240 is 36? _____

83. What is ½% of 48? _____   **84.** What is 6½% of 840? _____

85. What is 46% of 325? _____

Directions: Change the following fractions and decimals to ratios reduced to lowest terms.

86. $^{10}/_{45}$ _____   **87.** $1^{3}\!/_{4}/4^{2}\!/_{3}$ _____   **88.** 0.584 _____

89. $^{250}/_{375}$ _____   **90.** 0.48 _____

Directions: Find the value of x and round decimal answers to hundredths.

91. $8 : ^{4}\!/_{45} :: x : 3$ _____   **92.** $x : 34 :: 4 : 81$ _____   **93.** $4.6 : 3 :: 20 : x$ _____

94. $x : ½\% :: 4.5 : ^{1}\!/_{50}$ _____   **95.** $^{1}\!/_{300} : ^{1}\!/_{150} :: x : 300$ _____   **96.** $22 : x :: 4 : 88$ _____

97. $0.35 : 0.75 :: x : 425$ _____   **98.** $400 : x :: ^{1}\!/_{300} : ^{1}\!/_{225}$ _____   **99.** $x : 54 :: 4 : 8$ _____

100. $½/¾ : 8 :: x : 45$ _____

Answers on p. 479.

Units and Measurements for the Calculation of Drug Dosages

CHAPTERS

*P*art II is designed in the same way as Part I, Review of Mathematics. After completing Part I, you have validated that you do have the basic mathematical skills required to progress with Part II. A pretest precedes each of the three chapters in Part II. For some of you who have had experience in nursing and the administration of medications (such as a licensed practical nurse, licensed visiting nurse, or a registered nurse with an associate's degree), these pretests will allow you to assess your need for a more extensive review of the material. After completion of the test, check your answers with the key provided. A score of 95% correct as indicated on each test indicates a mastery of the material covered in that chapter. You may then skip to the next pretest and follow the same exercises until Part II has been completed.

For those of you who have *not* had experience in nursing and the administration of medications, the following chapters of Part II should be worked as written *without using the pretests preceding Chapters 6, 7, and 8.*

You are now ready to follow the path that matches your experience to ensure mastery of the following three chapters. Begin now, and good luck!

Metric and Household Measurements

Name _____

Date _____

ACCEPTABLE SCORE __29__

YOUR SCORE _____

PRETEST ✓

Directions: Change to equivalent metric or household measurements. Solve each problem by using a proportion. Show your work.

1. 800,000 mcg = _____ g

2. 3 mg = _____ mcg

3. 255 mg = _____ g

4. 46 mg = _____ mcg

5. 3000 mcg = _____ mg

6. 0.68 g = _____ mg

7. 326 mL = _____ L

8. 33 kg = _____ lb

9. 2.1 g = _____ mg

10. 3000 g = _____ kg

11. 0.1 L = _____ mL

12. 53 kg = _____ lb

13. 0.005 mg = _____ mcg

14. 0.8 kg = _____ g

15. 250 mcg = _____ mg

16. 1¼ cups = _____ mL

17. 22 lb = _____ g

18. 0.63 L = _____ mL

19. 733 g = _____ kg

20. 1.25 g = _____ mcg

21. 60 mg = _____ g

22. 0.25 mg = _____ mcg

23. 0.25 L = _____ mL

24. 45 lb = _____ kg

25. 10,000 mcg = _____ g

26. 1.2 kg = _____ g

27. 1⅔ Tbsp = _____ mL

28. 0.71 g = _____ mg

29. 480 mL = _____ L

30. 650 g = _____ lb

Answers on p. 480.

Metric and Household Measurements

LEARNING OBJECTIVES

On completion of the materials provided in this chapter, you will be able to perform computations accurately by mastering the following mathematical concepts:

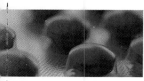

1 Recalling the metric measures of weight, volume, and length

2 Computing equivalents within the metric system by using a proportion

3 Recalling approximate equivalents between metric and household measures

4 Computing equivalents between the metric and household systems of measure by using a proportion

METRIC MEASUREMENTS

The metric system has become the system of choice for dealing with the weights and measures involved in the calculation of drug dosages. This is a result of its accuracy and simplicity because it is based on the decimal system. The use of decimals tends to eliminate errors made when working with fractions. Therefore **all answers within the metric system need to be expressed as decimals, not as fractions.**

Examples: 0.5, not ½

0.75, not ¾

0.007, not ⁷⁄₁₀₀₀

Certain prefixes identify the multiples of 10 that are being used. The four most commonly used prefixes of the metric system involved with the calculation of drug dosages are the following:

micro = 0.000001 or one millionth

milli = 0.001 or one thousandth

centi = 0.01 or one hundredth

kilo = 1000 or one thousand

These prefixes may be used with any of the base units of weight (gram), volume (liter), or length (meter). The nurse most often uses the following list of metric measures (Box 6-1). Memorize all the entries in the list.

BOX 6-1 ■ COMMON METRIC MEASURES

Metric Measure of Weight
1,000,000 micrograms (mcg) = 1 gram (g)
1000 micrograms (mcg) = 1 milligram (mg)
1000 milligrams (mg) = 1 gram (g)
1000 grams (g) = 1 kilogram (kg)

Metric Measure of Volume
1000 milliliters (mL) = 1 liter (L)
1 cubic centimeter (cc) = 1 milliliter (mL)*

Metric Measure of Length
1 meter (m) = 1000 mm or 100 cm
1 centimeter (cm) = 10 mm or 0.01 m
1 millimeter (mm) = 0.1 cm or 0.001 m

Sometimes, to compute drug dosages, the nurse must convert a metric measure to an equivalent measure within the system. This may be done easily by using a proportion.

Example: 300 mg equals how many grams?

a. On the left side of the proportion, place what you know to be an equivalent between milligrams and grams. From the preceding chart we know that there are 1000 mg in 1 g. Therefore the left side of the proportion would be

1000 mg : 1 g ::

b. The right side of the proportion is determined by the problem and by the abbreviations used on the left side of the proportion. Only *two* different abbreviations may be used in a single proportion. The abbreviations must also be in the same position on the right as they are on the left.

1000 mg : 1 g :: _____ mg : _____ g

From the problem we know we have 300 mg.

1000 mg : 1 g :: 300 mg : _____ g

We need to find the number of grams 300 mg equals, so we use the symbol x to represent the unknown. Therefore the full proportion would be

$$1000 \text{ mg} : 1 \text{ g} :: 300 \text{ mg} : x \text{ g}$$

c. Rewrite the proportion without using the abbreviations.

$$1000 : 1 :: 300 : x$$

d. Solve for x by multiplying the means and extremes. Write the answer as a decimal, since the metric system is based on decimals.

$$1000 : 1 :: 300 : x$$

$$1000x = 300$$

$$x = \frac{300}{1000}$$

$$x = 0.3$$

e. Label your answer, as determined by the abbreviation placed next to x in the original proportion.

$$300 \text{ mg} = 0.3 \text{ g}$$

Example 1: 2.5 L equals how many milliliters?

    a. 1000 mL : 1 L ::
    b. 1000 mL : 1 L :: _____ mL : _____ L
       1000 mL : 1 L :: x mL : 2.5 L
    c. 1000 : 1 :: x : 2.5
    d. 1x = 2500
       x = 2500
    e. 2.5 L = 2500 mL

Example 2: 180 mcg equals how many grams?

    a. 1,000,000 mcg : 1 g ::
    b. 1,000,000 mcg : 1 g :: _____ mcg : _____ g
       1,000,000 mcg : 1 g :: 180 mcg : x g
    c. 1,000,000 : 1 :: 180 : x
    d. 1,000,000x = 180

$$x = \frac{180}{1,000,000}$$

$$x = 0.00018$$

    e. 180 mcg = 0.00018 g

Example 3: 15 mm equals how many centimeters?

    a. 1 cm : 10 mm
    b. 1 cm : 10 mm :: _____ cm : _____ mm
       1 cm : 10 mm :: x cm : 15 mm
    c. 1 : 10 :: x : 15
    d. 10x = 1 × 15
       10x = 15

$$x = \frac{15}{10}$$

$$x = 1.5$$

    e. 15 mm = 1.5 cm

HOUSEHOLD MEASUREMENTS

Household measures are not accurate enough for the nurse to use in the calculation of drug dosages in the hospital. However, their metric equivalents are used in keeping a written record of a patient's "I" and "O," or intake and output. Always use your institution's conversions when documenting intake. For example, one cup of coffee at one institution may be 250 mL, and at another institution it may be 300 mL.

Memorize the following list of approximate equivalents between metric and household measurements (Box 6-2).

Box 6-2 ■ METRIC HOUSEHOLD EQUIVALENTS

Metric Measure = Household Measure

5 milliliters (mL) = 1 teaspoon (tsp)
15 milliliters (mL) = 1 tablespoon (Tbsp)
30 milliliters (mL) = 1 ounce (oz)
240 milliliters (mL) = 1 standard measuring cup
1 kilogram (kg) or 1000 grams (g) = 2.2 pounds (lb)
2.5 cm = 1 inch
1 foot = 12 inches

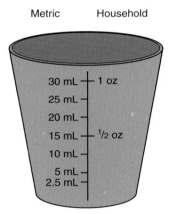

Conversion of measures between the metric and household systems of measure may also be done by using a proportion, as has been illustrated.

Example 1:   1½ cups equals how many milliliters?

   a. 1 cup : 240 mL ::

   b. 1 cup : 240 mL :: _____ cups : _____ mL
      1 cup : 240 mL :: 1½ cups : x mL

   c. 1 : 240 :: 1½ : x

   d. $x = \dfrac{240}{1} \times \dfrac{3}{2}$

   $x = \dfrac{720}{2} = 360$ mL

   e. 1½ cups = 360 mL

Example 2:   35 kg equals how many pounds?

      a. 1 kg : 2.2 lb ::

      b. 1 kg : 2.2 lb :: _____ kg : _____ lb
         1 kg : 2.2 lb :: 35 kg : x lb

      c. 1 : 2.2 :: 35 : x

      d. $1x = 2.2 \times 35$
         $x = 77$

      e. 35 kg = 77 lb

Example 3:   18 inches equals how many centimeters?

      a. 2.5 cm : 1 inch ::

      b. 2.5 cm : 1 inch :: _____ cm : _____ inch
         2.5 cm : 1 inch :: _____ cm : 18 inches

      c. 2.5 : 1 :: x : 18

      d. $x = 2.5 \times 18$
         $x = 45$ cm

      e. 18 inches = 45 cm

Memorize the tables of metric and household measurements. Study the material on forming proportions for the calculation of problems relating to the metric and household systems of measure. Complete the following work sheet, which provides for extensive practice in the manipulation of measurements within the metric and household systems. Check your answers. If you have difficulties, go back and review the necessary material. When you feel ready to evaluate your learning, take the first posttest. Check your answers. An acceptable score as indicated on the posttest signifies that you are ready for the next chapter. An unacceptable score signifies a need for further study before taking the second posttest.

WORK SHEET

Directions: Change to equivalents within the metric system. Solve the problems by using a proportion. Show your work.

1. 230 mcg = _____ g

2. 5 mg = _____ mcg

3. 2.5 g = _____ mcg

4. 4000 mcg = _____ mg

5. 0.33 g = _____ mg

6. 6 kg = _____ g

7. 725 mL = _____ L

8. 2000 mcg = _____ g

9. 3 cm = _____ mm

10. 620 g = _____ kg

11. 0.036 mg = _____ mcg

12. 460 mL = _____ L

13. 0.66 mg = _____ mcg   **14.** 0.5 g = _____ mcg   **15.** 18 inches = _____ cm

16. 350,000 mcg = _____ g   **17.** 25 mg = _____ g   **18.** 1.46 L = _____ mL

19. 2.5 kg = _____ g   **20.** 12 mg = _____ mcg   **21.** 3.4 kg = _____ g

22. 920 mcg = _____ g   **23.** 25 mm = _____ cm   **24.** 300 mcg = _____ mg

25. 0.16 L = _____ mL   **26.** 0.01 g = _____ mg   **27.** 500 mcg = _____ mg

28. 360 mg = _____ g   **29.** 1.7 L = _____ mL   **30.** 0.45 g = _____ mg

31. 240 mL = _____ L   **32.** 10 mcg = _____ mg

Directions: Change the following measurements into the approximate equivalents within the metric or household system, as indicated. Solve the problems by using a proportion. Show your work.

33. 3 inches = _____ cm   **34.** 2¼ cups = _____ mL   **35.** 2 tsp = _____ mL

36. 3 Tbsp = _____ mL   **37.** 1½ cups = _____ mL   **38.** 8 kg = _____ lb

39. 3825 g = _____ lb   **40.** 7 inches = _____ cm   **41.** 3 lb = _____ kg

42. 12 kg = _____ lb   **43.** 1400 g = _____ lb   **44.** 2½ feet = _____ inches

45. 150 lb = _____ kg

Answers on p. 480.

Name _____

Date _____

ACCEPTABLE SCORE __29__

YOUR SCORE _____

POSTTEST 1

Directions: Change to equivalent measurements. Solve each problem by using a proportion. Show your work.

1. 5000 mcg = _____ g

2. 10 mg = _____ mcg

3. 0.81 L = _____ mL

4. 35 mg = _____ g

5. 2½ feet = _____ inches

6. 0.12 g = _____ mcg

7. 16 kg = _____ lb

8. 280 mL = _____ L

9. 0.4 kg = _____ g

10. 42 inches = _____ feet

11. 28 lb = _____ g

12. 4 inches = _____ cm

13. 500,000 mcg = _____ g **14.** 37 mL = _____ L **15.** 20 mL = _____ cc

16. 1⅓ cups = _____ mL **17.** 2.5 g = _____ mg **18.** 350 mg = _____ g

19. 6700 g = _____ kg **20.** 0.3 L = _____ mL **21.** 4 mg = _____ mcg

22. 2600 g = _____ lb **23.** 1½ tsp = _____ mL **24.** 0.2 L = _____ mL

25. 533 mL = _____ L **26.** 1.5 g = _____ mcg **27.** 620 mg = _____ g

28. 2.3 kg = _____ g **29.** 15 inches = _____ feet **30.** 7 lb = _____ kg

Answers on p. 480.

Name _____

Date _____

ACCEPTABLE SCORE ___29___

YOUR SCORE _____

POSTTEST 2

Directions: Change to equivalent measurements. Solve each problem by using a proportion. Show your work.

1. 4000 mcg = _____ mg

2. 150 g = _____ kg

3. 2½ cups = _____ mL

4. 800 g = _____ lb

5. 44 kg = _____ lb

6. 760 mg = _____ g

7. 0.55 L = _____ mL

8. 35 mm = _____ cm

9. 4 Tbsp = _____ mL

10. 2⅛ lb = _____ g

11. 0.1 L = _____ mL

12. 32 mg = _____ mcg

13. 618 mL = _____ L

14. 100,000 mcg = _____ g

15. 28 inches = _____ feet

16. 714 mL = _____ L

17. 350 mg = _____ g

18. 250,000 mcg = _____ g

19. 0.87 g = _____ mg

20. 7 mg = _____ mcg

21. 37 mcg = _____ mg

22. 1.4 L = _____ mL

23. 0.78 g = _____ mg

24. 225 mcg = _____ mg

25. 4500 g = _____ kg

26. 0.2 L = _____ mL

27. 3⅓ feet = _____ inches

28. 420 mg = _____ g

29. 2.6 g = _____ mcg

30. 73 lb = _____ kg

Answers on p. 481.

 Refer to Introducing Drug Measures: Systems of Measurement on the enclosed CD for additional help.

Name _____

Date _____

ACCEPTABLE SCORE ___9___

YOUR SCORE _____

PRETEST ✓

Directions: Change to equivalents within the apothecary system. Solve by using proportions. Show your work.

1-2. 20 fl oz = _____ pt = _____ qt   **3-4.** 5 pt = _____ fl oz = _____ qt

5-6. 7 qt = _____ gal = _____ pt

Directions: Change the following household measurements into approximate equivalents within the apothecary system. Solve the problems by using proportions. Show your work.

7. 3 cups = _____ fl oz   **8.** 4 cups = _____ pt

9. 1½ cups = _____ fl oz   **10.** 2½ cups = _____ fl oz

Answers on p. 481.

Apothecary and Household Measurements

LEARNING OBJECTIVES

On completion of the materials provided in this chapter, you will be able to perform computations accurately by mastering the following mathematical concepts:

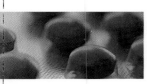

1 Converting Roman numerals to Arabic numerals

2 Converting Arabic numerals to Roman numerals

3 Adding and subtracting Roman numerals

4 Recalling the apothecary measures of weights and liquids

5 Computing equivalents within the apothecary system by using a proportion

6 Recalling approximate equivalents between apothecary and household measures

7 Computing equivalents between the apothecary and household measurement systems by using a proportion

The apothecary system of measure is a very old English system. It has slowly been replaced by the metric system. When writing orders in the apothecary system, physicians occasionally use Roman numerals. All parts of a whole are expressed as a fraction.

On the next page is a list of the more commonly used Roman numerals and their Arabic equivalents. Memorize the list.

Roman numeral	Arabic numeral
i	1
v	5
x	10
l	50
c	100

Only addition and subtraction may be performed in the Roman numeral system.

ADDITION OF ROMAN NUMERALS

1. Addition is performed when a smaller numeral follows a larger numeral.

Examples: xi = 11   xv = 15   li = 51

2. Addition is performed when a numeral is repeated. However, a numeral is *never* repeated more than three times.

Examples: viii = 8   xii = 12   ccxi = 211

SUBTRACTION OF ROMAN NUMERALS

1. Subtraction is performed when a smaller numeral is placed before a larger numeral.

Examples: ix = 9   iv = 4   ic = 99

2. Subtraction is performed when a smaller numeral is placed between two larger numerals. The smaller numeral is subtracted from the larger numeral that follows it.

Examples: xiv = 14   xxiv = 24   cxc = 190

APOTHECARY MEASUREMENTS

It is still important for a nurse to be knowledgeable about the apothecary system. Some of the older medications may still be ordered with the apothecary unit of measure.

Example: aspirin gr x

Some pharmaceutical companies label a drug using both the apothecary system and the metric system of measure.

A nurse is already familiar with many of the units of measure in the apothecary system because they are used every day. A nurse most commonly uses the apothecary system units of measure listed in Box 7-1. Memorize all entries in the list.

BOX 7-1 ■ COMMON APOTHECARY SYSTEM UNITS OF MEASURE

Apothecary Measure of Liquid
16 fluid ounces (fl oz) = 1 pint (pt)
32 fluid ounces (fl oz) = 2 pints (pt) or 1 quart (qt)
4 quarts (qt) = 1 gallon (gal)

Apothecary

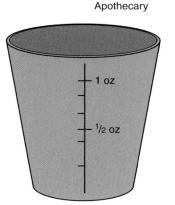

Sometimes, to compute drug dosages, the nurse must convert an apothecary measure to an equivalent measure within the same system. This may be done easily by using a proportion.

Example: 12 fl oz equals how many pints?

a. 16 fl oz : 1 pt ::

b. 16 fl oz : 1 pt :: _____ fl oz : _____ pt
    16 fl oz : 1 pt :: 12 fl oz : x pt

c. 16 : 1 :: 12 : x

d. 16x = 12

$$x = \frac{12}{16} = \frac{3}{4}$$

e. 12 fl oz = ¾ pt

Note that *fractions* (not decimals) are used when working with the apothecary system.

HOUSEHOLD MEASUREMENTS

Household measures are not accurate enough to be used by nurses in the calculation of drug dosages in the hospital. It is sometimes necessary to compute their approximate equivalents in the apothecary system of measure, especially when sending medicines home from the hospital.

Memorize the following approximate equivalent (Box 7-2).

BOX 7-2 ■ APOTHECARY/HOUSEHOLD EQUIVALENTS

Apothecary Measure = Household Measure
8 fluid ounces (fl oz) = 1 standard measuring cup

Conversion of measures between the apothecary and household systems of measure may also be made by using a proportion, as has been illustrated.

Example: 1½ cups equals how many fl oz?

    a. 8 fl oz : 1 cup ::
    b. 8 fl oz : 1 cup :: _____ fl oz : _____ cup
        8 fl oz : 1 cup :: x fl oz : 1½ cups
    c. 8 : 1 :: x : 1½
    d. $x = 8 \times 1\frac{1}{2}$

$$x = \frac{\cancel{8}^{4}}{1} \times \frac{3}{\cancel{2}_{1}}$$

$$x = \frac{12}{1} = 12$$

    e. 1½ cups = 12 fl oz

Memorize the tables for the apothecary and household measurements. Study the material on forming proportions for the calculation of problems relating to the apothecary and household systems of measure. Complete the following work sheet, which provides for extensive practice in the manipulation of measurements within the apothecary and household systems. Check your answers. If you have difficulties, go back and review the necessary material. When you feel ready to evaluate your learning, take the first posttest. Check your answers. An acceptable score as indicated on the posttest signifies that you are ready for the next chapter. An unacceptable score signifies a need for further study before you take the second posttest.

WORK SHEET

Directions: Express the following Arabic numerals as Roman numerals.

1. 22 _____

2. 9 _____

3. 3 _____

4. 30 _____

5. 14 _____

6. 6 _____

7. 15 _____

8. 12 _____

Directions: Express the following Roman numerals as Arabic numerals.

1. xxix _____

2. vii _____

3. xx _____

4. vi _____

5. xvi _____

6. iv _____

7. xxv _____

8. ccxl _____

Directions: Change to equivalents within the apothecary system. Solve by using proportions. Show your work.

1. 2½ fl oz = _____ pt

2. 15 fl oz = _____ pt

3. 4 pt = _____ fl oz = _____ qt

4. 2½ pt = _____ fl oz

5. 8 pt = _____ qt = _____ gal

6. ½ pt = _____ fl oz

7. 3 qt = _____ gal = _____ pt

8. 10 qt = _____ pt = _____ gal

Directions: Change the following household measurements into appropriate equivalents within the apothecary system. Solve the problems by using proportions. Show your work.

1. 2 cups = _____ fl oz

2. ½ cup = _____ fl oz

3. 3¼ cups = _____ fl oz

4. 1¾ cups = _____ fl oz

Answers on p. 481.

CHAPTER 7 **Apothecary and Household Measurements**

ACCEPTABLE SCORE ___10___

YOUR SCORE _____

POSTTEST 1

Directions: Change to equivalents within the apothecary system. Solve by using proportions. Show your work.

1-2. 24 fl oz = _____ qt = _____ pt

3-4. 48 fl oz = _____ pt = _____ qt

5-6. 5 qt = _____ gal = _____ pt

7-8. 1¾ gal = _____ qt = _____ fl oz

Directions: Change the following household measurements into approximate equivalents within the apothecary system. Solve the problems by using proportions. Show your work.

9-10. 1½ cups = _____ fl oz

= _____ pt

11. ¾ cup = _____ fl oz

Answers on p. 481.

Name _____

Date _____

ACCEPTABLE SCORE __10__

YOUR SCORE _____

POSTTEST 2

Directions: Change to equivalents within the apothecary system. Solve by using proportions. Show your work.

1-2. 48 fl oz = _____ pt = _____ qt

3-4. 4½ pt = _____ fl oz = _____ qt

5-6. 6 qt = _____ gal = _____ fl oz

7-8. 2½ gal = _____ qt = _____ pt

Directions: Change the following household measurements into approximate equivalents within the apothecary system. Solve the problems by using proportions. Show your work.

9-10. 2¼ cups = _____ fl oz

= _____ pt

11. ½ cup = _____ fl oz

Answers on p. 481.

Refer to Introducing Drug Measures: Systems of Measurement on the enclosed CD for additional help.

Equivalents between Apothecary and Metric Measurements

Name _____

Date _____

ACCEPTABLE SCORE __34__

YOUR SCORE _____

PRETEST ☑

Directions: Change to approximate equivalents as indicated. Solve the problems by using proportions. Show your work.

1. 110 lb = _____ kg

2. 500 mL = _____ qt

3. 36 kg = _____ lb

4. 5¼ qt = _____ mL

5. 90 mL = _____ fl oz

6. 1¾ qt = _____ L

7. 90 gr = _____ g

8. 8.2 kg = _____ lb

9. 8⅗ lb = _____ g

10. 2¼ pt = _____ mL

11. 7 fl oz = _____ mL

12. 10 gr = _____ g

13. 5.5 L = _____ qt

14. 1.6 kg = _____ lb

15. 4 gr = _____ mg

16. 360 mL = _____ fl oz

17. 600 mL = _____ pt

18. 5500 g = _____ lb

19. 20 mL = _____ fl oz

20. 12 mg = _____ gr

21. $\frac{1}{300}$ gr = _____ mg

22. 85 lb = _____ kg

23. 0.4 mg = _____ gr

24. 12¼ lb = _____ kg

25. 4200 mL = _____ qt

26. 1½ fl oz = _____ mL

27. $\frac{1}{5}$ gr = _____ mg

28. 4.6 g = _____ gr

29. 98.8° F = _____ ° C

30. 41° C = _____ ° F

31. 97.6° F = _____ ° C

32. 38.5° C = _____ ° F

33. 99.8° F = _____ ° C

34. 39.6° C = _____ ° F

35. 102.6° F = _____ ° C

36. 40.2° C = _____ ° F

Answers on p. 482.

CHAPTER 8 Equivalents between Apothecary and Metric Measurements

Equivalents between Apothecary and Metric Measurements

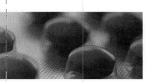

LEARNING OBJECTIVES

On completion of the materials provided in this chapter, you will be able to perform computations accurately by mastering the following mathematical concepts:

1 Recalling equivalent apothecary and metric measures

2 Computing equivalents between the apothecary and metric systems by using a proportion

3 Converting from the Fahrenheit scale to the Celsius scale

4 Converting from the Celsius scale to the Fahrenheit scale

One of a nurse's many responsibilities is the administration of medication. Historically, two different systems of measurements were used in the calculation of drug dosages: the apothecary system and the metric system. Currently, all hospitals and physicians use the metric system. However, rarely a physician may continue to write orders using the apothecary system of measure. Nurses must therefore be able to use both systems and know the approximate equivalents between the two systems. This brief chapter is devoted to the parts of the apothecary and metric systems that are found most often in physician orders.

APPROXIMATE EQUIVALENTS BETWEEN APOTHECARY AND METRIC MEASUREMENTS

A list of the most commonly used equivalents between apothecary and metric systems of measure is provided in Box 8-1. Memorize these equivalents. Sometimes a nurse will have to convert a medication order from one system to the other. This can be done by using a proportion, as shown in the examples on pp. 136-137.

```
┌─────────────────────────────────────────────────────────────────┐
│         BOX 8-1 ■ APOTHECARY/METRIC EQUIVALENTS                  │
│                                                                 │
│             Apothecary Measure = Metric Measure                 │
│            1 fluid ounce (fl oz) = 30 milliliters (mL)          │
│           6 fluid ounces (fl oz) = 180 milliliters (mL)         │
│           8 fluid ounces (fl oz) = 240 milliliters (mL)         │
│   16 fluid ounces (fl oz) or 1 pint (pt) = 500 milliliters (mL) │
│ 32 fluid ounces (fl oz) or 1 quart (qt) = 1000 milliliters (mL) or 1 liter (L) │
│            1 grain (gr) = 60 or 65 milligrams (mg)              │
│               15 grains (gr) = 1 gram (g)                       │
│    2.2 pounds (lb) = 1000 grams (g) or 1 kilogram (kg)          │
└─────────────────────────────────────────────────────────────────┘
```

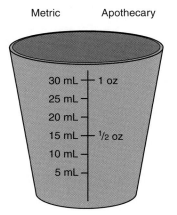

Example 1: 150 mL equals how many fluid ounces?

a. On the left side of the proportion, place what you know to be an equivalent between milliliters and fluid ounces. In this example the most appropriate equivalent is 30 mL = 1 fl oz. So the left side of the proportion would be

$$30 \text{ mL} : 1 \text{ fl oz} ::$$

b. The right side of the proportion is determined by the problem and by the abbreviations used on the left side. Only *two* different abbreviations may be used in a single proportion. The abbreviations must be in the same position on the right as they are on the left.

$$30 \text{ mL} : 1 \text{ fl oz} :: \underline{\hspace{1cm}} \text{ mL} : \underline{\hspace{1cm}} \text{ fl oz}$$

From the problem we know we have 150 mL.

$$30 \text{ mL} : 1 \text{ fl oz} :: 150 \text{ mL} : \underline{\hspace{1cm}} \text{ fl oz}$$

We need to find the number of fluid ounces in 150 mL, so we use the symbol x to represent the unknown. Therefore the full proportion would be

$$30 \text{ mL} : 1 \text{ fl oz} :: 150 \text{ mL} : x \text{ fl oz}$$

c. Rewrite the proportion without using the abbreviations.

$$30 : 1 :: 150 : x$$

    d. Solve for x.

$$30x = 1 \times 150$$

$$x = \frac{150}{30} = 5$$

    e. Label your answer, as determined by the abbreviation placed next to x in the original proportion.

150 mL = 5 fl oz

Example 2: 45 mg equals how many grains?

    a. 1 gr : 60 mg ::

    b. 1 gr : 60 mg :: _____ gr : _____ mg
       1 gr : 60 mg :: x gr : 45 mg

    c. 1 : 60 :: x : 45

    d. $60x = 1 \times 45$
       $60x = 45$

$$x = \frac{45}{60} = \frac{3}{4}$$

    e. 45 mg = ¾ gr

APPROXIMATE EQUIVALENTS BETWEEN CELSIUS AND FAHRENHEIT MEASUREMENTS

Hospitals and health care centers use the metric system of measurement, including thermometers calibrated in the Celsius scale. It may be necessary for the nurse to convert the Celsius, or centigrade, scale to the Fahrenheit scale for patient or family information. Because not everyone concerned with patient care uses the same scale, it is also important for the nurse to be able to convert the Fahrenheit scale to the Celsius scale.

    Most hospitals now use digital thermometers rather than mercury thermometers. The following thermometers are included for illustration purposes only. Digital thermometers are available in the Fahrenheit or Celsius scale. Patients frequently ask for conversion charts at the time of discharge so they can understand the readings when they take their hospital thermometers home. The conversion charts are helpful for the nurse as well. However, the nurse should be able to convert from one scale to the other if necessary.

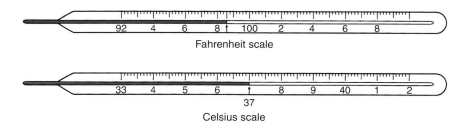

For conversion from one scale to another, the following proportion may be used:

> Celsius : Fahrenheit − 32 :: 5 : 9
> C : F − 32 :: 5 : 9

C or F will be the unknown.

Extend the decimal to hundredths; round to tenths.

Another means of converting Celsius and Fahrenheit temperatures to equivalents is given in Box 8-2.

BOX 8-2 ■ CONVERTING CELSIUS AND FAHRENHEIT TEMPERATURES

Fahrenheit to Celsius
Subtract 32
Divide by 1.8

Celsius to Fahrenheit
Multiply by 1.8
Add 32

The following examples illustrate each method.

Example 1: 100.6° F equals _____ ° C.

a. $C : F - 32 :: 5 : 9$

b. $C : 100.6 - 32 :: 5 : 9$

c. $9C = (100.6 - 32) \times 5$

d. $9C = 68.6 \times 5$

e. $9C = 343$

f. $C = \dfrac{343}{9}$

g. $C = 38.11$

h. $100.6° F = 38.1° C.$

    a. $100.6 - 32 = 68.6$

    b. $68.6 \div 1.8 = 38.111\ldots$
       or 38.1° C

Example 2: 37.6° C equals _____ ° F.

a. $C : F - 32 :: 5 : 9$

b. $37.6 : F - 32 :: 5 : 9$

c. $5(F - 32) = 9 \times 37.6$

d. $5F - 160 = 338.4$

e. $5F - 160 + 160 = 338.4 + 160$

f. $5F = 498.4$

g. $F = \dfrac{498.4}{5}$

h. $F = 99.68$

i. $37.6° C = 99.7° F.$

    a. $37.6 \times 1.8 = 67.68$

    b. $67.68 + 32 = 99.68$
       or 99.7° F

Memorize the table of approximate equivalents between the apothecary and the metric systems of measure. Study the material on forming proportions for the calculations of problems converting between the apothecary and metric systems. Complete the following work sheet, which provides for extensive practice in the manipulation of measurements between the apothecary and metric systems. Check your answers. If you have difficulties, go back and review the necessary material. When you feel ready to evaluate your learning, take the first posttest. Check your answers. An acceptable score as indicated on the posttest signifies that you are ready for the next chapter. An unacceptable score signifies a need for further study before you take the second posttest.

CHAPTER 8 Equivalents between Apothecary and Metric Measurements

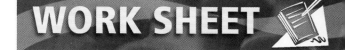

Directions: Change to approximate equivalents as indicated. Solve the problems by using a proportion. Show your work.

1. 200 mg = _____ gr

2. 22 lb = _____ kg

3. 150 gr = _____ g

4. 1¾ qt = _____ mL

5. 210 mL = _____ fl oz

6. 10 kg = _____ lb

7. 1750 mL = _____ pt

8. ½ fl oz = _____ mL

9. 4½ gr = _____ mg

10. 4200 g = _____ lb

11. 420 mg = _____ gr

12. 6 pt = _____ mL

13. 3500 mL = _____ qt

14. 5 gr = _____ mg

15. 150 mL = _____ fl oz

16. 3.3 kg = _____ lb

17. 6⅘ lb = _____ g

18. ⅜ fl oz = _____ mL

19. 2¾ gr = _____ mg

20. 5 lb = _____ kg

21. 2700 mL = _____ pt

22. 340 mg = _____ gr

23. 2½ qt = _____ L

24. 3650 g = _____ lb

25. 4 fl oz = _____ mL

26. 12 lb = _____ g

27. 75 lb = _____ kg

28. 2⅛ qt = _____ mL

29. 100 mg = _____ gr

30. 3.5 L = _____ qt

31. 1½ gr = _____ mg

32. 25 kg = _____ lb

33. 99.6° F = _____ ° C

34. 101.8° F = _____ ° C   **35.** 104.2° F = _____ ° C   **36.** 97.4° F = _____ ° C

37. 40.4° C = _____ ° F   **38.** 35.4° C = _____ ° F   **39.** 36.8° C = _____ ° F

40. 39.2° C = _____ ° F   **41.** 33° C = _____ ° F   **42.** 98.4° F = _____ ° C

43. 41.2° C = _____ ° F   **44.** 103.6° F = _____ ° C   **45.** 40.6° C = _____ ° F

46. 102.2° F = _____ ° C   **47.** 37.4° C = _____ ° F   **48.** 100.4° F = _____ ° C

Answers on p. 482.

Equivalents between Apothecary and Metric Measurements **CHAPTER 8**   141

Name _____

Date _____

ACCEPTABLE SCORE __29__

YOUR SCORE _____

POSTTEST 1

Directions: Change to approximate equivalents as indicated. Solve the problems by using proportions. Show your work.

1. 3 gr = _____ mg

2. 75 gr = _____ g

3. 3 fl oz = _____ mL

4. 1½ pt = _____ mL

5. 15 mg = _____ gr

6. 1500 mL = _____ qt

7. 7½ lb = _____ g

8. 1.7 L = _____ qt

9. 5 gr = _____ g

10. 20 lb = _____ kg

11. ⅙ gr = _____ mg

12. 1000 mL = _____ pt

13. 0.3 mg = _____ gr

14. 3 g = _____ gr

15. 60 mL = _____ fl oz

16. 2700 g = _____ lb

17. 5 fl oz = _____ mL

18. 32 kg = _____ lb

19. 0.5 mg = _____ gr

20. 80 gr = _____ g

21. 2¾ qt = _____ L

22. 540 mL = _____ fl oz

23. 95.4° F = _____ ° C

24. 35.6° C = _____ ° F

25. 103.2° F = _____ ° C

26. 40.8° C = _____ ° F

27. 104.2° F = _____ ° C

28. 37.2° C = _____ ° F

29. 99.4° F = _____ ° C

30. 33.8° C = _____ ° F

Answers on p. 482.

CHAPTER 8 Equivalents between Apothecary and Metric Measurements

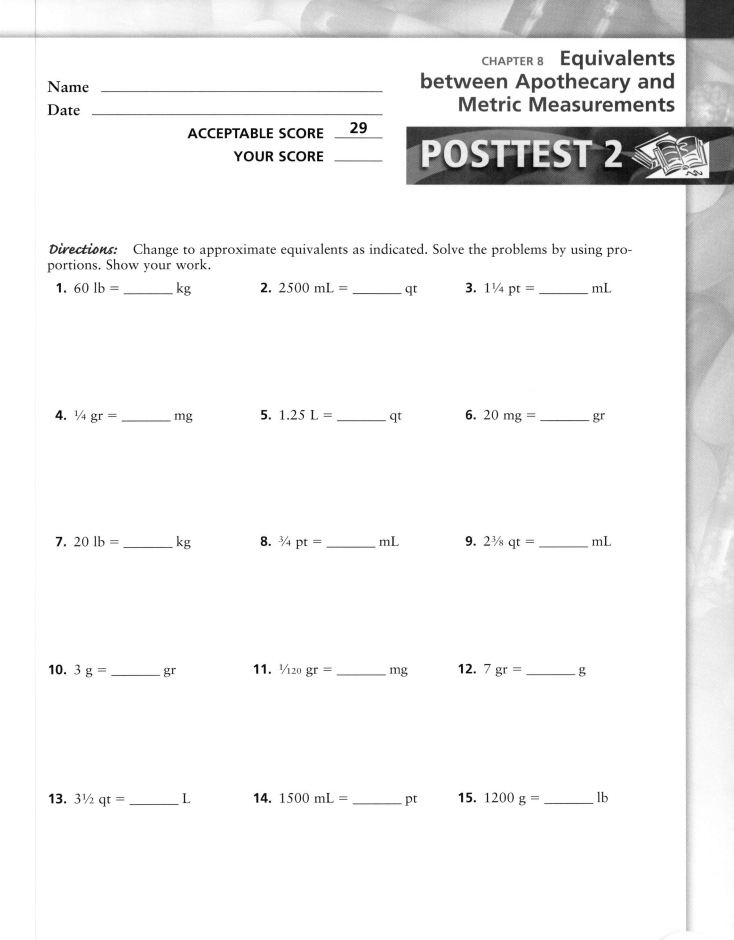

ACCEPTABLE SCORE ___29___

YOUR SCORE _____

POSTTEST 2

Directions: Change to approximate equivalents as indicated. Solve the problems by using proportions. Show your work.

1. 60 lb = _____ kg

2. 2500 mL = _____ qt

3. 1¼ pt = _____ mL

4. ¼ gr = _____ mg

5. 1.25 L = _____ qt

6. 20 mg = _____ gr

7. 20 lb = _____ kg

8. ¾ pt = _____ mL

9. 2⅜ qt = _____ mL

10. 3 g = _____ gr

11. ¹⁄₁₂₀ gr = _____ mg

12. 7 gr = _____ g

13. 3½ qt = _____ L

14. 1500 mL = _____ pt

15. 1200 g = _____ lb

16. 0.8 mg = _____ gr

17. 42 kg = _____ lb

18. ¹⁄₂₀ gr = _____ mg

19. 3⅓ lb = _____ g

20. 7 kg = _____ lb

21. 1.3 g = _____ gr

22. 3½ lb = _____ g

23. 96.2° F = _____ ° C

24. 38.2° C = _____ ° F

25. 36.8° C = _____ ° F

26. 97.8° F = _____ ° C

27. 40.4° C = _____ ° F

28. 100.8° F = _____ ° C

29. 41.4° C = _____ ° F

30. 103.2° F = _____ ° C

Answers on p. 483.

 Refer to Introducing Drug Measures: Systems of Measurement on the enclosed CD for additional help.

CHAPTER 8 Equivalents between Apothecary and Metric Measurements

Safety in Medication Administration

Ruth Anne Burris, MBA, RN

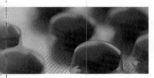

LEARNING OBJECTIVES

On completion of the materials provided in this chapter, you will be able to:

1 Understand the fundamental need for patient safety programs

2 Describe the impact of medical errors on patient outcomes

3 Relate patient safety to the calculation and delivery of medications

4 Determine individual responsibility in maintaining a safe patient environment

5 Define the types of injuries associated with medications for health care workers

6 List injury prevention strategies for health care workers

The concept of safety in health care is applicable to both patient populations and health care workers. Both groups are susceptible to injury unless measures are taken that maximize prevention while minimizing the likelihood that a medical error or injury will occur. The following sections relate to both patient and personal safety.

PATIENT SAFETY

Patient safety has never been more important. It is linked directly to a health care organization's ability to attract patients, to fund services that are market competitive, and to meet the requirements for accreditation by regulatory agencies. Additionally, it is also important in the delivery of high-quality patient care outcomes of interest to third-party payers for reimbursement and external agencies monitoring quality. These parties include the federal government through the Centers for Medicare & Medicaid Services (CMS), Joint Commission on Accreditation of Healthcare Organizations (JCAHO), the Leapfrog Group, and some state governments. All these agencies require reporting of significant or sentinel events that result in patient harm.

The risk associated with delivery of health services to patients creates a sense of urgency in monitoring safety. Health care, as an industry, is considered at high risk in regards to its ability to deliver safe patient care. In this people-to-people business, the likelihood of errors related to medications and procedures is greater than the likelihood of a product error in the manufacturing industry. This is believed to be due to many factors that are present in the health care culture today, such as

- The fast-paced environment in which patient care activities occur
- Advanced technologies that require more attention and skills
- Decreased staffing in critical positions, such as nursing
- A sicker and older patient population
- Declining financial resources

These factors create a more complex environment for both patients and health care workers. The potential for negative patient outcomes increases as workers become more stressed in terms of management of time, patient needs for medication and treatments, and equipment. Negative outcomes can result in

- Increasing costs of care
- Complications that affect patients' ability to get well and go home
- Serious physical or psychological harm
- Death

Safety Precautions for Patients

Health care workers who are administering medications to patients have a legal responsibility to ensure that the right medications are delivered to the right patient in the right dose and route at the right time, and that the administration is appropriately documented in the patient's medical record. A thorough knowledge of the patient's medical history, including drug allergies and medications that the patient has previously taken, is necessary to safeguard against medication interactions and anaphylactic reactions. It is extremely important that health care workers understand the intended action of the drug that has been ordered, how it is to be safely delivered, and the potential effects (both therapeutic and side effects) it can have on the patient. Additionally, health care workers involved in medication administration need to be aware of "do not use" abbreviations and look-alike/sound-alike medication names that can increase the potential for medication errors. Examples include q.d., q.o.d., cc, o.s., o.d., and o.u.

Patient safety outcomes are related to care processes that involve medical procedures, treatments, medications, documentation of care, and communication between care providers. The reduction in medical errors is highly reliant on each individual health care worker's commitment to practicing within the scope of his or her position, observing correct safety practices, and adhering to established standards of care. Medical errors are avoidable if the time is taken to provide the right care to the right patient at the right time.

How does this information relate to medication calculations and delivery? Let's examine the outcomes to three different scenarios in which a medication error has occurred. Each scenario describes the care that was ordered by a physician; the events that occurred; and the outcome for the patient in terms of recovery, cost, and long-term needs.

Scenario A: A 6-year-old girl has come into the hospital for a suspected infection in her kidneys that has caused her to become dehydrated and unable to keep down food or liquids. She complains of pain in her back and side and is unable to sit or lie down comfortably. The physician suspects a kidney stone may be present and wishes to run diagnostic tests to evaluate kidney function and to determine if there is blockage of the ureters. Tests are ordered that require a specific medication to be given before testing. The nurse assigned to this child gives the medication within the prescribed time frame before the test. However, she does not read the name of the drug correctly on the medication label (it is similar to a cardiac medication) and does not calculate the right dosage based on the child's weight. The child suffers a cardiac arrest after administration of the wrong medication at the wrong dose. The child survives but experiences severe brain damage and is determined to be mentally and physically disabled for life.

Scenario B: An 83-year-old man, Mr. Smith, is admitted from a nursing home to the medical/surgical unit for acute pneumonia with a high fever and delirium. His physician orders an antibiotic to be given four times a day through the intravenous (IV) line. The nurse assigned to his care is working a 12-hour shift and is also caring for five other patients, three of whom are high maintenance in terms of severity of illness, pain control, and care needs. The unit is short staffed so there is no one to assist her with her patient care responsibilities. Her attention is diverted by one patient in particular whose condition continues to deteriorate. This nurse is so distracted that she forgets to give three doses of the antibiotics to Mr. Smith during her shift. His condition deteriorates over the course of that day and the next, resulting in a transfer to the intensive care unit (ICU) for ventilation. This omission of treatment results in a transfer to the ICU, a prolonged recovery period of 2 weeks, and increased costs of care.

Scenario C: A 26-year-old woman comes into the hospital for surgery. Her admission history includes a list of allergies to medications, including antibiotics. Postoperative orders are written, which include an antibiotic to reduce surgical site infection. The nurse caring for this patient receives the order, but does not review the list of allergies before giving the medication. The patient has an allergic reaction that causes her to have a cardiac arrest and die.

All these scenarios are real-life events that have resulted in harm to a patient somewhere in the United States. There are no substitutes for attention to patient safety, since patients turn over their well-being to virtual strangers when they come into our institutions for care. With adverse drug events topping the list as the most frequently occurring type of medical error, JCAHO has taken a strong stance on establishing standards that address potential sources for error, especially abbreviations that are easily misread or confused in written form, and drug names that sound and look alike.

Health care workers owe it to their patients to be vigilant, detail oriented, and present mentally when directing or delivering care. This is especially true when calculating or administering medications. Medications that are inaccurately dosed, inaccurately delivered, or omitted create outcomes that may cost patients the ultimate price—their life. At the very least, these errors can affect the patient's ability to recover in a timely fashion and return to his or her life. Armed with this knowledge, each of us should begin and end our work shifts with one question in mind: Did I do all that I could from a safe practice perspective to protect my patients today?

PERSONAL SAFETY

Health care workers are at greater risk than other service workers of suffering an injury in the course of caring for patients. The risk is associated primarily with musculoskeletal injuries and delivery of medications. Injuries that are specifically related to medication delivery include eye splashes, splashes to the skin, and needlestick injuries. Each type of injury may occur because of a lack of personal protective equipment (PPE), end-user failure to adhere to practice or policy standards, equipment failure, and rarely, a twist of fate.

The use of PPE such as gloves, eye goggles, and gowns can directly protect an individual from exposure to bloodborne pathogens or a hazardous substance, such as a medication that may be toxic or damaging to the eyes, mucous membranes, or skin. The use of safety needles and safety devices during administration of injectable drugs or starting IV lines minimizes the likelihood of an injury from a contaminated needle. Practice standards—such as proper use and disposal of medications, their containers (especially glass), and delivery devices into specified containers such as needle boxes—provide a level of safety if stringent adherence is the normal pattern of practice (Figure 9-1). Workers experiencing any injury should implement first aid procedures and report it to their supervisor immediately.

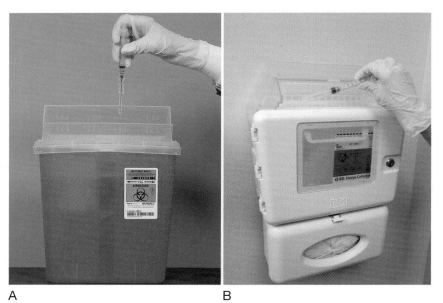

FIGURE 9-1   **A** and **B,** Examples of sharps disposal using only one hand. (**A,** From Potter PA, Perry AG: *Fundamentals of nursing,* ed 6, St Louis, 2005, Mosby. **B,** From Elkin MK, Perry PA, Potter AG: *Nursing interventions and clinical skills,* ed 3, St Louis, 2004, Mosby.)

Health care workers can significantly decrease their chances for injury by implementing practices that promote their personal safety, such as wearing PPE as needed, appropriately engaging safety devices (Figure 9-2), using approved disposal techniques, and monitoring their environment for potential hazards. Additionally, these same safety practices reduce the risk for their coworkers, physicians, patients, and visitors. It is the responsibility of every health care worker to work safely to protect himself or herself and others.

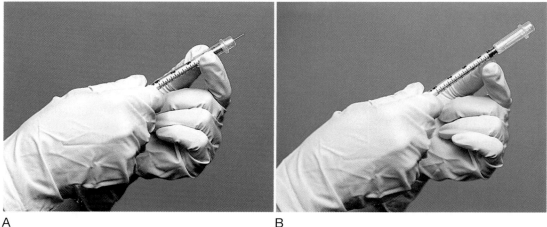

FIGURE 9-2   Needle with plastic guard to prevent needlesticks. **A,** Position of guard before injection. **B,** After injection the guard locks in place, covering the needle. (From Potter PA, Perry AG: *Fundamentals of nursing,* ed 6, St Louis, 2005, Mosby.)

Name _____

Date _____

ACCEPTABLE SCORE ___8___

YOUR SCORE _____

POSTTEST

Directions: Circle *True* for each correct statement and *False* for each incorrect statement.

1. A nurse checking a patient's medication record notices a change in the amount of a drug and the route of the drug, which is different from when she gave it earlier in the day. She should go ahead and give the drug as indicated on the medication record without checking the chart for new physician orders, since the medication record is the "one source of truth" for current medications.
True or False

2. While the nurse is giving medications to Mr. Jones, he asks what the pill is for. When his nurse tells him it is for his high cholesterol, he responds, "I have never had a problem with high cholesterol and I have never taken pills for it." The nurse should encourage Mr. Jones to take the pill and leave a note for the doctor in his chart to address in the morning.
True or False

3. Medication calculations that are incorrect are an example of a medical error.
True or False

4. Health care organizations are required to report sentinel events that result in patient harm to external agencies, such as JCAHO.
True or False

5. Safe patient care is the responsibility of every health care worker.
True or False

6. Health care workers are at risk of being injured by contaminated needles.
True or False

7. The use of personal protective equipment can reduce the risk of splashes by hazardous substances.
True or False

8. An injured health care worker does not have to report the injury to his or her supervisor.
True or False

Answers on p. 483.

Interpretation of the Physician's Orders

LEARNING OBJECTIVES

On completion of the materials provided in this chapter, you will be able to successfully complete a patient's medication administration record based on a physician's order.

Administration of medications is one of the nurse's most important responsibilities. For medications to be administered safely and effectively, the nurse must know how to interpret the physician's medication orders.

WRITTEN ORDERS

The physician prescribes medications. In hospitals and health care centers, the physician uses a physician's order sheet, which is part of the patient's hospital chart or record. The orders are written for a drug to be given until a stated date and time, until a certain amount of the medication has been given, or until the order is changed or discontinued.

The physician's order requires the date the order was written, the name and dosage of the drug, the route and frequency of administration, and any special instructions. For drugs ordered as needed (prn), the purpose for administration is also added. The physician's signature is required each time orders are written. In many institutions the time that the order is written is also preferred. However, if the time is not included, the order is still valid.

The nurse should review the policy and procedure for medication administration at each facility where he or she is employed to determine the appropriate schedule.

To interpret the medication order, the nurse must know the terminology, abbreviations, and symbols used in writing medical prescriptions and orders for medications. A list of the most frequently used abbreviations relating to medications can be found in Table 10-1. Memorize this list. Refer to the Glossary for help with unfamiliar terms.

In many states, other health care providers are legally authorized to prescribe medications. These may include a dentist, nurse practitioner, physician's assistant, or chiropractor. The nurse should always be knowledgeable about the laws governing practice in his or her own state and facility. In all institutions, nurses should have ready access to the most current listing of individuals credentialed for prescriptive authority.

TABLE 10-1 ■ Abbreviations and Examples of Times for Administering Medications

Abbreviations	Definition	Example Times of Administration
ac*	Before meals	0730-1130-1730
AM	Morning, before noon	0900
pc*	After meals	0830-1230-1830
PM	Evening, before midnight	2100
prn	As needed	
qh	Every hour	0800-0900-1000-etc.
q2 h	Every 2 hours	0800-1000-1200-etc.
q3 h	Every 3 hours	0900-1200-1500-etc.
q4 h	Every 4 hours	0800-1200-1600-etc.
q6 h	Every 6 hours	0600-1200-1800-2400
q8 h	Every 8 hours	0800-1600-2400
q12 h	Every 12 hours	0800-2000
stat	Immediately	

*Providing that meals are served at 0800, 1200, and 1800.

VERBAL ORDERS

Although verbal orders are discouraged as routine policy, certain situations or emergencies may require telephone orders. Such orders are generally initiated by the nurse. The order must include the same information as the written order: the date the order is recorded, the name and dosage of the drug, the route and frequency of administration, and any special instructions. After the nurse has recorded the orders on the patient's chart, the orders must be repeated to the physician for verification. The physician's name, a notation that this is a verbal order (VORB, verbal order read back), and the nurse's signature are required. The physician should sign the verbal orders as soon as possible. The nurse should follow his or her institution's policy.

Example: 1/18/11   Morphine sulfate 8 mg IM q4 h prn for pain
 1400   VORB Dr. James T. Smith/Helen Alexander, RN

SCHEDULING THE ADMINISTRATION OF MEDICATIONS

The physician's orders provide guidelines for the nurse in planning when each medication will be given to the patient. The purpose for prescribing the medication, drug interactions, absorption of the drug, or side effects caused by the drug may determine when the drug is given. The prescribed order may be very specific or may give the nurse latitude in scheduling.

Most hospitals and health care centers have routine times for administering medications. These times may differ from one hospital to another. The nurse should review the policy and procedure for medication administration at each facility where he or she is employed to determine the appropriate schedule. The guidelines assist the nurse in planning a medication routine that is safe for the patient. Table 10-1 provides examples of planning times for administering each medication at one institution.

The majority of hospitals use computer military time rather than ante meridiem (AM) and post meridiem (PM) time. Table 10-2 will assist in conversion from computer/military time. Computer/military time can be computed quickly by adding 12 to PM time—for example, 12 + 3 = 1500 hours.

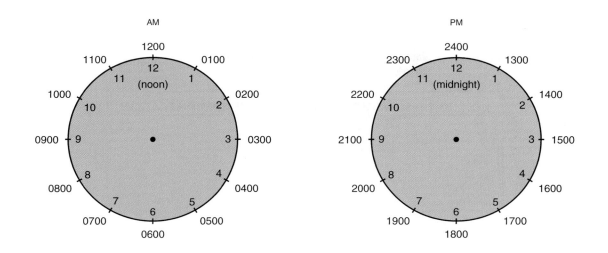

TABLE 10-2 ■ **Conversion from Computer/Military Time to AM–PM Time**

0100—1:00 AM	0900—9:00 AM	1700—5:00 PM
0200—2:00 AM	1000—10:00 AM	1800—6:00 PM
0300—3:00 AM	1100—11:00 AM	1900—7:00 PM
0400—4:00 AM	1200—12:00 noon	2000—8:00 PM
0500—5:00 AM	1300—1:00 PM	2100—9:00 PM
0600—6:00 AM	1400—2:00 PM	2200—10:00 PM
0700—7:00 AM	1500—3:00 PM	2300—11:00 PM
0800—8:00 AM	1600—4:00 PM	2400—12:00 midnight

INTRODUCTION TO DRUG DOSAGES

The nurse obtains the medication from the pharmacy or from an available supply in the clinical unit, prepares the dose, and administers the medication. Unit dosages are prepared in individual doses by the manufacturer or hospital pharmacy and are ready for the nurse to administer.

Most medications are secured in the required dosage. However, problems of drug calculation arise when a drug is not manufactured in the strength required by the patient, the drug is not available in the strength ordered, or the drug is ordered in one system of measurement but is available only in another system of measurement.

When you change from one system of measurement to another, you have an equivalent measure that may or may not be exact. Therefore the answer to your problem may vary according to the system of measurement used. For example, if you change the required dosage to the available dosage, the equivalent dosage may be different than if you changed the available dosage to the required dosage. All problems in this book are calculated by changing the required dosage to the available dosage. The answers reflect this method of calculation. This is good practice because you have the medication on hand in the dosage provided.

The nurse is ethically and legally responsible for the medications administered to the patient. Even though the physician writes the order for the medication to be given to the patient, and even though the pharmacy may prepare the wrong medication, the nurse who administers the medication is ultimately responsible for the error. Before preparing the drug, the nurse *must know* the maximum and minimum dosages and the actions of and contraindications for each administered drug. In addition, the nurse should consult the patient and the patient's medical record for any known allergies.

THE SIX RIGHTS OF MEDICATION ADMINISTRATION

Because the nurse is legally responsible for ensuring that medications are correctly administered, the six rights of medication administration listed in Box 10-1 must be diligently checked.

BOX 10-1 ■ SIX RIGHTS OF MEDICATION ADMINISTRATION

1. Drug
2. Dose
3. Patient
4. Route
5. Time
6. Documentation

Anytime these rights are not checked in the preparation and administration of medications, an error may occur for which the nurse is legally responsible.

When medications are prepared for administration, the information on the medication profile sheet or drug card should be checked *three* times:
1. As the medicine is taken from the drawer or shelf
2. As the medicine is prepared or opened
3. As the medicine is replaced or thrown out

If unit doses are used, the label should be checked three times. It is critical that all calculations be done accurately and checked. It is especially important to check computations involving fractions and decimals. Many nurses use calculators. In some institutions certain medications (e.g., heparin and insulin) are to be checked by another nurse before the medicine is administered to the patient. Always use the appropriate measuring devices.

When administering the medication, *ALWAYS* ask the patient his or her name and *ALWAYS* check the patient's identification armband and birthday.

Medications can be ordered to be administered by various routes. However, they must be administered only by the route included in the physician's order. Never assume the route by which the medication is to be given. If the route has not been included in the order, the physician must be notified and asked to clarify the route requested. The clarifying order needs to be written also.

Timing is very important—both the time of day and the interval between doses. With all medications, judgment and assessment by the nurse are required as to whether the medication should be given or withheld.

Medication Administration Record

Documentation has become more and more important for legal purposes. Remember that documentation of medications administered must include the five components of drug, dose, patient, route, and time. It is also necessary to document whether a medication has been withheld or refused. Each facility has its own policy concerning the full documentation of medications. The official medication administration record (commonly called *the patient's MAR*) varies in format from one institution to another but contains the same information. It is mandatory that all documentation be legible, and it is written in black ink or printed out from a computer.

In most institutions, personnel other than nurses transcribe the physician's orders to the patient's MAR. Nurses are then required to verify the transcription against the physician's order and to place their initials on the form indicating the transcription was correctly completed.

Figure 10-1 represents examples of, *A,* a physician's order and, *B,* a patient's MAR. Notice that the appropriate drug interpretations for the MAR include the patient's name, the medication name, the date, the drug dosage, the medication route, and the medication schedule.

PHYSICIAN'S ORDERS

1. ADDRESSOGRAPH BEFORE PLACING IN PATIENT'S CHART ▶
2. INITIAL AND DETACH COPY EACH TIME PHYSICIAN WRITES ORDERS
3. TRANSMIT COPY TO PHARMACY
4. ORDERS MUST BE DATED AND TIMED

Patient, James A.

DATE	ORDERS			TRANS BY
	Diagnosis:	Weight:	Height:	
	Sensitivities/Drug Allergies:			
1/12/11	0900	Lasix 80 mg. p.o. twice a day		
		Digoxin 0.125 mg. p.o. daily		
		Slow-K 10 mEq. p.o. with breakfast and lunch		
		A. Physician, M.D.		

A

MEDICAL RECORDS COPY	**PHYSICIAN'S ORDERS**	T-5

B-CLIN. NOTES	E-LAB	G-X-RAY	K-DIAGNOSTIC	M-SURGERY	Q-THERAPY	T-ORDERS	W-NURSING	Y-MISC.

Transcription of Med Sheet by: _____

Reviewed by: _____   Page _____ of _____

Initials	Signature
_____	_____
_____	_____
_____	_____
_____	_____
NJ	*N. Jones R.N.*
AN	*A. Nurse R.N.*

Allergies: ☑ NKDA

Injection Sites:
A = RUE
B = LUE E = Abdomen
C = RLE F = R Glut
D = LLE G = L Glut

Special Notes:

See Legend on Back

Patient, James A.

☐ Inpatient   ☐ Outpatient

DATE	DRUG				08 09 10 11	12 13 14 15	16 17 18 19	20 21 22 23	24 01 02 03	04 05 06 07	1/12/11	1/13/11	1/14/11	1/15/11	1/16/11
1 1/12	Lasix				09	17					09 AN / 21 NJ	09 AN / 21 NJ			
	80 mg dose	p.o. route	twice a day interval												
2 1/12	Digoxin				09						09 AN	09 AN			
	0.125 mg dose	p.o. route	once a day interval												
3 1/12	Slow-K				08	12					08 AN / 12 NJ	08 AN / 12 NJ			
	10 mEq dose	p.o. route	breakfast & lunch interval												
4															
	dose	route	interval												
5															
	dose	route	interval												

MEDICATION PROFILE

B-CLIN. NOTES	E-LAB	G-X-RAY	K-DIAGNOSTIC	M-SURGERY	Q-THERAPY	T-ORDERS	W-NURSING	Y-MISC.

B

FIGURE 10-1 Examples of physician's orders **(A)** and patient's medication administration record **(B)** with appropriate drug interpretations. (Forms courtesy Clarian Health, Indianapolis, Indiana.)

Name _____

Date _____

ACCEPTABLE SCORE ___18___

YOUR SCORE _____

POSTTEST

Directions: Copy the following physician's orders onto the medication administration record sheet below. Be sure to schedule the times for each drug administration.

PHYSICIAN'S ORDERS	Patient, James A.

1. ADDRESSOGRAPH BEFORE PLACING IN PATIENT'S CHART ▶
2. INITIAL AND DETACH COPY EACH TIME PHYSICIAN WRITES ORDERS
3. TRANSMIT COPY TO PHARMACY
4. ORDERS MUST BE DATED AND TIMED

DATE		ORDERS			TRANS BY
	Diagnosis:		Weight:	Height:	
	Sensitivities/Drug Allergies:				
1/12/11	0800	Cefuroxime 1 g IV q8 h			
		Lasix 40 mg po twice a day			
		Slow-K 10 mEq po twice a day			
		A. Physician, M.D.			

Transcription of Med Sheet by: _____

Reviewed by: _____   Page _____ of _____

Patient, James A.

Initials	Signature
_____	_____
_____	_____
_____	_____
_____	_____
_____	_____
_____	_____

Allergies: ☐ NKDA

Injection Sites:
A = RUE
B = LUE E = Abdomen
C = RLE F = R Glut
D = LLE G = L Glut

Special Notes:

☐ Inpatient ☐ Outpatient

See Legend on Back

DATE	DRUG	08 09 10 11	12 13 14 15	16 17 18 19	20 21 22 23	24 01 02 03	04 05 06 07	DATES					
1													
	dose route interval												
2													
	dose route interval												
3													
	dose route interval												
4													
	dose route interval												
5													
	dose route interval												

Answers on p. 483.

Refer to Safety in Medication Administration: Six Rights and MAR on the enclosed CD for additional help.

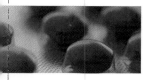

How to Read Drug Labels

LEARNING OBJECTIVES

On completion of the materials provided in this chapter, you will be able to identify the following parts of each drug label:

1 Trade name of the medication

2 Generic name of the medication

3 Strength of the medication dosage

4 Form in which the medication is provided

5 Route of administration

6 Total amount or volume of the medication provided in the container

7 Directions for mixing of the medication if required

The safe administration of medications to patients begins with the nurse accurately reading and interpreting the drug label. Thus it is important for the nurse to be familiar and comfortable with the information that is found on the drug label.

PARTS OF A DRUG LABEL

1. **TRADE NAME.** The trade name (also known as brand or proprietary name) is usually capitalized and written in bold print. It is the first name written on the label. The trade name is always followed by the ® registration symbol. Different manufacturers market the same medication under different trade names.

2. **GENERIC NAME.** The generic name is the official name of the drug. Each drug has only *one* generic name. This name appears directly under the trade name, usually in smaller or different type letters. Physicians may order a patient's medication by generic or trade name. Nurses need to be familiar with both names and cross-check references as needed. Occasionally, only the generic name will appear on the label.

3. DOSAGE STRENGTH. The strength indicates the amount or weight of the medication that is supplied in the specific unit of measure. This amount may be per capsule, tablet, or milliliter.
4. FORM. The form indicates how the drug is supplied. Examples of various forms are tablets, capsules, liquids, suppositories, and ointments.
5. ROUTE. The label will indicate how the drug is to be administered. The route can be oral, topical, injection (subcutaneous, intradermal, intramuscular), or intravenous.
6. AMOUNT. The total amount or volume of the medication may be indicated. Some examples are 250 mL of oral suspension and a bottle that contains 50 capsules.
7. DIRECTIONS. Some medications must be mixed before use. The amounts and types of diluent required will be listed along with the resulting strengths of the medication. This information may also be found on package inserts.

Other information may be found on drug labels: the name of the manufacturer, expiration date, special instructions for storage, and an NDC (National Drug Code) number.

EXAMPLES FOR PRACTICE IN READING DRUG LABELS

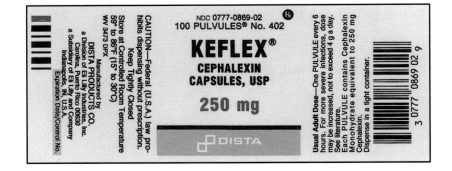

1. Trade name.................................Keflex
2. Generic name...........................cephalexin
3. Dosage strength ....250 mg
4. Form..Capsules
5. Amount 100
6. Directions ....Keep tightly closed. Store at controlled room temperature 59° to 86° F (15° to 30° C).
7. NDC number...........................0777-0869-02
8. Manufacturer...........................DISTA
9. Expiration date..........................(Yellow highlight)

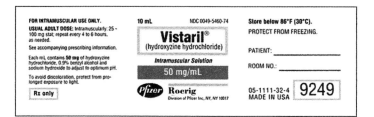

The first drug label image shows:

NDC 0005-3706-65

Erythromycin Ethylsuccinate
Oral Suspension, USP

200 mg/5 mL

Each 5 mL
(one teaspoonful)
contains: Erythromycin
Ethylsuccinate equivalent
to 200 mg Erythromycin.

USUAL DOSAGE:
See package circular.
CAUTION: Federal law
prohibits dispensing
without prescription.

Control No.

Exp. Date
ONE PINT (473 mL)

STANDARD Lederle PRODUCTS

14214-91 NA6

NDC 0005-3706-65

Erythromycin Ethylsuccinate
Oral Suspension, USP

200 mg/5 mL

SHAKE WELL BEFORE USING

STORAGE: Store in refrigerator to
preserve taste until dispensed.
Refrigeration by patient is not
required if used within 14 days.

This package not for
household dispensing.

Protect from light.
Dispense in amber bottles.

Manufactured by
BARRE-NATIONAL INC.
Baltimore, MD 21207
for
LEDERLE LABORATORIES
DIVISION
American Cyanamid Company,
Pearl River, NY 10965

1. Trade name...............................Erythromycin
2. Generic name...........................erythromycin ethylsuccinate
3. Dosage strength.......................200 mg/5 mL
4. Form..Suspension
5. Route......................................Oral
6. Amount...................................1 pint (473 mL)
7. Directions...............................Shake well before using. Storage: Store in refrigerator to preserve taste until dispensed. Refrigeration by patient is not required if used within 14 days. Protect from light. Dispense in amber bottles.
8. NDC number...........................0005-3706-65
9. Manufacturer.........................Barre-National Inc., Lederle Laboratories Division
10. Expiration date......................(Yellow highlight)

The second drug label image shows:

FOR INTRAMUSCULAR USE ONLY.

USUAL ADULT DOSE: Intramuscularly: 25 -
100 mg stat; repeat every 4 to 6 hours,
as needed.

See accompanying prescribing information.

Each mL contains 50 mg of hydroxyzine
hydrochloride, 0.9% benzyl alcohol and
sodium hydroxide to adjust to optimum pH.

To avoid discoloration, protect from prolonged exposure to light.

Rx only

10 mL   NDC 0049-5460-74

Vistaril®
(hydroxyzine hydrochloride)

Intramuscular Solution

50 mg/mL

Pfizer **Roerig**
Division of Pfizer Inc, NY, NY 10017

Store below 86°F (30°C).
PROTECT FROM FREEZING.

PATIENT: _____

ROOM NO.: _____

05-1111-32-4   **9249**
MADE IN USA

1. Trade name.................................Vistaril
2. Generic name..............................hydroxyzine hydrochloride
3. Dosage strength..........................50 mg/mL
4. Form..Intramuscular solution
5. Route......................................Intramuscular injection
6. Amount...................................Total amount of 10 mL in vial
7. Directions...............................Storage: Store below 86° F (30° C). Protect from freezing. To avoid discoloration, protect from prolonged exposure to light.
8. NDC.......................................0049-5460-74

Occasionally, a drug label will only have one name listed. The one name is the generic name. These are drugs that have been in use for many years and are very well known. The drug companies do not market them under different trade names. They all simply use the generic name.

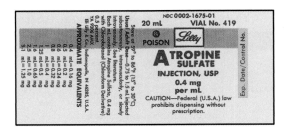

1. Trade name .... None
2. Generic name .... atropine sulfate
3. Dosage strength .... 0.4 mg per mL
4. Form .... Solution
5. Route .... Injection
6. Amount .... 20 mL
7. NDC number 0002-1675-01
8. Expiration date .... (Yellow highlight)

Study the material and examples for practice in reading drug labels. When you feel ready to evaluate your learning, take the first posttest. Check your answers. An acceptable score as indicated on the posttest signifies that you are ready for the next chapter. An unacceptable score signifies a need for further study before you take the second posttest.

Name _____

Date _____

ACCEPTABLE SCORE ___19___

YOUR SCORE _____

POSTTEST 1

Directions: Identify the requested parts of each of the following medication labels.

500 Tablets   NDC 0087-**6060-10**

N3 0087-6060-10 9

Each tablet contains 500 mg of metformin hydrochloride.
See enclosed package insert for dosage information.
Caution: Federal law prohibits
dispensing without prescription.
Store between 15°–30° C (59°–86° F).
Dispense in light resistant container.
Glucophage is a registered trademark of LIPHA s.a.
Licensed to Bristol-Myers Squibb Company.
Distributed by
Bristol-Myers Squibb Company   606010DRL-2
Princeton, NJ 08543 USA   34-007102-01

GLUCOPHAGE®
(metformin hydrochloride
tablets)

500
mg

⬡ Bristol-Myers Squibb Company

1. Trade name _____
   Generic name _____
   Dosage strength _____
   Form _____
   Amount _____

NDC 0663-3940-71

250 Tablets

6505-00-817-2279

Diabinese®
chlorpropamide

250 mg

CAUTION: Federal law prohibits
dispensing without prescription.

Pfizer Distributed by
LABORATORIES DIVISION
New York, N.Y. 10017

2. Trade name _____
   Generic name _____
   Dosage strength _____
   Form _____
   Amount _____

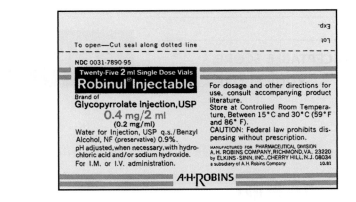

3. Trade name   _____
   Generic name   _____
   Dosage strength   _____
   Form   _____
   Route   _____

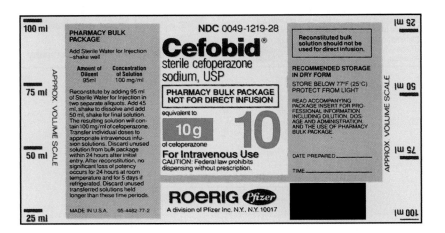

4. Trade name   _____
   Generic name   _____
   Dosage strength   _____
   Form   _____
   Route   _____

Answers on p. 483.

Name _____

Date _____

ACCEPTABLE SCORE __19__

YOUR SCORE _____

POSTTEST 2

Directions: Identify the requested parts of each of the following medication labels.

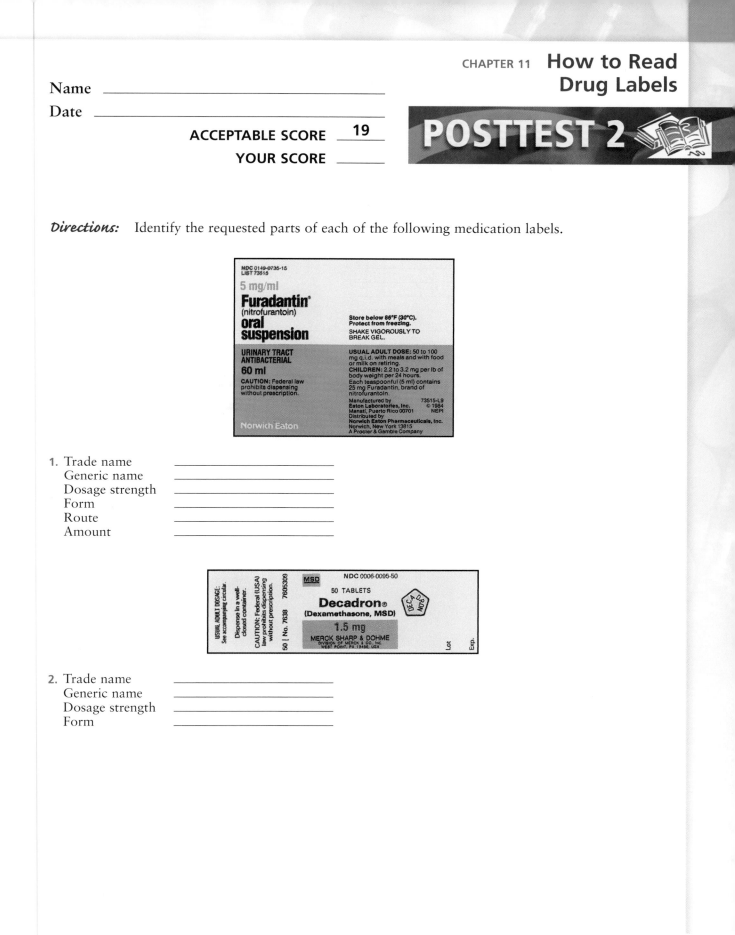

NDC 0149-0735-15
LIST 73515

5 mg/ml

Furadantin®
(nitrofurantoin)
oral suspension

URINARY TRACT ANTIBACTERIAL
60 ml

CAUTION: Federal law prohibits dispensing without prescription.

Norwich Eaton

Store below 86°F (30°C). Protect from freezing.
SHAKE VIGOROUSLY TO BREAK GEL.

USUAL ADULT DOSE: 50 to 100 mg q.i.d. with meals and with food or milk on retiring.
CHILDREN: 2.2 to 3.2 mg per lb of body weight per 24 hours.
Each teaspoonful (5 ml) contains 25 mg Furadantin, brand of nitrofurantoin.

Manufactured by
Eaton Laboratories, Inc.   73515-L9
Manati, Puerto Rico 00701   © 1984
Distributed by   NEPI
Norwich Eaton Pharmaceuticals, Inc.
Norwich, New York 13815
A Procter & Gamble Company

1. Trade name   _____
    Generic name   _____
    Dosage strength   _____
    Form   _____
    Route   _____
    Amount   _____

USUAL ADULT DOSAGE:
See accompanying circular.

Dispense in a well-closed container.

CAUTION: Federal (USA) law prohibits dispensing without prescription.

50 | No. 7638   7605309

MSD   NDC 0006-0095-50

50 TABLETS

Decadron®
(Dexamethasone, MSD)

DECADRON

1.5 mg

MERCK SHARP & DOHME
DIVISION OF MERCK & CO., INC.
WEST POINT, PA 19486, USA

Lot   Exp.

2. Trade name   _____
    Generic name   _____
    Dosage strength   _____
    Form   _____

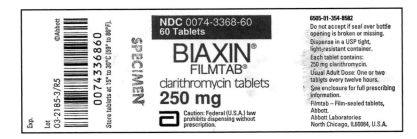

3. Trade name   _____
    Generic name   _____
    Dosage strength   _____
    Form   _____
    Amount   _____

4. Trade name   _____
    Generic name   _____
    Dosage strength   _____
    Form   _____
    Route   _____

Answers on p. 484.

Refer to Safety in Medication Administration: Parts of a Drug Label and Reading Drug Labels on the enclosed CD for additional help.

Dimensional Analysis and the Calculation of Drug Dosages*

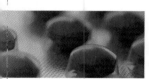

LEARNING OBJECTIVES

On completion of the materials provided in this chapter, you will be able to perform computations accurately by mastering the following mathematical concepts:

1 Using the dimensional analysis format to solve oral dosage problems

2 Using the dimensional analysis format to solve parenteral dosage problems

3 Using the dimensional analysis format to solve problems of intravenous flow rate in drops per minute

4 Using the dimensional analysis format to solve problems involving administration of medications in units per hour

5 Using the dimensional analysis format to solve problems involving administration of medications in milligrams per minute, micrograms per minute, and micrograms per kilogram per minute

Dimensional analysis is another format for setting up problems to calculate drug dosages. The advantage of dimensional analysis is that only one equation is needed. This is true even if the information supplied indicates a need to convert to like units before setting up the proportion to perform the actual calculation of the amount of medication to be given to the patient.

*Linda K. Fluharty, MSN, RN, and Mary Ann Reklau, MSN, RN, CPNP, contributed practice problems to this chapter.

Example: The order states Augmentin 500 mg po daily. The drug is supplied in 250-mg tablets. How many tablets will the nurse administer?

    a. On the left side of the equation, place the name or abbreviation of the drug form of x, or what you are solving for.

$$x \text{ tablet} =$$

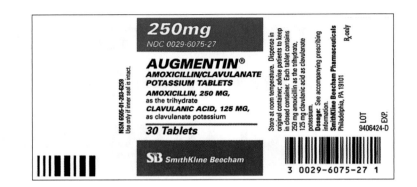

    b. On the right side of the equation, place the available information related to the measurement or abbreviation that was placed on the left side. In this example that is *tablet*. This information is placed in the equation as a common fraction; match the appropriate abbreviation or measurement. Thus the abbreviation that matches the x quantity must be placed in the numerator. We also know from the problem that each tablet contains 250 mg of Augmentin. This information is the denominator of our fraction.

$$x \textbf{ tablet} = \frac{1 \textbf{ tablet}}{250 \text{ mg}}$$

    c. Next, find the information that matches the measurement or abbreviation used in the denominator of the fraction you created. In this example *mg* is in the denominator and our order is for 500 mg. Therefore the full proportion is

$$x \text{ tablet} = \frac{1 \text{ tablet}}{250 \text{ mg}} \times \frac{500 \text{ mg}}{1}$$

    d. Now cancel out the like abbreviations on the right side of the equation. If you have set up the problem correctly, the remaining measurement or abbreviation should match that used on the left side of the equation. You are now ready to solve for x.

$$x \text{ tablet} = \frac{1 \text{ tablet}}{250 \text{ m\hspace{-0.6em}\diagup g}} \times \frac{500 \text{ m\hspace{-0.6em}\diagup g}}{1}$$

$$x = \frac{500}{250}$$

$$x = 2 \text{ tablets}$$

The answer to the problem is 2 tablets.

As stated earlier, the advantage of this method is not having to convert into like systems of measurement as would be required if the usual proportion method were used. With dimensional analysis, remember that only one equation is necessary. Let's look at another example.

Example: The order states Kantrex 400 mg IM q12 h. The drug is supplied as 0.5 g/2 mL. How many milliliters will the nurse administer?

a. On the left side of the equation, place the name or abbreviation of the drug form for which you are solving, or *x*.

$$x \text{ mL} =$$

b. On the right side of the equation, place the available information related to the measurement or abbreviation that was placed on the left side. In this example that is *mL*. This information is placed in the equation as part of a fraction; match the appropriate abbreviation. Remember that the abbreviation that matches the *x* quantity must be placed in the numerator. We know from the problem that each 2 mL contains 0.5 g of Kantrex.

$$x \text{ mL} = \frac{2 \text{ mL}}{0.5 \text{ g}}$$

c. Because the order is for 400 mg and the medication is supplied to us as 0.5 g/2 mL, a conversion would normally be required. However, with the dimensional analysis method, an additional fraction is added on the right side of the equation. From information supplied in earlier chapters, we know that 1 g equals 1000 mg. This information is then placed in the equation next in the form of the fraction $\frac{1 \text{ g}}{1000 \text{ mg}}$. Note that the abbreviation or measurement in the *numerator* of this fraction must match the abbreviation or measurement in the *denominator* of the immediate previous fraction. The equation now looks like

$$x \text{ mL} = \frac{2 \text{ mL}}{0.5 \text{ g}} \times \frac{1 \text{ g}}{1000 \text{ mg}}$$

d. Next, place the amount of drug ordered in the equation. Note that this will once again match the measurement or abbreviation of the denominator of the fraction immediately before. In this example, that is 400 mg. Therefore the full equation is

$$x \text{ mL} = \frac{2 \text{ mL}}{0.5 \text{ g}} \times \frac{1 \text{ g}}{1000 \text{ mg}} \times \frac{400 \text{ mg}}{1}$$

e. For the final step, cancel out the like abbreviations on the right side of the equation. If the equation has been set up correctly, the remaining abbreviation should match that located on the left side. Now solve for *x*.

$$x \text{ mL} = \frac{2 \text{ mL}}{0.5 \cancel{\text{g}}} \times \frac{1 \cancel{\text{g}}}{1000 \cancel{\text{mg}}} \times \frac{400 \cancel{\text{mg}}}{1}$$

$$x = \frac{2 \times 400}{0.5 \times 1000}$$

$$x = \frac{800}{500}$$

$$x = 1.6 \text{ mL}$$

The answer to the problem is 1.6 mL.

USING DIMENSIONAL ANALYSIS TO CALCULATE IV FLOW RATES

The dimensional analysis method can also be used to calculate intravenous (IV) flow rates. The following formulas demonstrate how to calculate drops per minute (gtt/min) and milliliters per hour (mL/h). These formulas can be used to solve IV problems in Chapters 16 and 17.

Example 1: A patient has an order for enalaprilat 0.625 mg daily IVPB (intravenous piggyback). The enalaprilat is diluted in 50 mL of D_5W (dextrose 5% in water) and is to be infused over 20 minutes. The tubing drop factor is 60 gtt/mL. At what rate, in drops per minute, should the IVPB be programmed?

  a. On the left side of the equation, place what you are solving for.

$$x \text{ gtt/min} =$$

  b. On the right side of the equation, place the available information related to the measurement that was placed on the left side of the equation. In this example the measurement we are solving for is *gtt/min*. We will deal with the numerator portion of our answer first: the gtt. This information is placed in the equation as a common fraction; match the appropriate measurement. Thus the abbreviation that matches the x quantity must be placed in the numerator. We also know from the problem that each milliliter contains 60 gtt. This information is the denominator of our fraction.

$$x \textbf{ gtt}/\text{min} = \frac{60 \textbf{ gtt}}{1 \text{ mL}}$$

  c. Next, find the information that matches the measurement used in the denominator of the fraction you created. In this example mL is in the denominator and our order is for 50 mL. We also know that the enalaprilat should be infused over 20 minutes. The equation now looks like

$$x \textbf{ gtt/min} = \frac{60 \text{ gtt}}{1 \text{ mL}} \times \frac{50 \textbf{ mL}}{20 \textbf{ min}}$$

  d. Then cancel out the like abbreviations on the right side of the equation. If you have set up the problem correctly, the remaining measurement should match the measurement on the left side of the equation. Now solve for x.

$$x \text{ gtt/min} = \frac{60 \text{ gtt}}{1 \text{ mL}} \times \frac{50 \text{ mL}}{20 \text{ min}}$$

$$x \text{ gtt/min} = \frac{60 \text{ gtt} \times 50}{20 \text{ min}}$$

$$x = \frac{3000 \text{ gtt}}{20 \text{ min}}$$

$$x = 150 \text{ gtt/min}$$

Therefore the nurse will regulate the IVPB for 150 gtt/min, and the enalaprilat will be infused over 20 minutes.

Example 2: A postoperative patient has an order for 200 mL 0.9% normal saline solution (NS) over 2 hours. The tubing drop factor is 10 gtt/mL. At what rate, in drops per minute, should the NS be infused?

  a. On the left side of the equation, place what you are solving for.

$$x \text{ gtt/min} =$$

b. On the right side of the equation, place the available information related to the measurement that was placed on the left side of the equation. In this example, the measurement we are solving for is *gtt/min*. We will deal with the numerator portion of our answer first: the gtt. This information is placed in the equation as a common fraction; match the appropriate measurement. Thus the abbreviation that matches the x quantity must be placed in the numerator on the right side of the equation. We know from the problem that each milliliter contains 10 gtt. This information is the denominator of our fraction.

$$x \text{ gtt/min} = \frac{10 \text{ gtt}}{1 \text{ mL}}$$

c. Next, find the information that matches the measurement used in the denominator of the fraction you created. In this example mL is in the denominator and our order is for 200 mL. We also know that this 200 mL should be infused over 2 hours. The equation now looks like

$$x \text{ gtt/min} = \frac{10 \text{ gtt}}{1 \text{ mL}} \times \frac{200 \text{ mL}}{2 \text{ h}}$$

d. Now, we need to solve for minutes, but the order is for hours. So, the equivalent of *1 h : 60 min* must be added to the equation as a fraction. The equation would now look like this.

$$x \text{ gtt/min} = \frac{10 \text{ gtt}}{1 \text{ mL}} \times \frac{200 \text{ mL}}{2 \text{ h}} \times \frac{1 \text{ h}}{60 \text{ min}}$$

e. Then cancel out the abbreviations on the right side of the equation. If you have set up the problem correctly, the remaining measurement should match that used on the left side of the equation. Now solve for x.

$$x \text{ gtt/min} = \frac{10 \text{ gtt}}{1 \text{ mL}} \times \frac{200 \text{ mL}}{2 \text{ h}} \times \frac{1 \text{ h}}{60 \text{ min}}$$

$$x \text{ gtt/min} = \frac{10 \times 200 \text{ gtt}}{2 \times 60 \text{ min}}$$

$$x = \frac{2000 \text{ gtt}}{120 \text{ min}}$$

$$x = 16.6 \text{ or } 17 \text{ gtt/min}$$

Therefore the nurse will regulate the IV for 17 gtt/min, and 200 mL of 0.9% NS will be infused over 2 hours.

Example 3: A patient has an order for regular insulin IV at a rate of 5 units/h. The concentration is insulin 100 units/100 mL 0.9% NS. At what rate, in milliliters per hour, should the IV pump be programmed?

a. On the left side of the equation, place what you are solving for.

$$x \text{ mL/h} =$$

b. On the right side of the equation, place the available information related to the measurement that was placed on the left side of the equation. In this example the measurement we are solving for is *mL/h*. We will deal with the numerator portion of our answer first: the mL. This information is placed in the equation as a common fraction; match the appropriate measurement. Thus the abbreviation that matches the x quantity must be placed in the numerator on the right side of the equation. We know from the problem that 100 units of insulin are diluted in the 100 mL; this information becomes the denominator of our fraction.

$$x \text{ mL/h} = \frac{100 \text{ mL}}{100 \text{ units}}$$

c. Next, find the information that matches the measurement used in the denominator of the fraction you created. In this example, *units* is the denominator and our order is for 5 units/h. The equation now looks like

$$x \text{ mL/h} = \frac{100 \text{ mL}}{100 \text{ \textbf{units}}} \times \frac{5 \text{ \textbf{units}}}{1 \text{ h}}$$

d. Then cancel out the abbreviations on the right side of the equation. If you have set up the problem correctly, the remaining measurement should match the measurement on the left side of the equation. Now solve for *x*.

$$x \text{ mL/h} = \frac{100 \text{ mL}}{100 \text{ \cancel{units}}} \times \frac{5 \text{ \cancel{units}}}{1 \text{ h}}$$

$$x = \frac{500 \text{ mL}}{100 \text{ h}}$$

$$x = 5 \text{ mL/h}$$

Therefore the nurse will program the IV pump for 5 mL/h, and the insulin will be infused at a rate of 5 units/h.

Example 4: A patient with a femoral thrombus has an order for heparin IV at 1200 units/h. The concentration is heparin 20,000 units in 250 mL of D_5W. At what rate, in milliliters per hour, should the IV pump be programmed?

a. On the left side of the equation, place what you are solving for.

$$x \text{ mL/h} =$$

b. On the right side of the equation, place the available information related to the measurement that was placed on the left side of the equation. In this example the measurement we are solving for is *mL/h*. We will deal with the numerator portion of our answer first: the mL. This information is placed in the equation as a common fraction; match the appropriate measurement. Thus the abbreviation that matches the *x* quantity must be placed in the numerator. We also know from the problem that there are 20,000 units of heparin in 250 mL. This information becomes the denominator of our fraction.

$$x \text{ mL/h} = \frac{250 \text{ mL}}{20,000 \text{ units}}$$

c. Next, find the information that matches the measurement used in the denominator of the fraction you created. In this example, *units* is the denominator. The order is for 1200 units/h. The equation now looks like

$$x \text{ mL/h} = \frac{250 \text{ mL}}{20,000 \text{ \textbf{units}}} \times \frac{1200 \text{ \textbf{units}}}{1 \text{ h}}$$

d. Then cancel out the like abbreviations on the right side of the equation. If you have set up the problem correctly, the remaining measurement should match the measurement on the left side of the equation. Now solve for x.

$$x \text{ mL/h} = \frac{250 \text{ mL}}{20,000 \text{ units}} \times \frac{1200 \text{ units}}{1 \text{ h}}$$

$$x = \frac{250 \text{ mL} \times 1200}{20,000 \text{ h}}$$

$$x = \frac{300,000 \text{ mL}}{20,000 \text{ h}}$$

$$x = 15 \text{ mL/h}$$

Therefore the nurse will program the IV pump for 15 mL/h, and the heparin will be infused at a rate of 1200 units/h.

Example 5: The order is to start a heparin infusion using the heparin protocol. The patient's weight is 143 lb. Using the weight-based heparin protocol example below, the nurse needs to do two calculations: the heparin bolus and the rate, in milliliters per hour, at which to program the IV pump.

Weight-Based Heparin Protocol (Example)

An order is received to begin IV heparin per facility protocol. The patient's weight is 143 lb.

Facility Protocol (Sample)

PTT Result	Heparin Dosing
<35	Bolus 70 units/kg and increase drip by 4 units/kg/h
35–54	Bolus 35 units/kg and increase drip by 3 units/kg/h
55–85	Therapeutic—no change
86–100	Decrease drip by 2 units/kg/h
>100	Hold infusion 1 hour; decrease drip by 3 units/kg/h, then restart drip

1. Bolus dose of 70 units/kg, rounded to the nearest 100 units (e.g., 6850 units would be rounded to 6900 units).
2. Begin infusion of heparin at 17 units/kg/h (25,000 units/250 mL = 100 units/mL).
3. Obtain partial thromboplastin time (PTT) every 6 hours and adjust the infusion using the following scale:

Bolus. The protocol calls for 70 units/kg, rounded to the nearest hundreds.

a. On the left side of the equation, place what you are solving for.

$$x \text{ units} =$$

b. On the right side of the equation, place the available information related to the measurement that was placed on the left side of the equation. In this example the measurement we are solving for is *units*. We will deal with the numerator portion of our answer first: the *units*. This information is placed in the equation as a common fraction, matching the appropriate measurement. Thus the abbreviation that matches the x quantity must be placed in the numerator. We know from the protocol that 70 units/kg is needed. This information becomes the denominator of our fraction.

$$x \text{ units} = \frac{70 \text{ units}}{1 \text{ kg}}$$

c. Next, find the information that matches the measurement used in the denominator of the fraction you created. In this example, *kg* is the denominator. The conversion of 1 kg = 2.2 lb is used as the next fraction. The equation now looks like

$$x \text{ units} = \frac{70 \text{ units}}{1 \text{ kg}} \times \frac{1 \text{ kg}}{2.2 \text{ lb}}$$

d. Next, the *lb* in the denominator must be cancelled out. We know from the problem that the patient weighs 143 lb.

$$x \text{ units} = \frac{70 \text{ units}}{1 \text{ kg}} \times \frac{1 \text{ kg}}{2.2 \text{ lb}} \times \frac{143 \text{ lb}}{1}$$

e. Then cancel out the like abbreviations on the right side of the equation. If you have set up the problem correctly, the remaining measurement should match the measurement on the left side of the equation. Now solve for *x*.

$$x \text{ units} = \frac{70 \text{ units}}{1 \text{ \cancel{kg}}} \times \frac{1 \text{ \cancel{kg}}}{2.2 \text{ \cancel{lb}}} \times \frac{143 \text{ \cancel{lb}}}{1}$$

$$x \text{ units} = \frac{70 \times 143}{2.2}$$

$$x \text{ units} = \frac{10,010}{2.2}$$

$$x = 4550 \text{ or } 4600 \text{ units IV bolus}$$

IV Infusion. The health care provider needs to calculate how many milliliters are needed to deliver 17 units/kg (protocol states 17 units/kg/h, rounded to the nearest tenth).

a. On the left side of the equation, place what you are solving for.

$$x \text{ mL} =$$

b. On the right side of the equation, place the available information related to the measurement that was placed on the left side of the equation. In this example the measurement we are solving for is *mL*. This information is placed in the equation as a common fraction, matching the appropriate measurement. Thus the abbreviation that matches the *x* quantity must be placed in the numerator. We know from the protocol that there are 100 units of heparin in 1 mL. This information becomes the first fraction of our equation.

$$x \text{ mL} = \frac{1 \text{ mL}}{100 \text{ units}}$$

c. Next, find the information that matches the measurement used in the denominator of the fraction you created. In this example, *units* is the denominator. The order is for 17 units/kg/h. The equation now looks like

$$x \text{ mL} = \frac{1 \text{ mL}}{100 \text{ units}} \times \frac{17 \text{ units}}{1 \text{ kg}}$$

d. Now, the kg is the denominator that needs to be cancelled. The conversion of 1 kg = 2.2 lb is used as the next fraction. Continue this process until all the denominators can be cancelled.

$$x \text{ mL} = \frac{1 \text{ mL}}{100 \text{ units}} \times \frac{17 \text{ units}}{1 \text{ kg}} \times \frac{1 \text{ kg}}{2.2 \text{ lb}} \times \frac{143 \text{ lb}}{1}$$

CHAPTER 12 Dimensional Analysis and the Calculation of Drug Dosages

e. Then cancel out the like abbreviations on the right side of the equation. If you have set up the problem correctly, the remaining measurement should match the measurement on the left side of the equation. Now solve for x.

$$x \text{ mL} = \frac{1 \text{ mL}}{100 \text{ units}} \times \frac{17 \text{ units}}{1 \text{ kg}} \times \frac{1 \text{ kg}}{2.2 \text{ lb}} \times \frac{143 \text{ lb}}{1}$$

$$x \text{ mL} = \frac{17 \times 143}{100 \times 2.2}$$

$$x \text{ mL} = \frac{2431}{220}$$

$$x = 11.05 \text{ or } 11.1 \text{ mL}$$

Therefore the nurse will program the IV pump for 11.1 mL/h, and the heparin will be infused at a rate of 17 units/kg/h.

Example 6: Lidocaine 1 g has been added to 500 mL of D_5W. The order states to infuse the lidocaine at 2 mg/min. The nurse needs to calculate the rate, in milliliters per hour, at which the IV pump should be set (rounded to the nearest tenth).

a. On the left side of the equation, place what you are solving for.

$$x \text{ mL/h} =$$

b. On the right side of the equation, place the available information related to the measurement that was placed on the left side of the equation. In this example the measurement we are solving for is *mL/h*. We will deal with the numerator portion of our answer first: the *mL*. This information is placed in the equation as a common fraction, matching the appropriate measurement. Thus the abbreviation that matches the x quantity must be placed in the numerator. We know from the problem that there is 1 g of lidocaine in 500 mL of D_5W. This information becomes the first fraction of our equation.

$$x \text{ mL/h} = \frac{500 \text{ mL}}{1 \text{ g}}$$

c. Next, find the information that matches the measurement used in the denominator of the fraction you created. In this example, g is the denominator. The conversion of 1 g = 1000 mg is used. The equation now looks like

$$x \text{ mL/h} = \frac{500 \text{ mL}}{1 \text{ g}} \times \frac{1 \text{ g}}{1000 \text{ mg}}$$

d. Now, the *mg* is the denominator that needs to be cancelled. The order for 2 mg/min is used as the next fraction. Continue this process until all the denominators except for hour can be cancelled.

$$x \text{ mL/h} = \frac{500 \text{ mL}}{1 \text{ g}} \times \frac{1 \text{ g}}{1000 \text{ mg}} \times \frac{2 \text{ mg}}{1 \text{ min}} \times \frac{60 \text{ min}}{1 \text{ h}}$$

e. Then cancel out the like abbreviations on the right side of the equation. If you have set up the problem correctly, the remaining measurement should match the measurement on the left side of the equation. Now solve for x.

$$x \text{ mL/h} = \frac{500 \text{ mL}}{1 \cancel{g}} \times \frac{1 \cancel{g}}{1000 \cancel{mg}} \times \frac{2 \cancel{mg}}{1 \cancel{min}} \times \frac{60 \cancel{min}}{1 \text{ h}}$$

$$x \text{ mL/h} = \frac{500 \times 2 \times 60}{1000}$$

$$x \text{ mL/h} = \frac{60,000}{1000}$$

$$x = 60 \text{ mL/h}$$

Therefore the nurse will program the IV pump for 60 mL/h, and the lidocaine will be infused at a rate of 2 mg/min.

Example 7: The order is to infuse the nitroglycerin at 5 mcg/min; 50 mg of nitroglycerin has been added to 500 mL of 0.9% NS. The nurse needs to calculate the rate, in milliliters per hour, at which to set the IV pump.

a. On the left side of the equation, place what you are solving for.

$$x \text{ mL/h} =$$

b. On the right side of the equation, place the available information related to the measurement that was placed on the left side of the equation. In this example the measurement we are solving for is *mL/h*. We will deal with the numerator portion of our answer first: the *mL*. This information is placed in the equation as a common fraction, matching the appropriate measurement. Thus the abbreviation that matches the x quantity must be placed in the numerator. We know from the problem that there are 50 mg of nitroglycerin in 500 mL of 0.9% NS. This information becomes the first fraction of our equation.

$$x \text{ mL/h} = \frac{500 \text{ mL}}{50 \text{ mg}}$$

c. Next, find the information that matches the measurement used in the denominator of the fraction you created. In this example, *mg* is the denominator. The conversion of 1 mg = 1000 mcg is used. The equation now looks like

$$x \text{ mL/h} = \frac{500 \text{ mL}}{50 \text{ mg}} \times \frac{1 \text{ mg}}{1000 \text{ mcg}}$$

d. Now, the *mcg* is the denominator that needs to be cancelled. The order for 5 mcg/min is used as the next fraction. Continue this process until all the denominators except for hour can be cancelled.

$$x \text{ mL/h} = \frac{500 \text{ mL}}{50 \text{ mg}} \times \frac{1 \text{ mg}}{1000 \text{ mcg}} \times \frac{5 \text{ mcg}}{1 \text{ min}} \times \frac{60 \text{ min}}{1 \text{ h}}$$

e. Then cancel out the like abbreviations on the right side of the equation. If you have set up the problem correctly, the remaining measurement should match the measurement on the left side of the equation. Now solve for x.

$$x \text{ mL/h} = \frac{500 \text{ mL}}{50 \text{ mg}} \times \frac{1 \text{ mg}}{1000 \text{ mcg}} \times \frac{5 \text{ mcg}}{1 \text{ min}} \times \frac{60 \text{ min}}{1 \text{ h}}$$

$$x \text{ mL/h} = \frac{500 \times 5 \times 60}{50 \times 1000}$$

$$x \text{ mL/h} = \frac{150,000}{50,000}$$

$$x = 3 \text{ mL/h}$$

Therefore the nurse will program the IV pump for 3 mL/h, and the nitroglycerin will be infused at a rate of 5 mcg/min.

Example 8: The order is to begin the infusion of 3 mcg/kg/min; 800 mg of dopamine is added to 250 mL of 0.9% NS. The patient's weight is 70 kg. The nurse needs to calculate the rate, in milliliters per hour, at which to set the IV pump.

a. On the left side of the equation, place what you are solving for.

$$x \text{ mL/h} =$$

b. On the right side of the equation, place the available information related to the measurement that was placed on the left side of the equation. In this example the measurement we are solving for is *mL/h*. We will deal with the numerator portion of our answer first: the *mL*. This information is placed in the equation as a common fraction, matching the appropriate measurement. Thus the abbreviation that matches the x quantity must be placed in the numerator. We know from the problem that there are 800 mg of dopamine in 250 mL of 0.9% NS. This information becomes the first fraction of our equation.

$$x \text{ mL/h} = \frac{250 \text{ mL}}{800 \text{ mg}}$$

c. Next, find the information that matches the measurement used in the denominator of the fraction you created. In this example *mg* is the denominator. The conversion of 1 mg = 1000 mcg is used. The equation now looks like

$$x \text{ mL/h} = \frac{250 \text{ mL}}{800 \text{ mg}} \times \frac{1 \text{ mg}}{1000 \text{ mcg}}$$

d. Now, the mcg is the denominator that needs to be cancelled. The order for 3 mcg/kg/min is used as the next fraction. Continue this process until all the denominators except for hour can be cancelled.

$$x \text{ mL/h} = \frac{250 \text{ mL}}{800 \text{ mg}} \times \frac{1 \text{ mg}}{1000 \text{ mcg}} \times \frac{3 \text{ mcg/kg}}{1 \text{ min}} \times \frac{60 \text{ min}}{1 \text{ h}} \times \frac{70 \text{ kg}}{1}$$

e. Then cancel out the like abbreviations on the right side of the equation. If you have set up the problem correctly, the remaining measurement should match the measurement on the left side of the equation. Now solve for x.

$$x \text{ mL/h} = \frac{250 \text{ mL}}{800 \text{ mg}} \times \frac{1 \text{ mg}}{1000 \text{ mcg}} \times \frac{3 \text{ mcg/kg}}{1 \text{ min}} \times \frac{60 \text{ min}}{1 \text{ h}} \times \frac{70 \text{ kg}}{1}$$

$$x \text{ mL/h} = \frac{250 \times 3 \times 60 \times 70}{800 \times 1000}$$

$$x \text{ mL/h} = \frac{3,150,000}{800,000}$$

$$x = 3.93 \text{ or } 3.9 \text{ mL/h}$$

Therefore the nurse will program the IV pump for 3.9 mL/h, and the dopamine will be infused at a rate of 3 mcg/kg/min.

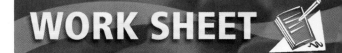

Directions: Calculate the following drug doses by using the dimensional analysis method. Show your work and check your answers.

1. Your patient with diabetes receives glipizide 10 mg po every morning. The drug is supplied in 5-mg scored tablets. How many tablets will you administer? _____

2. Mr. Theson receives Vistaril 60 mg po q6 h for relief of nausea after his acoustic neuroma revision. Vistaril oral suspension, 25 mg/5 mL, is supplied. How many milliliters will the nurse administer? _____

3. A patient who has undergone a lumbar laminectomy receives Demerol 0.025 g po q4 h prn for relief of pain. Demerol 50-mg tablets are available. How many tablets will the nurse administer? _____

4. Mrs. Fare receives codeine 30 mg po q3 h prn for pain relief after knee replacement surgery. How many tablets will you administer? _____

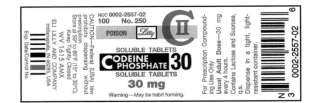

5. Your patient receives Keflex 0.5 g po four times a day. You have Keflex 250-mg capsules available. How many capsules will you administer? _____

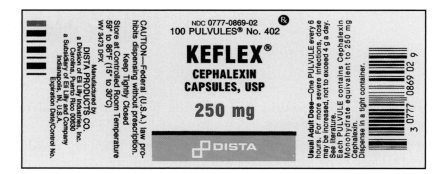

6. Your patient may receive Dilaudid 3 mg IM q3 h for relief of pain caused by a total hip replacement. Dilaudid is supplied in 1-mL ampules containing 4 mg. How many milliliters will you administer? _____

7. Johnny receives Lanoxin 40 mcg po q12 h for treatment of cardiac dysrhythmias. Lanoxin, 0.05 mg/mL, is available. How many milliliters will the nurse administer? _____

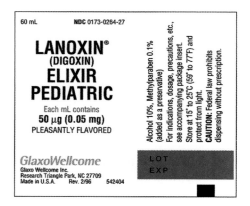

8. The physician prescribes Stadol 1 mg IV q4 h for a patient with a below-the-knee amputation. Stadol, 2 mg/mL, is available. How many milliliters will the nurse administer? _____

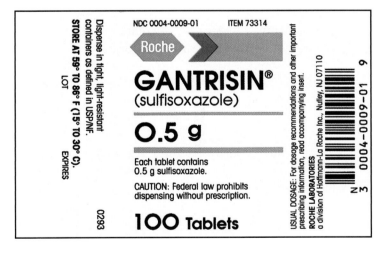

9. The physician orders heparin 2500 units subcutaneous q12 h for your patient with a jejunostomy. You have heparin, 5000 units/mL, available. How many milliliters will you administer? _____

10. The physician orders Gantrisin 2 g po stat. Gantrisin is supplied in 0.5-g tablets. How many tablets will the nurse administer? _____

11. A patient with an infection has an order for Timentin 3.1 g q6 h IVPB. The Timentin is dissolved in 100 mL of D$_5$W and is to be infused over 1 hour. The tubing drop factor is 20 gtt/mL. At what rate, in drops per minute, should the IVPB be programmed? _____

12. A patient with anuria has an order for 500 mL of 0.9% NS over 2 hours. The tubing drop factor is 10 gtt/mL. At what rate, in drops per minute, should the IV pump be programmed? _____

13. A patient who takes Coumadin at home is admitted to the hospital before surgery to receive a regulated infusion of heparin. The heparin is ordered for 1400 units/h. The heparin bag concentration is heparin, 25,000 units in 250 mL of D_5W. At what rate, in milliliters per hour, should the IV pump be programmed? _____

14. A patient with hyperglycemia has an order for regular insulin IV at a rate of 8 units/h. The concentration is insulin 50 units in 100 mL of 0.9% NS. At what rate, in milliliters per hour, will the IV pump be programmed? _____

15. Using the heparin protocol example on p. 177, calculate the heparin IV bolus and infusion rate for a patient weighing 132 lb. _____

16. The physician orders dobutamine at 12 mcg/kg/min for a patient weighing 75 kg. The concentration is dobutamine 1 g in 250 mL of D_5W. At what rate, in milliliters per hour, will the IV pump be programmed? _____

17. Mr. Perez is having chest pain and has an order for nitroglycerin at 10 mcg/min. The concentration is nitroglycerin 100 mg in 500 mL of D_5W. At what rate, in milliliters per hour, will the IV pump be programmed? _____

18. The physician orders amiodarone at 0.5 mg/min. The concentration of amiodarone is 900 mg in 500 mL of D$_5$W. At what rate, in milliliters per hour, will the IV pump be set? _____

19. a. Calculate the acetaminophen dose range for a child who weighs 14.5 kg. The recommended dose for acetaminophen is 10 to 15 mg/kg/dose q4-6 h. _____

b. What milliliter range is needed to deliver the calculated dose range? Acetaminophen is available as Tylenol elixir 160 mg/5 mL. _____

20. The doctor orders Lanoxin elixir 20 mcg po now. You have Lanoxin 0.1 mg/mL. What is the amount to be given? _____

21. Amoxil 500 mg po q6 h is ordered for a child weighing 50 kg. The recommended high dosage of Amoxil is 80 to 100 mg/kg/24 h q12.

a. What is the single dose range for this child? _____

b. Is the ordered dose safe to administer? Prove your response. _____

22. Phenobarbital elixir comes in 4 mg/mL. How many milliliters are needed to deliver 7.5 mg? _____

Answers on pp. 484-486.

Refer to Methods of Calculating Dosages: Dimensional Analysis on the enclosed CD for additional help and practice problems.

Calculation of Drug Dosages

Oral Dosages

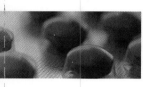

LEARNING OBJECTIVES

On completion of the materials provided in this chapter, you will be able to perform computations accurately by mastering the following mathematical concepts:

1 Converting all measures within the problem to equivalent measures in one system of measurement

2 Using a proportion to solve problems of oral dosage involving tablets, capsules, or liquid medications

3 Using a proportion to solve problems of oral dosages of medications measured in milliequivalents

4 Using the stated formula as an alternative method of solving oral-drug dosage problems

Oral drugs are preferred for administration of medications because they are easy to take and convenient for the patient. Oral medications are absorbed through the gastrointestinal tract; therefore the skin is not interrupted. Oral medications may be more economical because the production cost is usually lower than for other forms of medication.

Oral medications are absorbed primarily in the small intestine. Because of the differences in absorption factors, they might not be as effective as other forms of medication. Some oral medications are irritating to the alimentary canal and must be given with meals or a snack. Others may be harmful to the teeth and should be taken through a straw or feeding tube.

Oral medications are supplied in a variety of forms (Figure 13-1). The most common form is a tablet. Tablets come in many colors, sizes, and shapes. A tablet is produced from a drug powder. The tablet may be grooved for ease in administering only a fraction of the whole tablet. Some tablets are scored into halves, and others are divided into fourths (Figure 13-2).

If a patient has difficulty swallowing pills, some pills may be crushed using a mortar and pestle or a device that is specifically made for crushing pills (Figure 13-3). Before crushing any medication in pill form, verify the medication can be crushed. Some medications, such as those that are enteric coated or sustained or extended release, should not be crushed.

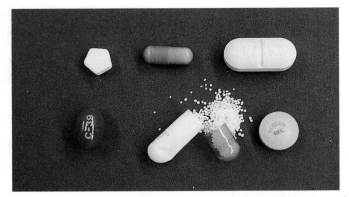

FIGURE 13-1 Forms of solid oral medication. *Top row:* Uniquely shaped tablet, capsule, scored tablet. *Bottom row:* Gelatin-coated liquid, extended-release capsule, and enteric-coated tablet. (From Potter PA, Perry AG: *Fundamentals of nursing,* ed 6, St Louis, 2005, Mosby.)

FIGURE 13-2 Scored medication tablet. (From *1999 Mosby's GenRx,* St Louis, 1999, Mosby.)

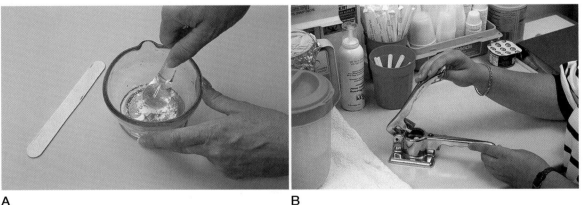

A   B

FIGURE 13-3 **A,** Mortar and pestle. **B,** Pill crusher. (From Elkin MK, Perry PA, Potter AG: *Nursing interventions and clinical skills,* ed 3, St Louis, 2004, Mosby.)

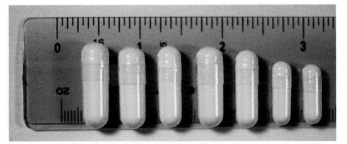

FIGURE 13-4 Various sizes and numbers of gelatin capsules (actual size). (From Clayton BD, Stock YN: *Basic pharmacology for nurses,* ed 13, St Louis, 2004, Mosby. Courtesy Oscar H. Allison, Jr.)

Oral medications may also be supplied in capsule form. A capsule is a hard or soft gelatin that houses a powder, liquid, or granular form of a specific medicine(s). Capsules are produced in a variety of sizes and colors (Figure 13-4). Capsules cannot be divided or crushed.

Oral medications may also be administered in liquid form such as an elixir or an oral suspension. Oral liquid medications can be measured with a medication cup, oral syringe (syringe without the needle attached), or dropper (Figures 13-5 to 13-7).

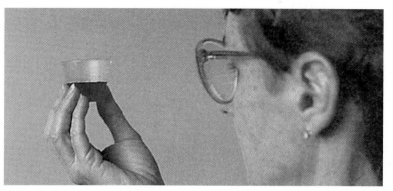

FIGURE 13-5 Oral liquid medication measured with a medication cup. (From Potter PA, Perry AG: *Fundamentals of nursing,* ed 6, St Louis, 2005, Mosby.)

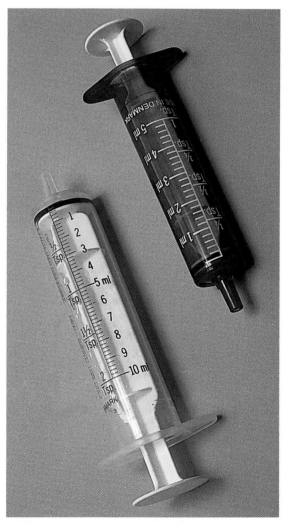

FIGURE 13-6 Plastic oral syringe. (From Clayton BD, Stock YN: *Basic pharmacology for nurses,* ed 13, St Louis, 2004, Mosby. Courtesy Chuck Dresner.)

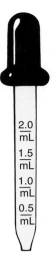

FIGURE 13-7 Medicine dropper. (From Clayton BD, Stock YN: *Basic pharmacology for nurses,* ed 13, St Louis, 2004, Mosby. Courtesy Chuck Dresner.)

Table 13-1 describes the forms of a variety of medications.

TABLE 13-1 ■ Forms of Medication

Forms	Description
Caplet	Solid dosage form for oral use; shaped like capsule and coated for ease of swallowing
Capsule	Solid dosage form for oral use; medication in powder, liquid, or oil form encased by gelatin shell; capsule colored to aid in product identification
Elixir	Clear fluid containing water and/or alcohol; designed for oral use; usually has sweetener added
Enteric-coated tablet	Tablet for oral use coated with materials that do not dissolve in stomach; coatings dissolve in intestine, where medication is absorbed
Extract	Concentrated medication form made by removing active portion of medication from its other components (e.g., fluid extract is medication made into solution from vegetable source)
Glycerite	Solution of medication combined with glycerin for external use; contains at least 50% glycerin
Intraocular disk	Small, flexible oval consisting of two soft, outer layers and a middle layer containing medication; when moistened by ocular fluid, releases medication for up to 1 week
Liniment	Preparation usually containing alcohol, oil, or soapy emollient that is applied to skin
Lotion	Medication in liquid suspension applied externally to protect skin
Ointment (salve, cream, or unguent)	Semisolid, externally applied preparation, usually containing one or more medications
Paste	Semisolid preparation, thicker and stiffer than ointment, absorbed through skin more slowly than ointment
Pill	Solid dosage form containing one or more medications, shaped into globules, ovoids, or oblong shapes; true pills rarely used because they have been replaced by tablets

TABLE 13-1 ■ Forms of Medication—cont'd

Forms	Description
Solution	Liquid preparation that may be used orally, parenterally, or externally; can also be instilled into body organ or cavity (e.g., bladder irrigations); contains water with one or more dissolved compounds; must be sterile for parenteral use
Suppository	Solid dosage form mixed with gelatin and shaped in form of pellet for insertion into body cavity (rectum or vagina); melts when it reaches body temperature, releasing medication for absorption
Suspension	Finely divided drug particles dispersed in liquid medium; when suspension is left standing, particles settle to bottom of container; commonly oral medication and not given intravenously
Syrup	Medication dissolved in concentrated sugar solution; may contain flavoring to make medication more palatable
Tablet	Powdered dosage form compressed into hard disks or cylinders; in addition to primary medication, contains binders (adhesive to allow powder to stick together), disintegrators (to promote tablet dissolution), lubricants (for ease of manufacturing), and fillers (for convenient tablet size)
Tincture	Alcohol or water-alcohol medication solution
Transdermal disk or patch	Medication contained within semipermeable membrane disk or patch, which allows medications to be absorbed through skin slowly over long period
Troche (lozenge)	Flat, round dosage form containing medication, flavoring, sugar, and mucilage; dissolves in mouth to release medication

From Potter PA, Perry AG: *Fundamentals of nursing*, ed 6, St Louis, 2005, Mosby.

Oral Dosages Involving Capsules and Tablets: Proportion Method

Sometimes the physician's order is in one system of measurement, and the drug is supplied in another system of measurement. It is therefore necessary to convert one of the measurements so that they are both in either the apothecary or the metric system of measurement. After this is done, another proportion will be written to calculate the actual drug dosage.

Example 1:   The physician orders ampicillin 0.5 g po four times a day. The drug is supplied in 250-mg capsules. How many capsules will the nurse administer? _____

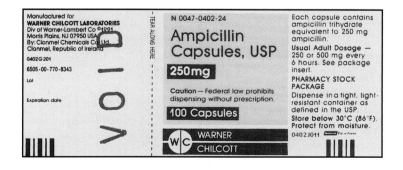

The physician's order is in grams and the drug is supplied in milligrams. The order and the supplied drug must be in the same metric measurement because only two different abbreviations can be used in each proportion. Therefore first convert 0.5 g to milligrams.

$$1000 \text{ mg} : 1 \text{ g} :: x \text{ mg} : 0.5 \text{ g}$$

$$1000 : 1 :: x : 0.5$$

$$1x = 1000 \times 0.5$$

$$x = 500 \text{ mg}$$

$$0.5 \text{ g} = 500 \text{ mg}$$

Now that once the order and the supplied drug are in the same metric measurement, a proportion may be written to calculate the amount of the drug to be given.

    a. $250 \text{ mg} : 1 \text{ capsule} ::$

    b. $250 \text{ mg} : 1 \text{ capsule} ::$ _____ mg : _____ capsule

       $250 \text{ mg} : 1 \text{ capsule} :: 500 \text{ mg} : x \text{ capsule}$

    c. $250 : 1 :: 500 : x$

    d. $250x = 1 \times 500$

       $250x = 500$

$$x = \frac{500}{250}$$

       $x = 2$

    e. $x = 2$ capsules. Therefore to give 0.5 g of the medication, the nurse will administer 2 capsules.

How many capsules will be given in 1 day? _____

The drug is to be given four times a day.

    a. 2 capsules : 1 dose ::

    b. 2 capsules : 1 dose :: _____ capsules : _____ dose

       2 capsules : 1 dose :: x capsules : 4 doses

    c. $2 : 1 :: x : 4$

    d. $1x = 2 \times 4$

       $x = 8$

    e. 8 capsules will be given each day.

Example 2: The physician orders aspirin gr xv po four times a day. Aspirin tablets gr v are available. How many tablets will the nurse administer? _____

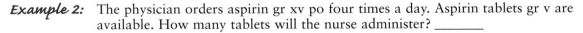

a. On the left side of the proportion place what you know or have available. In this example, each tablet contains gr v, or 5 gr. So the left side of the proportion would be

$$1 \text{ tablet} : 5 \text{ gr} ::$$

b. The right side of the proportion is determined by the physician's order and the abbreviations used on the left side of the proportion. Only *two* different abbreviations may be used in a single proportion. The abbreviations must be in the same position on the right as they are on the left.

$$1 \text{ tablet} : 5 \text{ gr} :: \underline{\hspace{1cm}} \text{ tablet} : \underline{\hspace{1cm}} \text{ gr}$$

In the example, the physician has ordered gr xv, or 15 gr.

$$1 \text{ tablet} : 5 \text{ gr} :: \underline{\hspace{1cm}} \text{ tablet} : 15 \text{ gr}$$

We need to find the number of tablets to be given, so we use the symbol x to represent the unknown. Therefore the full proportion would be

$$1 \text{ tablet} : 5 \text{ gr} :: x \text{ tablet} : 15 \text{ gr}$$

c. Rewrite the proportion without using the abbreviations.

$$1 : 5 :: x : 15$$

d. Solve for x.

$$5x = 1 \times 15$$
$$5x = 15$$
$$x = \frac{15}{5}$$
$$x = 3$$

e. Label your answer, as determined by the abbreviation placed next to x in the original proportion.

$$15 \text{ gr} = 3 \text{ tablets}$$

Oral Dosages Involving Liquids: Proportion Method

Example 1: The physician orders phenobarbital gr ¾ po two times a day. Phenobarbital elixir, 20 mg/5 mL, is available. How many milliliters will the nurse administer? _____

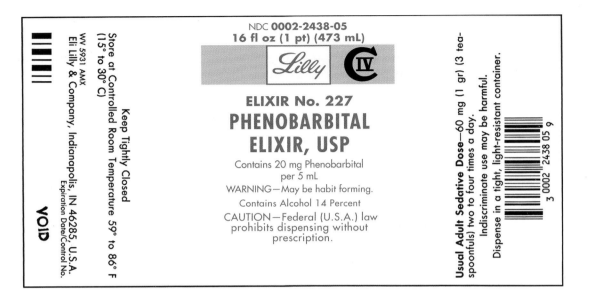

The physician's order is in the apothecary system and the drug is available in the metric system. Both the order and the available drug must be in the same system of measurement. Therefore convert gr ¾ to milligrams.

$$60 \text{ mg} : 1 \text{ gr} :: x \text{ mg} : \frac{3}{4} \text{ gr}$$

$$60 : 1 :: x : \frac{3}{4}$$

$$x = \frac{\overset{15}{\cancel{60}}}{1} \times \frac{3}{\underset{1}{\cancel{4}}}$$

$$x = \frac{15 \times 3}{1 \times 1}$$

$$x = \frac{45}{1}$$

$$x = 45 \text{ mg}$$

$$\frac{3}{4} \text{ gr} = 45 \text{ mg}$$

Now that the order and available drug are in the same system of measurement, a proportion can be written to calculate the actual amount of the drug to be administered.

a. 20 mg : 5 mL ::

b. 20 mg : 5 mL :: _____ mg : _____ mL
    20 mg : 5 mL :: 45 mg : x mL

c. 20 : 5 :: 45 : x

d. $20x = 5 \times 45$

$20x = 225$

$x = \dfrac{225}{20}$

$x = 11.25$

e. $x = 11.25$ mL. Therefore 11.25 mL is the amount of each individual dose twice a day.

Example 2: The physician orders Thorazine 20 mg po q4 h. The drug is available in iv oz bottles of Thorazine syrup containing 10 mg/5 mL. How many milliliters will the nurse administer? _____ How many doses are available in iv oz? _____

1. a. 10 mg : 5 mL ::
   b. 10 mg : 5 mL :: _____ mg : _____ mL
      10 mg : 5 mL :: 20 mg : x mL
   c. 10 : 5 :: 20 : x
   d. $10x = 5 \times 20$

   $10x = 100$

   $x = \dfrac{100}{10}$

   $x = 10$

   e. $x = 10$ mL. Therefore 10 mL is the amount of each individual dose q4 h.

2. The physician's order is in the metric system and the drug is supplied in the apothecary system. Both the order and the available drug must be in the same system of measurement. Therefore convert 10 mL to ounces, or the iv oz to milliliters, whichever is easier.

$$30 \text{ mL} : 1 \text{ fl oz} :: x \text{ mL} : 4 \text{ fl oz}$$

$$30 : 1 :: x : 4$$

$$x = 120$$

$$\text{iv oz bottle} = 120 \text{ mL}$$

Now that the order and available drug are in the same system of measurement, a proportion can be written to calculate the number of doses in a iv oz bottle.

a. 10 mL : 1 dose ::
b. 10 mL : 1 dose :: _____ mL : _____ dose
   10 mL : 1 dose :: 120 mL : x dose
c. 10 : 1 :: 120 : x
d. $10x = 120$

$x = \dfrac{120}{10}$

$x = 12$

e. $x = 12$ doses. Therefore each iv oz bottle contains 12 doses.

Oral Dosages Involving Milliequivalents: Proportion Method

Example: The physician orders potassium chloride (KCl) 60 mEq three times a day with meals. KCl 40 mEq/30 mL is available. How many milliliters will the nurse administer? _____

A **milliequivalent** is the number of grams of a solute contained in 1 mL of a normal solution. The milliequivalent is used in a drug dosage proportion, the same as a form of measurement in the apothecary or metric system.

    a. $40 \text{ mEq} : 30 \text{ mL} ::$

    b. $40 \text{ mEq} : 30 \text{ mL} ::$ _____ $\text{mEq} :$ _____ mL

        $40 \text{ mEq} : 30 \text{ mL} :: 60 \text{ mEq} : x \text{ mL}$

    c. $40 : 30 :: 60 : x$

    d. $40x = 30 \times 60$

        $40x = 1800$

        $x = \dfrac{1800}{40}$

        $x = 45$

    e. $x = 45$ mL. Therefore, to give 60 mEq of the medication, the nurse will administer 45 mL.

Alternative Formula Method of Oral Drug Dosage Calculation

A formula has been used for many years in the calculation of drug dosages by nurses. The formula method may be the method that some students learned first in an earlier nursing role (e.g., for a nurse who was a licensed practical nurse or who is returning to work in the area of direct patient care). If this is the case and the student accurately uses the formula method, I do not recommend changing to the proportion method. However, if calculations have frequently been difficult or incorrect, I recommend using the proportion method. Remember, choose the method that you feel is best for you and consistently use the chosen method. I do not recommend switching back and forth between the formula method and the proportion method. When you use the formula method, the *desired and available amounts must be in the same units of measurement.*

$$\text{Formula: } \frac{D}{A} \times Q = x$$

D represents the **desired** amount of the medication that has been ordered by the physician.

A represents the strength of the medication that is **available.**

Q represents the **quantity** or amount of the medication that contains the available strength. (NOTE: *When the medication is a solid such as a tablet, capsule, or caplet, the quantity will always be 1. If the medication is in liquid form, the number will vary. Remember from the math review, the denominator of a whole number is always one:* $\frac{1}{1}$, $\frac{2}{1}$, $\frac{3}{1}$, *etc.*)

x represents the dose that is unknown.

This formula can be read as:

Desired over (or divided by) available multiplied by the quantity available equals *x*, or the amount to be given to the patient.

200   **CHAPTER 13** Oral Dosages

Oral Dosages Involving Capsules and Tablets: Alternative Formula

If the physician's order is in one system of measurement and the drug is supplied in another system of measurement, it will still be necessary to convert one of the measurements so that both are expressed in the same system. After this is done, the formula may be used to calculate the drug dose to be administered.

Example 1: The physician orders ampicillin 0.5 g po four times a day. The drug is supplied in 250-mg capsules. How many capsules will the nurse administer? _____

The physician's order is expressed in grams and the drug is supplied in milligrams. Therefore convert the order to milligrams as outlined in Chapter 8.

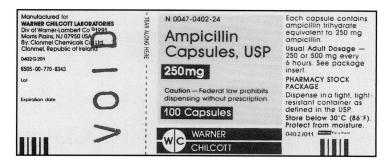

$$1000 \text{ mg} : 1 \text{ g} :: x \text{ mg} : 0.5 \text{ g}$$

$$1000 : 1 :: x : 0.5$$

$$x = 1000 \times 0.5$$

$$x = 500 \text{ mg}$$

Now the numbers may be filled into the formula $\dfrac{D}{A} \times Q = x$

    a. The desired amount of ampicillin is 500 mg. The available amount or strength of ampicillin supplied is 250 mg.

$$\frac{500}{250}$$

    b. The quantity available is in capsule form, or 1.

$$\frac{500 \text{ mg}}{250 \text{ mg}} \times \frac{1 \text{ capsule}}{1 \text{ capsule}}$$

    c. Rewrite the problem with the abbreviations cancelled.

$$\frac{500 \cancel{\text{ mg}}}{250 \cancel{\text{ mg}}} \times \frac{1 \cancel{\text{ capsule}}}{1 \cancel{\text{ capsule}}}$$

    d. Solve for x.

$$x = \frac{500 \times 1}{250 \times 1}$$

$$x = \frac{500}{250}$$

$$x = 2$$

    e. Label your answer as determined by the quantity.

$$500 \text{ mg} = 2 \text{ capsules}$$

Example 2: The physician orders aspirin gr xv po four times a day. Aspirin tablets gr v are available. How many tablets will the nurse administer? _____

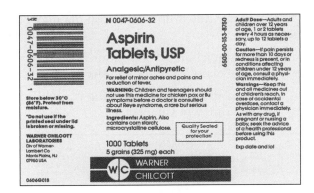

$$\frac{D}{A} \times Q = x$$

a. The desired amount of aspirin is gr xv, or 15 gr. The available amount or strength of the aspirin supplied is gr v, or 5 gr.

$$\frac{15 \text{ gr}}{5 \text{ gr}}$$

b. The quantity of the medication for gr v is 1 tablet.

$$\frac{15 \text{ gr}}{5 \text{ gr}} \times \frac{1 \text{ tablet}}{1 \text{ tablet}}$$

c. Rewrite the problem with the abbreviations cancelled.

$$\frac{15 \text{ \cancel{gr}}}{5 \text{ \cancel{gr}}} \times \frac{1 \text{ \cancel{tablet}}}{1 \text{ \cancel{tablet}}}$$

d. We can now solve for *x*.

$$x = \frac{15}{5} \times \frac{1}{1}$$

$$x = \frac{15 \times 1}{5 \times 1}$$

$$x = \frac{15}{5}$$

$$x = 3$$

e. Label your answer as determined by the quantity.

$$15 \text{ gr} = 3 \text{ tablets}$$

Oral Dosages Involving Liquids: Alternative Formula

Example: The physician orders phenobarbital gr ¾ po twice a day. Phenobarbital elixir 20 mg/5 mL is available. How many milliliters will the nurse administer? _____

The physician's order is in the apothecary system and the drug is available in the metric system. Change the order to an equivalent within the metric system of measure as outlined in Chapter 8.

$$60 \text{ mg} : 1 \text{ gr} :: x \text{ mg} : \tfrac{3}{4} \text{ gr}$$

$$60 : 1 :: x : \tfrac{3}{4}$$

$$x = \frac{\overset{15}{\cancel{60}}}{1} \times \frac{3}{\underset{1}{\cancel{4}}}$$

$$x = 45$$

$$\tfrac{3}{4} \text{ gr} = 45 \text{ mg}$$

Now the numbers may be filled into the formula $\dfrac{D}{A} \times Q = x$.

a. The desired amount is 45 mg. The available amount or strength of phenobarbital is 20 mg.

$$\frac{45 \text{ mg}}{20 \text{ mg}}$$

b. The quantity available is 5 mL.

$$\frac{45 \text{ mg}}{20 \text{ mg}} \times \frac{5 \text{ mL}}{1 \text{ mL}}$$

c. Rewrite the problem with the abbreviations cancelled.

$$\frac{45 \cancel{\text{mg}}}{20 \cancel{\text{mg}}} \times \frac{5 \cancel{\text{mL}}}{1 \cancel{\text{mL}}}$$

d. Solve for *x*.

$$x = \frac{45}{20} \times \frac{5}{1}$$

$$x = \frac{45}{\underset{4}{\cancel{20}}} \times \frac{\overset{1}{\cancel{5}}}{1}$$

$$x = \frac{45 \times 1}{4 \times 1}$$

$$x = \frac{45}{4}$$

$$x = 11.25$$

e. Label your answer as determined by the quantity.

$$45 \text{ mg} = 11.25 \text{ mL}$$

Complete the following work sheet, which provides for extensive practice in the calculation of oral dosage problems. Use either the proportion or formula method. Check your answers. It is sometimes impossible to administer the exact amount ordered. All capsules and tablets that are not scored are impossible to divide accurately. If you have difficulties, go back and review the necessary material. When you feel ready to evaluate your learning, take the first posttest. Check your answers. An acceptable score as indicated on the posttest signifies that you are ready for the next chapter. An unacceptable score signifies a need for further study before taking the second posttest.

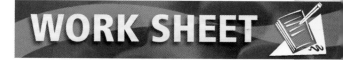

Directions: The medication order is listed at the beginning of each problem. Calculate the oral doses. Show your work. Shade each medicine cup or oral syringe when provided to indicate the correct dose.

1. The physician orders Minipress 2 mg po two times a day for Mr. Shaw's high blood pressure. How many capsules will the nurse administer per dose? _____

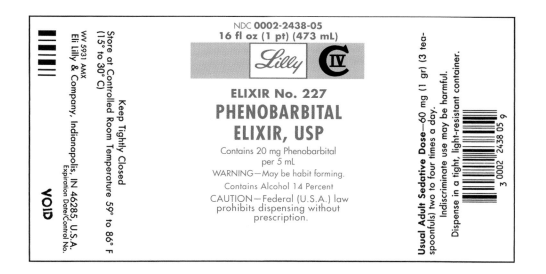

2. Mrs. Taylor has a long history of seizures. Elixir of phenobarbital 30 mg po q12 h is ordered. How many milliliters will the nurse administer per dose? _____

3. The physician orders Crystodigin 0.2 mg po two times a day for 4 days, then 0.15 mg po two times a day. You have Crystodigin 0.05-mg tablets available. How many tablets will you give for each dose the first 4 days? _____ How many tablets will you give for each dose thereafter? _____

4. Mr. Davis has a diagnosis of acute maxillary sinusitis. His physician orders Biaxin 500 mg q12 h × 10 days. How many tablets will the nurse administer per dose? _____

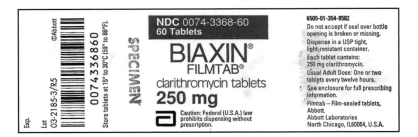

5. Mrs. Rios complains of nausea. Compazine 2.5 mg po three times a day is ordered. The stock supply is Compazine syrup 5 mg/5 mL. How many milliliters will the nurse administer per dose? _____

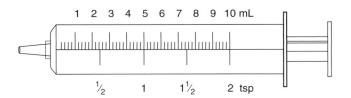

6. The physician orders Ativan 2 mg at bedtime. How many tablets will the nurse administer per dose? _____

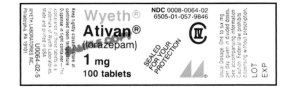

7. The physician orders Pravachol 20 mg po at bedtime. How many tablets will the nurse administer per dose? _____

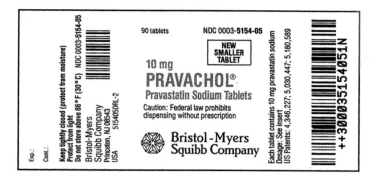

8. Mandelamine 1 g po four times a day is scheduled for Mr. Eaton to treat his urinary tract infection. You have 0.5-g tablets available. How many tablets will you administer per dose? _____

9. The physician orders Prozac 40 mg po daily in AM. How many milliliters will the nurse administer per dose? _____

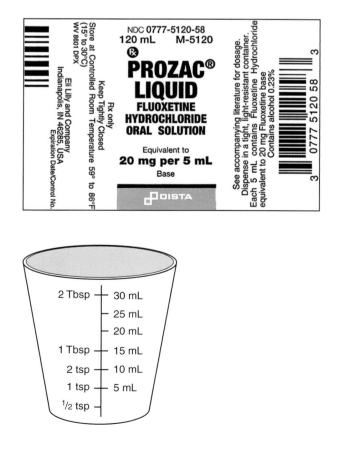

10. Mr. Chang has Parkinson's disease and is to receive Cogentin 1 mg po at 1900. How many tablets will the nurse administer per dose? _____

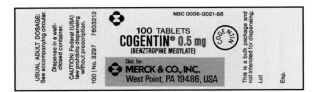

11. Mrs. Martin receives Motrin 800 mg po three times a day for arthritis pain. The drug is supplied in 400-mg tablets. How many tablets will the nurse administer per dose? _____

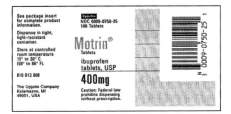

12. The physician orders lithium carbonate 0.6 g po two times a day. The drug is supplied in 300-mg scored tablets. How many tablets will the nurse administer per dose? _____ How many milligrams will be given each day? _____

13. Your patient is taking minoxidil 30 mg daily for hypertension. How many tablets will you administer per dose? _____

14. Mr. Hill is to receive Cipro 0.75 g q12 h for a knee infection. How many tablets will the nurse administer per dose? _____

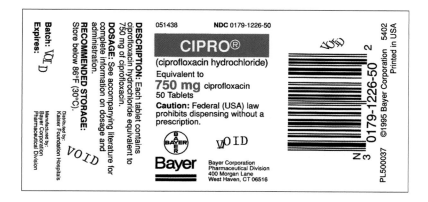

15. The physician orders ferrous sulfate ($FeSO_4$) 324 mg po daily to treat Mrs. Basey's anemia. You have $FeSO_4$ 0.324-g tablets available. How many tablets will you administer per dose? _____

16. The physician orders Gantrisin 4 g po stat, then 2 g q6 h. How many tablets will be given for the stat dose? _____ How many tablets will be given for each of the 2-g doses? _____

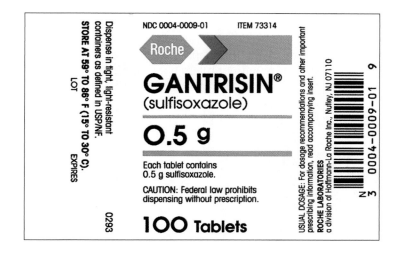

17. The physician orders acyclovir 800 mg po q4 h while the patient is awake. Acyclovir 400-mg tablets are available. How many tablets will the nurse administer per dose? _____

18. The physician orders Gaviscon 30 mL po four times a day. Gaviscon is supplied in xii oz bottles. Each dose is equal to _____ oz. How many ounces will be given in 1 day? _____

19. Ms. Vega complains of a rash on her abdomen, and the physician orders Benadryl 30 mg po three times a day. How many milliliters will the nurse administer per dose? _____

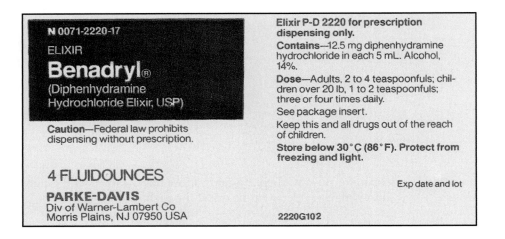

20. Mr. Gifford has had a lumbar laminectomy and requires pain medication. The patient has an order for codeine 60 mg po q3 h prn. How many tablets will the nurse administer per dose? _____

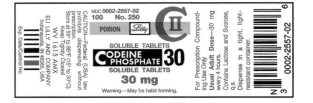

21. The physician orders Amoxil suspension 5.5 mL (125 mg/5 mL strength) po q6 h for your patient who had a tonsillectomy. How many milligrams will you administer every 6 hours? _____

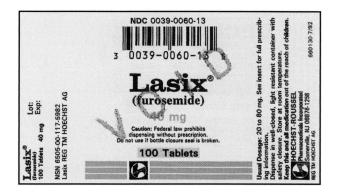

22. Mr. Sawyer is admitted with congestive heart failure. His orders require Lasix 80 mg po daily. How many tablets will the nurse administer per dose? _____

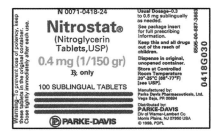

23. The physician orders nitroglycerin gr $\frac{1}{150}$ sublingual prn for angina. The patient should take no more than three tablets in 15 minutes. Mr. Cane took two tablets 5 minutes apart. How many milligrams did he receive? _____

24. Mr. Koehler has rheumatoid arthritis and has Decadron 1.5 mg po q12 h ordered. You have Decadron elixir 0.5 mg/5 mL. How many milliliters will you administer per dose? _____ How many ounces will you administer per dose? _____

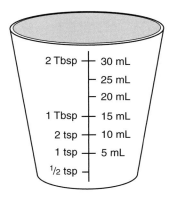

25. Your adult patient has acute bronchitis and has cefaclor 500 mg po q12 h ordered. How many milliliters will you administer per dose? _____

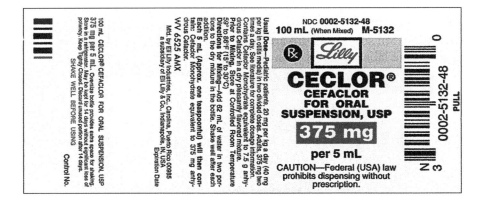

26. Mrs. Turner is admitted with hypertension. Apresoline 25 mg po four times a day is ordered. You have 50-mg scored tablets available. How many tablets will you administer per dose? _____

27. Your patient complains of indigestion during meals. Mylanta 30 mL po pc four times a day is ordered. Mylanta is supplied in a 12-oz bottle. There are _____ doses in one 12-oz bottle. How many ounces will you administer per dose? _____

28. The physician orders Halcion 0.25 mg po at bedtime. How many tablets will the nurse administer per dose? _____

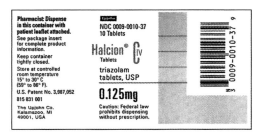

29. Mr. Bates has a history of seizure activity. Phenobarbital 15 mg po q3 h is ordered. How many tablets will the nurse administer per dose? _____

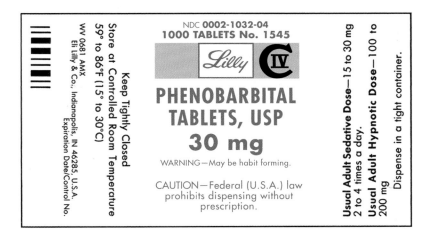

30. Mrs. Ortega has chronic sinusitis. Her physician orders amoxicillin 125 mg po q8 h. How many milliliters will the nurse administer per dose? _____

31. The physician prescribes Tenormin 25 mg po q4 h for Mr. Hutton's high blood pressure. You have Tenormin 50-mg scored tablets available. How many tablets will you administer per dose? _____

32. The physician orders quinidine 0.6 g po q4 h. Quinidine is supplied in 200-mg tablets. How many tablets will you give for one dose? _____ How many tablets will you give in 24 hours? _____

33. Mrs. Farmer has Phenergan 12.5 mg po three times a day ordered for relief of nausea. The drug is available in syrup containing 6.25 mg/5 mL. How many milliliters will the nurse administer per dose? _____

34. Your patient has Cipro 750 mg po q12 h ordered for a severe respiratory tract infection. You have Cipro oral suspension 500 mg/5 mL available. How many milliliters will you administer per dose? _____

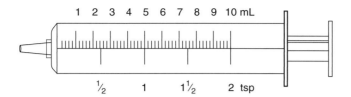

35. Mr. Golden, recovering from a left great toe amputation, has Colace elixir 100 mg po at bedtime ordered for constipation. How many milliliters will the nurse administer per dose? _____

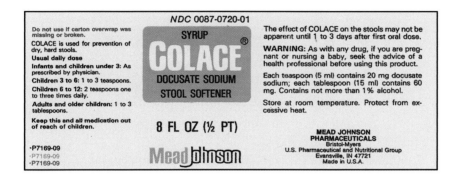

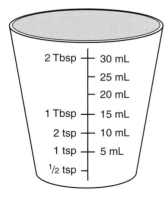

36. Mr. Malito is to receive Procanbid 1 g po now. How many tablets will you administer per dose? _____

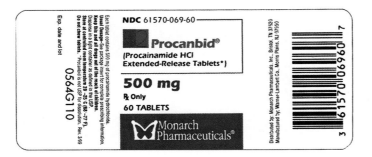

37. Mr. Mikal was admitted for treatment of leukemia and receives Deltasone 7.5 mg po three times a day as part of his chemotherapy. The drug is available in 2.5-mg tablets. How many tablets will the nurse administer per dose? _____

38. The physician orders Tegretol 0.2 g po three times a day for Mr. Pine's epilepsy. How many tablets will the nurse administer per dose? _____

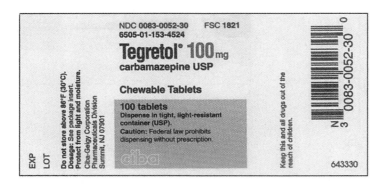

39. Lortab 5/500 po now is ordered for Mrs. Lindl for pain. How many tablets will she receive per dose? _____ How much acetaminophen is in each tablet? _____

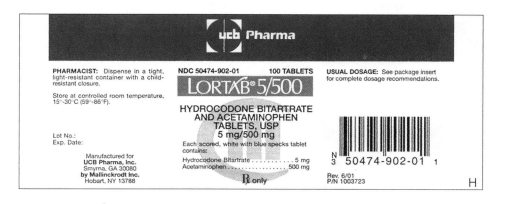

40. Mrs. Cross was admitted with a myasthenia crisis. Decadron 0.5 mg po q12 h is ordered. How many tablets will the nurse administer per dose? _____

41. Mr. Cook requires medication for nausea. Compazine 10 mg po q4 h prn is ordered. You have Compazine 5-mg tablets available. How many tablets will you administer per dose? _____

42. Mr. Pace receives Atarax 100 mg po at bedtime prn to relieve anxiety. You have 50-mg tablets available. How many tablets will you administer per dose? _____

43. The physician orders Rifadin 600 mg po 1 hour before dinner daily. How many capsules will the nurse administer per dose? _____

44. Mr. Day receives Lanoxin 0.25 mg po daily for atrial fibrillation. How many tablets will the nurse administer per dose? _____

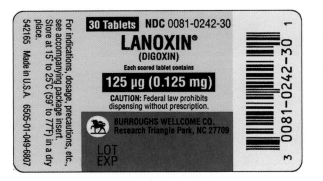

45. Mr. Payne receives Keflex 500 mg po four times a day before his dental extraction. How many capsules will the nurse administer in each dose? _____ How many capsules will the nurse administer for 1 day? _____

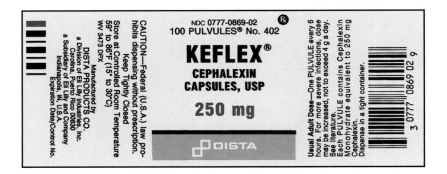

46. Mr. Tune is experiencing gastroesophageal reflux. The physician orders Nexium 40 mg po daily for 3 days. How many capsules will the nurse administer per dose? _____

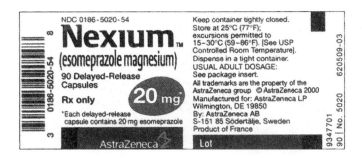

47. Mrs. Graves receives phenobarbital tablets gr 1½ po q3 h prn for seizure activity. How many tablets will the nurse administer per dose? _____

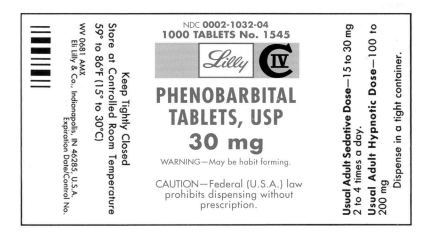

48. Mr. Vee is enrolled in a smoking cessation program. He is to begin with Wellbutrin 150 mg po daily for 3 days. How many tablets will the nurse administer per dose? _____

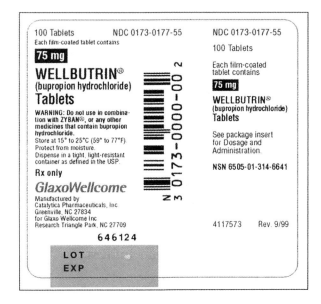

49. Mr. Sahl, recovering from a coronary artery bypass graft, receives aspirin gr x po twice a day. How many tablets will the nurse administer per dose? _____

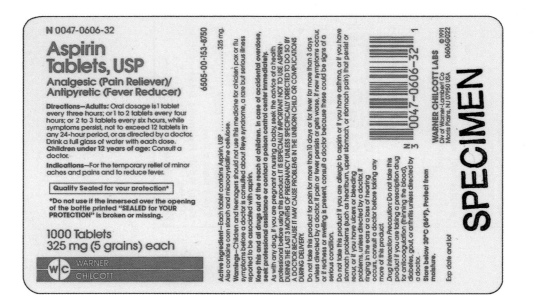

50. Mr. Dale receives Zantac 150 mg two times a day as part of his treatment for esophagitis. How many milliliters will the nurse administer per dose? _____

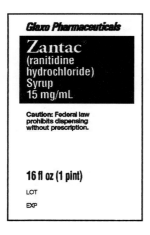

51. Mrs. Line has erythromycin 500 mg po q6 h prescribed for treatment of her strep throat. How many tablets will you administer per dose? _____

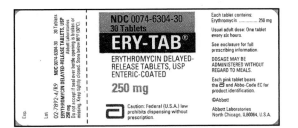

52. The physician prescribes FeSO₄ gr v po three times a day as a supplement for Mr. Bay, a patient who has undergone cardiac catheterization. How many tablets will the nurse administer per dose? _____ How many milligrams will be given per dose? _____

53. Mr. Romero, admitted with chronic obstructive lung disease, takes Bentyl 20 mg po three times a day ac. The drug is available in 10-mg capsules. How many capsules will the nurse administer per dose? _____

54. Mrs. Tyth has pruritic dermatosis. The physician prescribes Atarax 30 mg po two times daily as part of her therapy. The drug is supplied in syrup containing 10 mg/5 mL. How many milliliters will the nurse administer per dose? _____

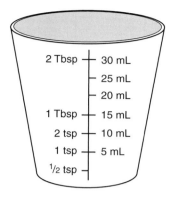

55. Mrs. Gale, admitted for alcohol abuse, has an order for ascorbic acid 0.75 g po daily while hospitalized. You have 250-mg tablets available. How many tablets will you administer per dose? _____

56. Your patient who is receiving chemotherapy has an order for Zofran 8 mg po ½ hour before chemotherapy for relief of nausea. The drug is supplied in 4-mg tablets. How many tablets will the nurse administer per dose? _____

57. Mr. Nade, hospitalized for a radical neck dissection, has Vistaril 15 mg po four times a day ordered to suppress nausea. You have Vistaril 25 mg/5 mL available. How many milliliters will you administer per dose? _____

58. Mrs. Snell requires Lopressor 100 mg po two times daily. How many tablets will the nurse administer per dose? _____

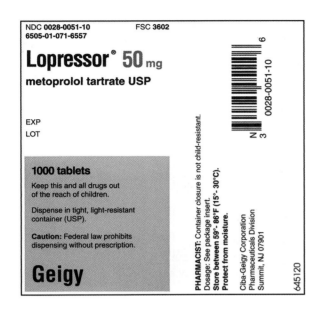

59. Your patient with type 2 adult-onset diabetes mellitus receives metformin hydrochloride 1 g po twice daily. How many tablets will the nurse administer per dose? _____

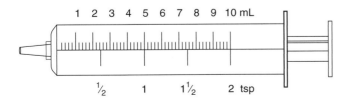

60. Mr. Aden requires Chloromycetin 250 mg po q6 h for treatment of a *Salmonella* infection. You have Chloromycetin 150 mg/5 mL available. How many milliliters will you administer per dose? _____

Oral Dosages **CHAPTER 13**   223

61. Mr. Scheottle receives Vibramycin 100 mg po q12 h for treatment of inclusion conjunctivitis. How many milliliters will the nurse administer per dose? _____

Vibramycin® Calcium
SYRUP
doxycycline calcium
oral suspension
50 mg / 5 ml†
1 PINT (473 ml)
†Each teaspoonful (5 ml) contains
doxycycline calcium equivalent
to 50 mg of doxycycline.
USUAL DOSAGE:
Adults: 200 mg on the first day
(100 mg every 12 hours) followed by
a maintenance dose of 100 mg a day.
Children above eight years of age:
Under 100 lbs.—2 mg/lb. of body
weight daily divided in two doses
on the first day, followed by
1 mg/lb. of body weight on
subsequent days in one or two doses.
Over 100 lbs.—See adult dosage.
doxycycline U.S. Pat. No. 3,200,149
READ ACCOMPANYING
PROFESSIONAL INFORMATION
RECOMMENDED STORAGE
STORE BELOW 86° F. (30° C.)
Dispense in tight, light resistant
containers (USP).
CAUTION: Federal law prohibits
dispensing without prescription.
Pfizer LABORATORIES DIVISION
PFIZER INC.,
NEW YORK, N.Y. 10017

MADE IN U.S.A. 2

Pfizer
NDC 0069-0971-93
6188
Vibramycin® Calcium
SYRUP
doxycycline calcium
oral suspension
50 mg/5ml†
1 PINT
(473 ml)
RASPBERRY/APPLE
FLAVORED
For oral use
only
SHAKE WELL
BEFORE USING
IMPORTANT:
This closure is
not child-resistant.

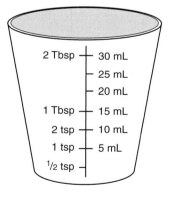

62. Your patient, admitted for cardiac catheterization, receives HydroDIURIL 25 mg po two times a day for hypertension. You have 50-mg scored tablets available. How many tablets will you administer per dose? _____

63. Tylenol 240 mg po q4 h is ordered for a temperature of 38.9° C. You have Tylenol 80-mg chewable tablets available. How many tablets will be required for each dose? _____

64. The physician prescribes Lanoxin elixir 90 mcg po two times a day for your patient with atrial fibrillation. How many milliliters will you administer per dose? _____

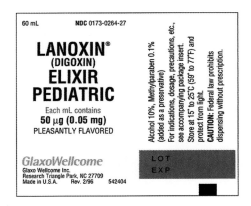

60 mL NDC 0173-0264-27

LANOXIN®
(DIGOXIN)
ELIXIR
PEDIATRIC
Each mL contains
50 µg (0.05 mg)
PLEASANTLY FLAVORED

GlaxoWellcome
Glaxo Wellcome Inc.
Research Triangle Park, NC 27709
Made in U.S.A.   Rev. 2/96   542404

Alcohol 10%, Methylparaben 0.1% (added as a preservative)
For indications, dosage, precautions, etc., see accompanying package insert.
Store at 15° to 25°C (59° to 77°F) and protect from light.
CAUTION: Federal law prohibits dispensing without prescription.

LOT
EXP

65. Mr. Ceney, admitted for contact dermatitis, receives elixir of Benadryl 10 mL po q6 h prn for relief of itching. The drug is supplied as 12.5 mg/5 mL. This dose delivers _____ mg.

66. The physician orders Indocin 50 mg po twice a day. How many capsules will the nurse administer per dose? _____

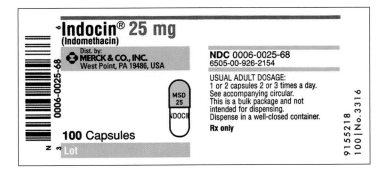

Indocin® 25 mg
(Indomethacin)
Dist. by:
⊕ **MERCK & CO., INC.**
West Point, PA 19486, USA

0006-0025-68

MSD
25

NDOCI

100 Capsules

N Lot

NDC 0006-0025-68
6505-00-926-2154

USUAL ADULT DOSAGE:
1 or 2 capsules 2 or 3 times a day.
See accompanying circular.
This is a bulk package and not intended for dispensing.
Dispense in a well-closed container.

Rx only

9155218
100 | No. 3316

67. Your patient receives Dilantin gr i ss po three times a day for past seizure activity. How many capsules will you administer per dose? _____

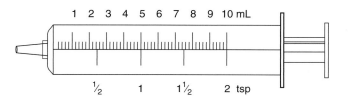

68. The physician orders Lipitor 40 mg po daily. You have available 10-mg, 20-mg, and 40-mg tablets. Which tablet would be most appropriate? _____ How many tablets will you administer per dose? _____

69. Your patient, admitted with a small-bowel obstruction, has KCl 10 mEq po daily ordered for his low potassium level. The drug is available as a liquid in KCl 20 mEq/15 mL. How many milliliters will you administer per dose? _____

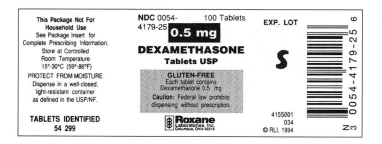

70. Mr. Brown receives dexamethasone 1.5 mg po q12 h for inflammation. How many tablets will the nurse administer per dose? _____

71. Mrs. Roget has been receiving digoxin 0.5 mg po daily for her cardiac dysrhythmia. The drug is available in 0.25-mg tablets. How many tablets will the nurse administer per dose? _____

72. Acetaminophen 650 mg po q4 h is prescribed for a temperature of more than 38.5° C × 24 h. How many tablets will the nurse administer every 4 hours? _____

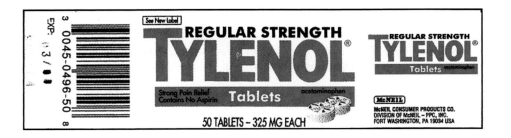

73. The physician prescribes Decadron 0.5 mg po q12 h for your patient's keratitis. How many tablets will you administer per dose? _____

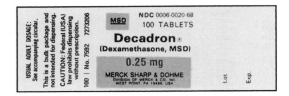

74. The physician orders Keflex 375 mg po q6 h for Mr. Pein after his thyroidectomy. How many milliliters will the nurse administer per dose? _____

75. Your postoperative patient receives Demerol 30 mg po q4 h prn for pain relief. The drug is supplied 50 mg/5 mL. How many milliliters will you administer per dose? _____

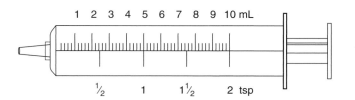

76. The physician orders Crystodigin gr $\frac{1}{200}$ po daily. You have Crystodigin in 0.05-mg, 0.15-mg, and 0.2-mg tablets. The best way to administer this drug is to give _____ tablets of _____ mg each.

77. Mr. Zeman has prednisone 7.5 mg po daily ordered for exfoliative dermatitis. Prednisone is supplied in 5-mg scored tablets. How many tablets will the nurse administer per dose? _____

78. Your patient who has had a partial craniotomy has Ceclor suspension 250 mg po four times a day ordered. How many milliliters will you administer per dose? _____

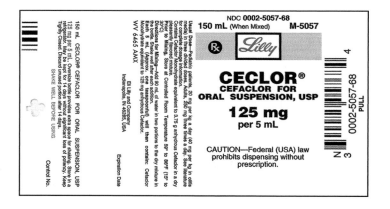

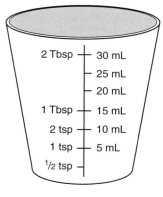

79. Your patient, who has undergone a coronary artery bypass graft, receives Surfak 250 mg po daily as a stool softener. How many capsules will you administer per dose? _____

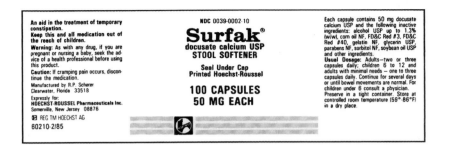

80. The physician orders 20 mEq KCl elixir po three times a day. Elixir of KCl 15 mEq/11.25 mL is available. How many milliliters will you administer per dose? _____

81. Your patient with epilepsy receives phenobarbital 55 mg po two times a day. How many milliliters will you administer per dose? _____

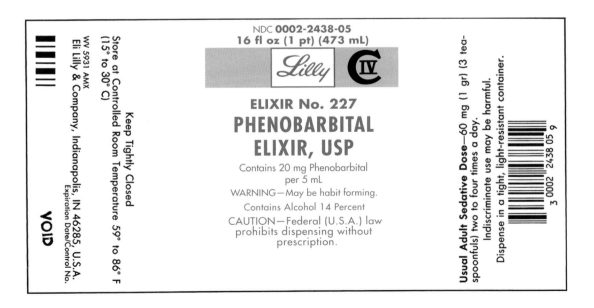

82. The physician orders Aldomet 250 mg po two times a day. How many tablets will the nurse administer per dose? _____

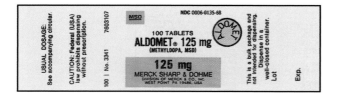

83. Mrs. Richardson, a patient who had a thyroidectomy, receives Synthroid 0.05 mg po daily in the morning. How many tablets will the nurse administer per dose? _____

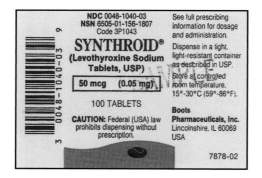

84. The physician orders Theo-Dur 0.2 g po q8 h. Theo-Dur is supplied in 100-mg, 200-mg, and 300-mg sustained-action tablets. Give _____ tablets of _____ mg. How many milligrams will be given per day? _____

85. Your patient who had a valve repair begins receiving Coumadin 15 mg po stat. Coumadin 5-mg scored tablets are available. How many tablets will you administer per dose? _____

86. Your patient, who has an ulcer, receives cimetidine 800 mg po at bedtime. How many tablets will you administer each night? _____

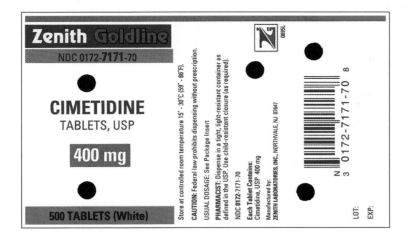

87. The physician prescribes Restoril 30 mg po at bedtime prn for a patient who has insomnia before surgery. How many capsules will the nurse administer at bedtime? _____

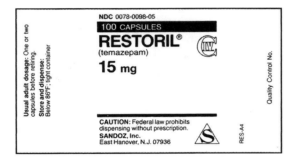

88. The physician orders imipramine 50 mg po once in the morning and once at bedtime. The drug is supplied in 25-mg tablets. How many tablets will the nurse administer per dose? _____

89. Your patient with depression receives Prozac 30 mg po twice a day. How many pills will you administer per dose? _____

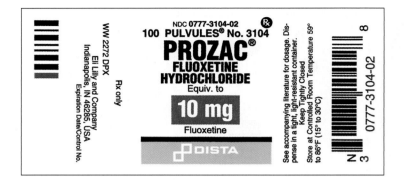

90. A patient receives Lasix 6 mg po twice a day with meals. Lasix is available in an oral solution of 10 mg/mL. How many milliliters will be given per dose? _____

91. Mrs. Adams receives Cleocin 150 mg po q6 h for her upper respiratory tract infection. Cleocin is supplied in 75-mg capsules. How many capsules will the nurse administer per dose? _____

92. Your patient receives Dilantin 200 mg po three times a day for seizures. How many capsules will you administer per dose? _____

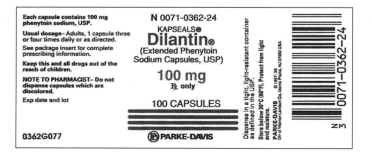

93. The physician orders Coumadin 10 mg po at 1800 today. How many tablets will the nurse administer per dose? _____

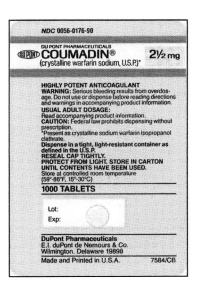

94. Your patient with diabetes receives Diabinese 0.25 g po daily in the morning. How many tablets will you administer per dose? _____

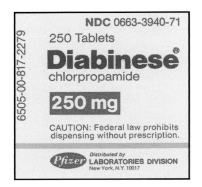

95. The physician prescribes Apresoline 25 mg po two times a day for Mr. Yu's hypertension. You have Apresoline scored tablets gr ⅙ available. How many tablets will you administer per dose? _____

96. The physician orders Flexeril 30 mg po at bedtime. Flexeril 10-mg tablets are available. How many tablets will the nurse administer per dose? _____

97. Your patient has begun receiving prednisone 15 mg po daily for asthma. Prednisone is available in 5-mg tablets. How many tablets will you administer per dose? _____

98. Mr. Gray, who has undergone cervical discectomy, receives Restoril 0.015 g po at bedtime for insomnia. How many capsules will the nurse administer per dose? _____

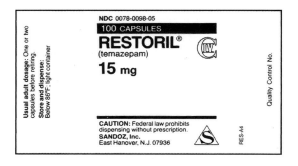

99. A patient receives KCl elixir 30 mEq po three times a day with juice. KCl 6.7 mEq/5 mL is available. How many milliliters will the nurse administer per dose? _____

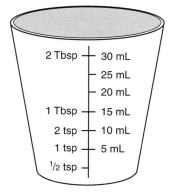

100. Mrs. Endres receives furosemide 20 mg po q8 h for congestive heart failure. How many tablets will the nurse administer per dose? _____

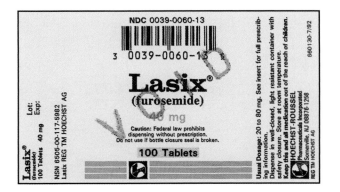

Answers on pp. 486–507.

Name _____

Date _____

ACCEPTABLE SCORE __24__

YOUR SCORE _____

POSTTEST 1

Directions: The medication order is listed at the beginning of each problem. Calculate the oral doses. Show your work. Shade each medicine cup or oral syringe when provided to indicate the correct dose.

1. The physician orders aspirin gr xv po four times a day for a patient who had a mitral valve repair. How many tablets will the nurse administer per dose? _____

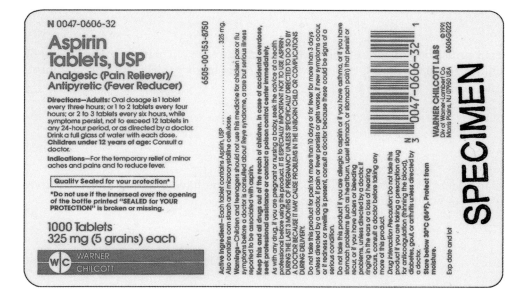

2. Mr. Clay receives tetracycline 0.5 g po four times a day for a gastrointestinal infection. How many capsules will the nurse administer per dose? _____

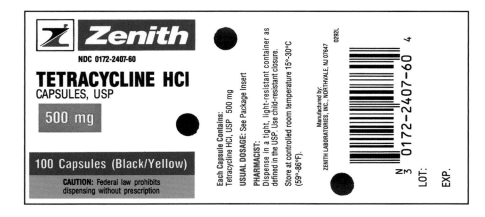

3. The physician orders ampicillin 1 g po q6 h for treatment of shigellosis. How many capsules will the nurse administer per dose? _____

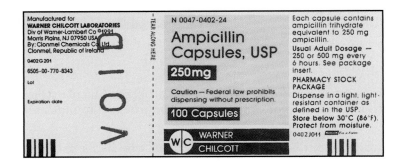

4. The physician prescribes Allegra 60 mg two times a day for your patient's complaints of allergic rhinitis. You have 0.03-g tablets available. How many tablets will you administer per dose? _____

5. The physician orders levothyroxine 100 mcg po daily. You have 0.05-mg tablets available. How many tablets will you administer per dose? _____

6. Mr. Shen, admitted with a psychoneurotic disorder, receives Atarax 25 mg po daily in the morning. You have Atarax 10 mg/5 mL. How many milliliters will you administer per dose? _____

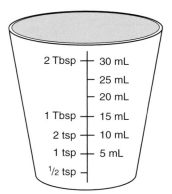

7. Your cardiac patient has Cardizem 60 mg four times a day ordered. How many tablets will you administer per dose? ____

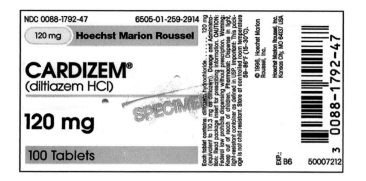

8. The physician prescribes codeine 30 mg po q3 h prn for pain relief for your patient with a total hip replacement. How many tablets will you administer per dose? _____

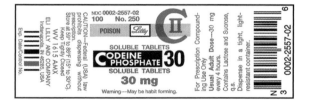

9. Your patient receives Vistaril 50 mg po three times a day for preoperative anxiety. Vistaril oral suspension 25 mg/5 mL is available. How many milliliters will you administer per dose? _____

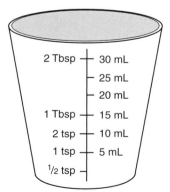

10. The physician orders Prozac liquid 30 mg po twice a day. How many milliliters will you administer per dose? _____

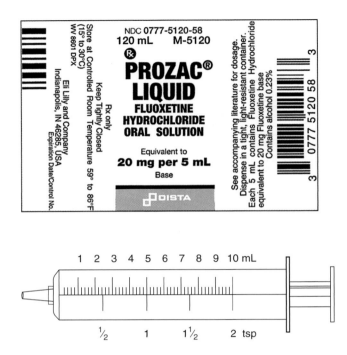

11. Your patient receives Crystodigin gr ¹⁄₆₀₀ po daily for an atrial arrhythmia. Crystodigin tablets gr ¹⁄₃₀₀ are available. How many tablets will you administer per dose? _____

12. The physician prescribes KCl 20 mEq po twice a day for hypokalemia. KCl liquid is supplied 30 mEq/22.5 mL. How many milliliters will the nurse administer per dose? _____

13. The physician orders Lipitor 40 mg po daily. How many tablets will you give per dose? _____

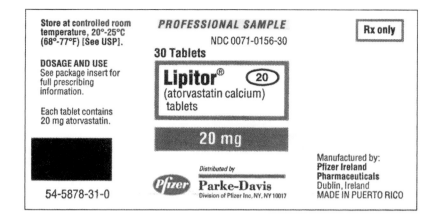

14. Your patient with a lumbar laminectomy has Benadryl 100 mg po at bedtime prn ordered for insomnia. How many capsules will you administer per dose? _____

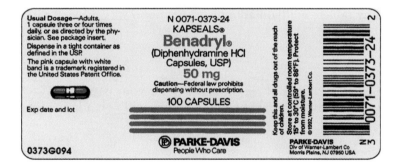

15. Your patient has Lasix 38 mg po q12 h ordered for hypercalcemia. You have Lasix 10 mg/mL. How many milliliters will you administer per dose? _____

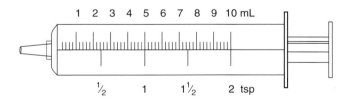

16. Mrs. Cook receives Keflex 100 mg po q6 h for a sinus infection. How many milliliters will the nurse administer per dose? _____

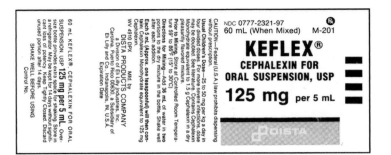

17. The physician orders Mevacor 30 mg po daily to be given with evening meal. You have 10-mg tablets available. How many tablets will you administer per dose? _____

18. Mr. Jones receives Inderal 80 mg po two times a day for a dysrhythmia. You have Inderal 40-mg scored tablets. How many tablets will you administer per dose? _____

19. The physician prescribes Apresoline 20 mg po three times a day for your patient's hypertension. You have 10-mg tablets available. How many tablets will you administer per dose? _____

20. Your patient with epilepsy receives phenobarbital gr i ss po three times a day. How many tablets will you administer in each dose? _____ How many tablets will you administer in 1 day?

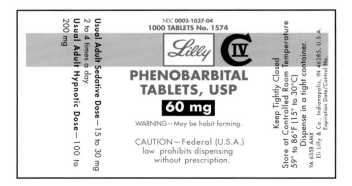

21. Mrs. Luther has alprazolam 0.5 mg po three times a day prescribed for her panic disorder. You have 0.25-mg tablets available. How many tablets will you administer per dose? _____

22. Mr. Barry has Ambien 10 mg po at bedtime ordered for insomnia. How many tablets will the nurse administer per dose? _____

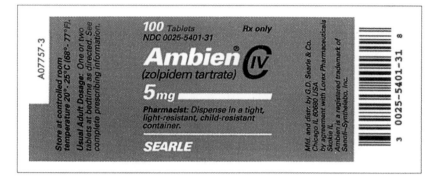

23. Mrs. Torres has metoprolol 150 mg po twice daily ordered for hypertension. You have metoprolol 100-mg scored tablets available. How many tablets will you administer per dose? _____

24. The physician orders Zocor 30 mg po daily in the evening. How many tablets will you administer per dose? _____

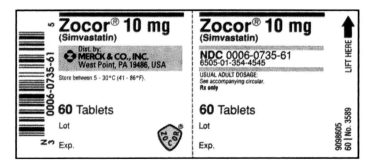

25. Mr. Bond has Allegra 60 mg po twice a day ordered. Allegra 30-mg tablets are available. How many tablets will you administer per dose? _____

Answers on pp. 507–512.

Name _____

Date _____

ACCEPTABLE SCORE __24__

YOUR SCORE _____

POSTTEST 2

Directions: The medication order is listed at the beginning of each problem. Calculate the oral doses. Show your work. Shade each medicine cup or oral syringe when provided to indicate correct dose.

1. Your patient receives Feldene 20 mg po daily for gouty arthritis. Feldene 10-mg capsules are available. How many capsules will you administer per dose? _____

2. The physician orders Zofran 8 mg po before chemotherapy. How many milliliters will the nurse administer per dose? _____

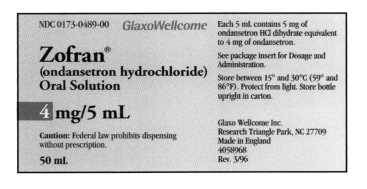

NDC 0173-0489-00   *GlaxoWellcome*

Zofran®
(ondansetron hydrochloride)
Oral Solution

4 mg/5 mL

Caution: Federal law prohibits dispensing without prescription.

50 mL

Each 5 mL contains 5 mg of ondansetron HCl dihydrate equivalent to 4 mg of ondansetron.

See package insert for Dosage and Administration.

Store between 15° and 30°C (59° and 86°F). Protect from light. Store bottle upright in carton.

Glaxo Wellcome Inc.
Research Triangle Park, NC 27709
Made in England
4058968
Rev. 3/96

3. A patient who has undergone cleft palate revision requires Tylenol elixir 30 mg po stat. How many milliliters will you administer per dose? _____

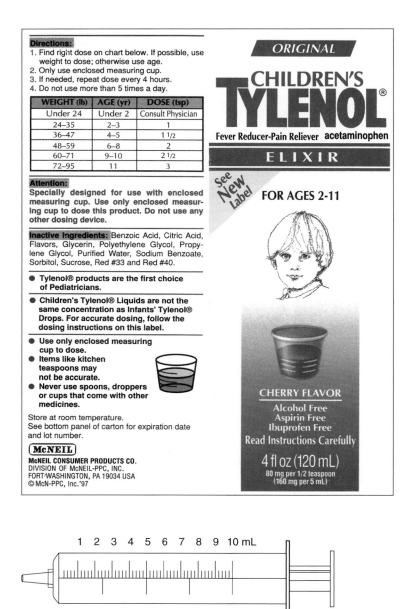

Directions:
1. Find right dose on chart below. If possible, use weight to dose; otherwise use age.
2. Only use enclosed measuring cup.
3. If needed, repeat dose every 4 hours.
4. Do not use more than 5 times a day.

WEIGHT (lb)	AGE (yr)	DOSE (tsp)
Under 24	Under 2	Consult Physician
24–35	2–3	1
36–47	4–5	1 1/2
48–59	6–8	2
60–71	9–10	2 1/2
72–95	11	3

Attention:
Specially designed for use with enclosed measuring cup. Use only enclosed measuring cup to dose this product. Do not use any other dosing device.

Inactive Ingredients: Benzoic Acid, Citric Acid, Flavors, Glycerin, Polyethylene Glycol, Propylene Glycol, Purified Water, Sodium Benzoate, Sorbitol, Sucrose, Red #33 and Red #40.

● Tylenol® products are the first choice of Pediatricians.

● Children's Tylenol® Liquids are not the same concentration as Infants' Tylenol® Drops. For accurate dosing, follow the dosing instructions on this label.

● Use only enclosed measuring cup to dose.
● Items like kitchen teaspoons may not be accurate.
● Never use spoons, droppers or cups that come with other medicines.

Store at room temperature.
See bottom panel of carton for expiration date and lot number.

McNEIL
McNEIL CONSUMER PRODUCTS CO.
DIVISION OF McNEIL-PPC, INC.
FORT WASHINGTON, PA 19034 USA
© McN-PPC, Inc.'97

ORIGINAL
CHILDREN'S TYLENOL®
Fever Reducer-Pain Reliever acetaminophen
ELIXIR
See New Label
FOR AGES 2-11
CHERRY FLAVOR
Alcohol Free
Aspirin Free
Ibuprofen Free
Read Instructions Carefully
4 fl oz (120 mL)
80 mg per 1/2 teaspoon
(160 mg per 5 mL)

1 2 3 4 5 6 7 8 9 10 mL

1/2   1   1 1/2   2 tsp

4. The physician orders Glucotrol 15 mg daily. Glucotrol 10-mg scored tablets are available. How many tablets will the nurse administer per dose? _____

5. Your patient who is being treated for congestive heart failure requires KCl 5 mEq po two times a day for hypokalemia. KCl 20 mEq/30 mL is available. How many milliliters will you administer per dose? _____

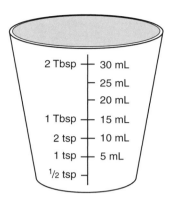

6. Your patient who has had a tonsillectomy receives Keflex 250 mg po four times a day. How many capsules will you administer per dose? _____

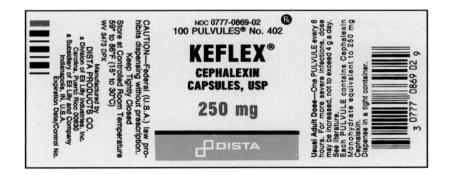

7. Mrs. Pace receives prednisone 7.5 mg po four times a day for asthma. Prednisone is supplied as 2.5-mg tablets. How many tablets will the nurse administer per dose? _____

8. Your patient receives Lanoxin 0.05 mg po daily for cardiac arrhythmia. How many milliliters will you administer per dose? _____

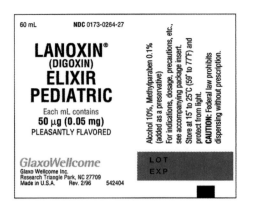

9. The physician orders Macrodantin 0.1 g po four times a day. How many capsules will the nurse administer per dose? _____

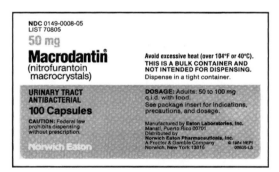

10. Your patient who had a bilateral turbinate reduction receives acetaminophen 650 mg po q4 h for pain relief. Acetaminophen is supplied in 325-mg tablets. How many tablets will you administer per dose? _____

11. The physician prescribes Dilantin 100 mg po twice a day for seizure activity in your patient with epilepsy. Dilantin 50-mg Infatabs are available. How many tablets will you administer per dose? _____

12. Mr. Bales requires Pen-V K 250 mg po q6 h for bacterial endocarditis. Pen-Vee K solution 125 mg/5 mL is available. How many milliliters will the nurse administer per dose? _____

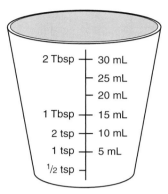

13. The physician orders Deltasone 20 mg po four times a day. Deltasone is supplied in 2.5-mg, 5-mg, and 50-mg tablets. The nurse will give _____ tablets of _____ mg.

14. Mr. Cy, who has had mitral valve repair, receives Lanoxin 0.25 mg po daily. How many tablets will the nurse administer per dose? _____

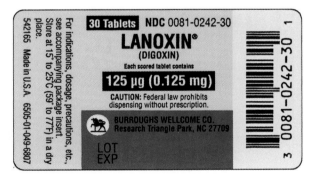

15. Colace syrup 25 mg po three times a day prn for constipation is ordered for your patient after an ethmoidectomy. How many milliliters will you administer per dose? _____

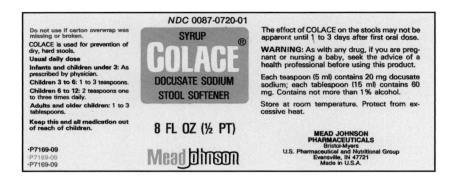

16. Mr. Tate, who has undergone left leg debridement, receives aspirin 0.6 g po q3 h prn for relief of pain. How many tablets will the nurse administer per dose? _____

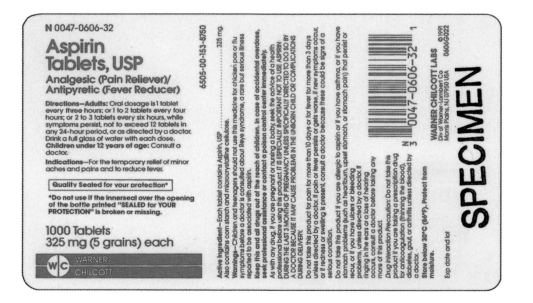

17. Your patient with hypertension has verapamil 80 mg po three times a day ordered. You have 40-mg tablets. How many tablets will you administer per dose? _____

18. The physician orders Zyprexa 15 mg po daily for bipolar mania. How many tablets will the nurse administer per dose? _____

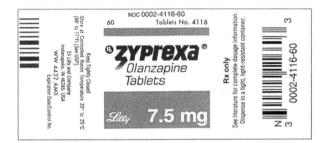

19. Your patient was admitted with seizure activity. The physician orders phenobarbital 30 mg po q8 h. How many tablets will you administer per dose?

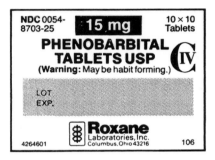

20. The physician orders Flagyl 750 mg po three times a day for 5 days for a yeast infection. Flagyl is supplied in 250-mg tablets. How many tablets will the nurse administer per dose? _____

21. Mr. Luke's physician has ordered Norvasc 10 mg po daily for hypertension. Norvasc 5-mg tablets are available. How many tablets will you administer per dose? _____

22. Mrs. Martin is prescribed Tofranil-PM 0.225 g po at bedtime for depression. How many capsules will you administer per dose? _____

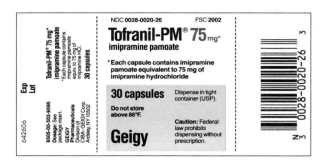

23. The physician orders Vibramycin 100 mg po daily. You have Vibramycin syrup 50 mg/5 mL. How many milliliters will you administer per dose? _____

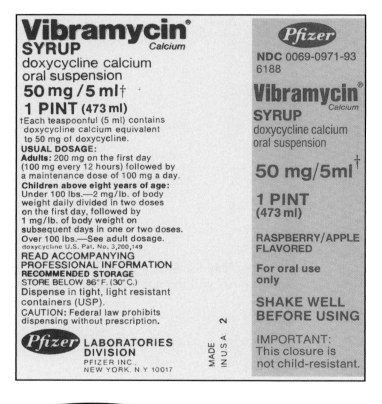

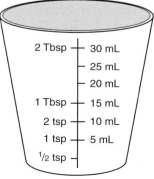

24. Vasotec 5 mg po twice a day is ordered for Mr. Butter's congestive heart failure. How many tablets will the nurse administer per dose? _____

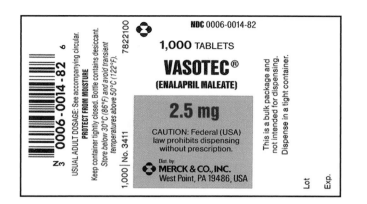

25. Ms. Wang is to receive Zithromax oral suspension 1 g po now. How many milliliters will you administer per dose? _____

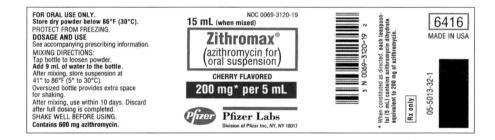

Answers on pp. 512–517.

Refer to Methods of Calculating Dosages: Basic Formula, Ratio, and Proportion; and Basic Calculations: Oral Dosages for additional help and practice problems.

Parenteral Dosages

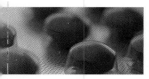

LEARNING OBJECTIVES

On completion of the materials provided in this chapter, you will be able to perform computations accurately by mastering the following mathematical concepts:

1 Converting the measure within the problem to equivalent measures in one system of measurement

2 Using a proportion to solve problems of parenteral dosages when medication is in liquid or reconstituted powder form

3 Using a proportion to solve problems of parenteral dosages of medications measured in milliequivalents

4 Using the stated formula as an alternative method of solving parenteral drug dosage problems

Parenteral refers to outside the alimentary canal or gastrointestinal tract. Medications may be given parenterally when they cannot be taken by mouth or when rapid action is desired. Parenteral medications are absorbed directly into the bloodstream; therefore the amount of drug needed can be determined more accurately. This type of administration of medications is necessary for the uncooperative or unconscious patient, or for a patient who has been designated *NPO* (nothing by mouth). An advantage of intravenous (IV) parenteral medications is that the patient does not have to endure the discomfort of multiple injections, especially when the medications are used for pain control.

Parenteral medications are administered by (1) subcutaneous injection—beneath the skin, in fat; (2) intramuscular (IM) injection—within the muscle; or (3) intradermal injection—within the skin (Figure 14-1). Parenteral medications may also be given intravenously—within the vein. IV drugs may be diluted and administered by themselves, in conjunction with existing IV fluids, or in addition to IV fluids (Figure 14-2). Any time that the integrity of the skin—the body's prime defense against microorganisms—is threatened, infection may occur. Thus the nurse must use sterile technique when preparing and administering parenteral medications.

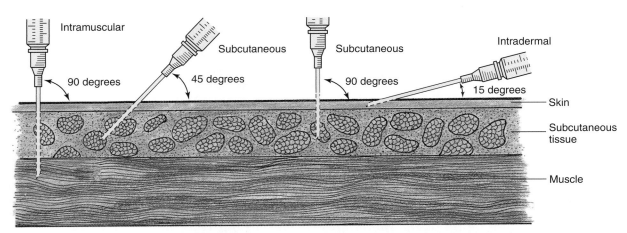

FIGURE 14–1 Intramuscular, subcutaneous, and intradermal injections, with comparison of the angles of insertion. (From Potter PA, Perry AG: *Fundamentals of nursing,* ed 6, St Louis, 2005, Mosby.)

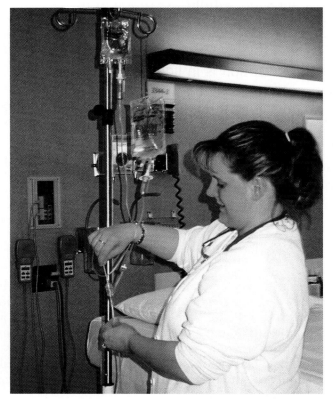

FIGURE 14–2 Intravenous drug administered with existing intravenous fluids. (From Potter PA, Perry AG: *Fundamentals of nursing,* ed 6, St Louis, 2005, Mosby.)

Drugs for parenteral use are supplied as liquids or powders. The medications are packaged in a variety of forms. A liquid may be contained in an ampule, which is a single-dose container that must be broken at the neck to withdraw the drug (Figures 14-3 and 14-4).

Vials are also used to package parenteral medications in liquid or powder form. A vial is a glass or plastic container that is sealed with a rubber stopper (Figure 14-5). Because vials usually

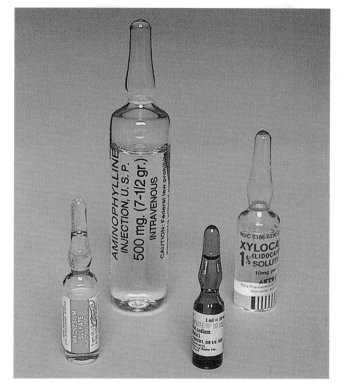

FIGURE 14–3 Examples of ampules. (From Potter PA, Perry AG: *Fundamentals of nursing*, ed 6, St Louis, 2005, Mosby.)

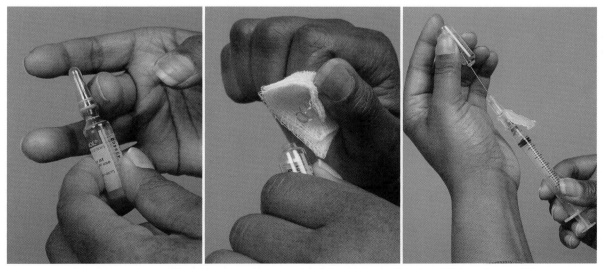

FIGURE 14–4 Breaking the ampule to withdraw the medication. (From Potter PA, Perry AG: *Fundamentals of nursing*, ed 6, St Louis, 2005, Mosby.)

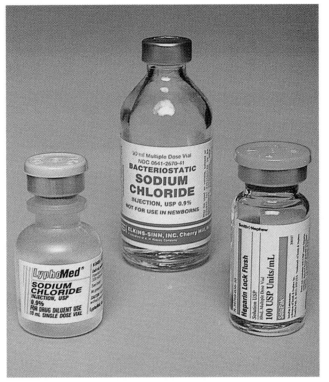

FIGURE 14–5 Examples of vials. (From Potter PA, Perry AG: *Fundamentals of nursing,* ed 6, St Louis, 2005, Mosby.)

contain more than one dose of a medication, the amount desired is withdrawn by inserting a needle through the rubber stopper and removing the required amount (Figure 14-6). If the medication is in powder form, the drug must be reconstituted before withdrawal and administration. The **diluent** in which to dissolve the powder is usually sterile water or normal saline solution.

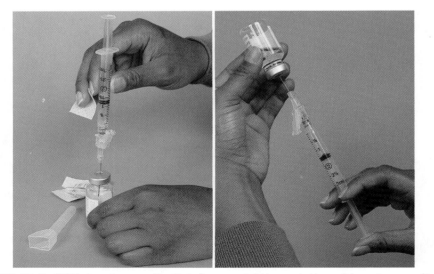

FIGURE 14–6 Withdrawing medication from a vial through the rubber stopper. (From Potter PA, Perry AG: *Fundamentals of nursing,* ed 6, St Louis, 2005, Mosby.)

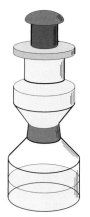

FIGURE 14–7 A Mix-O-Vial. (From Clayton BD, Stock YN: *Basic pharmacology for nurses,* ed 13, St Louis, 2004, Mosby.)

The amount of diluent recommended is normally printed on the vial; however, if it is not, no less than 1 mL is used for a single-dose vial. The powder must be completely dissolved. If the nurse is using a multiple-dose vial, the date and time of mixing should be noted on the vial's label. Also, some drugs supplied in liquid form must be further diluted before injecting intravenously.

Some of the more unstable drugs may be supplied in vials that have a compartment containing the liquid diluent. Pressure applied to the top of the vial releases the stopper between the compartments and allows the drug to be dissolved. These are called *Mix-O-Vials* (Figure 14-7).

Medications may also be supplied in either prefilled disposable syringes or a plastic reusable syringe with a disposable cartridge and a needle unit. Such units contain a specific amount of medication. If the medication order is less than the amount supplied, discard the unneeded portion before administering the medication to the patient.

Syringes

For accurate measurement of medications that are to be administered by the parenteral route, a syringe must be used. Each syringe is supplied in a sterile package. Although syringes may be made of glass or plastic, plastic syringes are more commonly used. All are designed to be used only once and then discarded. The syringe that is used to withdraw and measure the medication from its container may also be used to administer the medication to the patient.

Figure 14-8 shows the parts of a syringe.

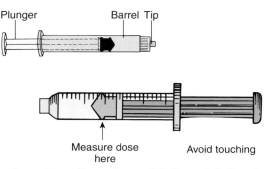

FIGURE 14–8 Parts of a syringe. (From Potter PA, Perry AG: *Fundamentals of nursing,* ed 6, St Louis, 2005, Mosby.)

1. TIP. The tip is located at the end of the syringe. This is the part that holds the needle.

2. BARREL. This is the outer part of the syringe, which holds the medication. The various calibrations are printed on the outside of the barrel.

3. PLUNGER. This is the interior part of the syringe, which slides within the barrel. The plunger is moved backward to withdraw and measure the medication. Then it is pushed forward to inject the medication into the patient. Avoid touching the main stem of the plunger.

Syringes come in a variety of sizes. The size used depends on the amount and type of medication to be administered. There are three types of syringes: hypodermic, tuberculin, and insulin syringes.

Hypodermic Syringes. Hypodermic syringes vary in size as to the amount of fluid they can measure. The most commonly used sizes are 2-, 2½-, 3-, and 5-mL syringes (Figure 14-9). Hypodermic syringes are also available in 10-, 20-, 30-, and 50-mL sizes.

Syringes that are smaller capacity can easily be used to measure decimal fractions of a milliliter. Longer lines mark the half and whole number mL, and shorter lines mark the decimal fractions. Each line indicates one tenth of a milliliter. With larger-capacity syringes, each mark may represent a 0.2-mL increment, or whole mL increments. The larger-capacity syringes would not

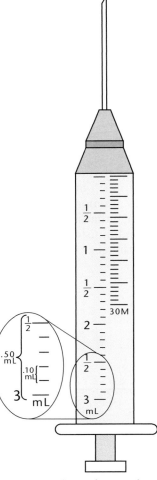

FIGURE 14–9 Calibrations on a 3-mL syringe. (From Clayton BD, Stock YN: *Basic pharmacology for nurses,* ed 13, St Louis, 2004, Mosby.)

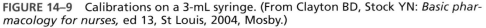

be appropriate for measuring smaller quantities of medication for administration. The nurse must select the proper size syringe for the calculated volume of medication.

Tuberculin Syringes. A tuberculin syringe is a thin, 1-mL syringe (Figure 14-10). The mL side of the syringe includes markings for hundredths of a mL. The other side of the syringe is calibrated in minims. These syringes are commonly used in pediatrics and also to measure medications given in very small amounts, such as heparin. Tuberculin syringes should not be confused with insulin syringes.

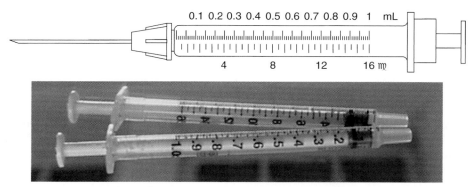

FIGURE 14–10   BD tuberculin syringes. (From Becton, Dickinson and Company, Franklin Lakes, NJ.)

Insulin Syringes. Insulin syringes were developed specifically for the administration of insulin. They are calibrated in units (U). These syringes were designed to be used with U-100 insulin. There are three types of insulin syringes.

1. The Lo-Dose syringe is used for administration of 50 units or less of insulin. The syringe is marked for each unit, with longer lines for each 5 units (Figure 14-11).

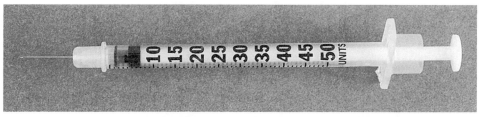

FIGURE 14–11   BD Lo-Dose insulin syringe. (From Becton, Dickinson and Company, Franklin Lakes, NJ.)

2. The 30-unit syringe is used for insulin doses that equal less than 30 units of U-100 insulin only (Figure 14-12).

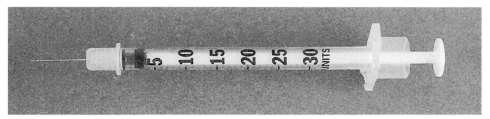

FIGURE 14–12   BD 30-unit insulin syringe. (From Becton, Dickinson and Company, Franklin Lakes, NJ.)

3. The U-100/1-mL syringe is used for the administration of up to 100 units of U-100 insulin (Figure 14-13).

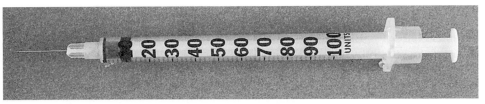

FIGURE 14–13 BD 100-unit (U-100) insulin syringe. (From Becton, Dickinson and Company, Franklin Lakes, NJ.)

Remember, when preparing medication for administration, it is important to choose the correct size of syringe for accurate measurement of the medication.

Needleless System. The Occupational Safety and Health Administration has recommended administration of parenteral medications with the use of a needleless system. This recommendation is for the protection of both patients and nurses from needlesticks. Needleless systems provide a shield that protects the needle device (Figure 14-14).

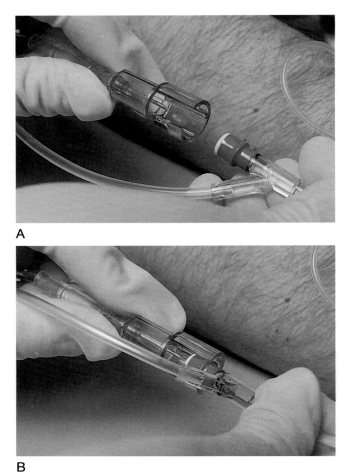

FIGURE 14–14 **A,** Needleless infusion system. **B,** Connection into an injection port. (From Elkin MK, Perry PA, Potter AG: *Nursing interventions and clinical skills,* ed 3, St Louis, 2004, Mosby.)

Calculation of Parenteral Drug Dosages: Proportion Method

Parenteral drug dosages may also be calculated by using a proportion. The physician's order and the available medication must be in the same system of measurement to write a proportion for the actual amount of medication to be administered. Examples of parenteral drug dosage problems follow.

Example 1: The physician orders Apresoline 30 mg IM. Apresoline 20 mg/mL is available. How many milliliters will the nurse administer?

 a. On the left side of the proportion, place what you know or have available. In this example, there are 20 mg/mL. Therefore the left side of the proportion would be

$$20 \text{ mg} : 1 \text{ mL} ::$$

 b. The right side of the proportion is determined by the physician's order and the abbreviations placed on the left side of the proportion. Remember, only *two* different abbreviations may be used in a single proportion.

$$20 \text{ mg} : 1 \text{ mL} :: \underline{\hspace{1cm}} \text{ mg} : \underline{\hspace{1cm}} \text{ mL}$$

The physician ordered 30 mg.

$$20 \text{ mg} : 1 \text{ mL} :: 30 \text{ mg} : \underline{\hspace{1cm}} \text{ mL}$$

The symbol x is used to represent the unknown number of milliliters.

$$20 \text{ mg} : 1 \text{ mL} :: 30 \text{ mg} : x \text{ mL}$$

 c. Rewrite the proportion without the abbreviations.

$$20 : 1 :: 30 : x$$

 d. Solve for x.

$$20x = 30$$
$$x = \frac{30}{20}$$
$$x = 1.5$$

 e. Label your answer as determined by the abbreviation placed next to x in the original proportion.

$$1.5 \text{ mL}$$

The patient would receive 1.5 mL of Apresoline containing 30 mg.

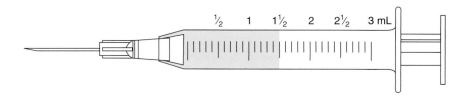

Example 2: The physician orders meperidine 30 mg IM q4 h prn. Demerol 25 mg/mL is available. How many milliliters will the nurse administer?

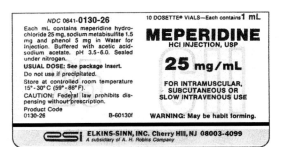

a. On the left side of the proportion, place what you know or have available. In this example, each milliliter contains 25 mg. So the left side of the proportion would be

$$25 \text{ mg} : 1 \text{ mL} ::$$

b. The right side of the proportion is determined by the physician's order and the abbreviations on the left side of the proportion. Only *two* different abbreviations may be used in a single proportion. The abbreviations must be in the same position on the right side as they are on the left.

$$25 \text{ mg} : 1 \text{ mL} :: \underline{\hspace{1cm}} \text{ mg} : \underline{\hspace{1cm}} \text{ mL}$$

In this example the physician ordered 30 mg.

$$25 \text{ mg} : 1 \text{ mL} :: 30 \text{ mg} : \underline{\hspace{1cm}} \text{ mL}$$

We need to find the number of milliliters to be given, so we use the symbol x to represent the unknown.

$$25 \text{ mg} : 1 \text{ mL} :: 30 \text{ mg} : x \text{ mL}$$

c. Rewrite the proportion without using the abbreviations.

$$25 : 1 :: 30 : x$$

d. Solve for x.

$$25x = 1 \times 30$$
$$25x = 30$$
$$x = \frac{30}{25}$$
$$x = 1.2$$

e. Label your answer as determined by the abbreviation placed next to x in the original proportion.

The nurse would measure 1.2 mL to administer 30 mg of Demerol.

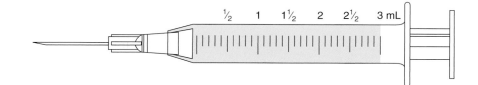

Example 3: The physician orders Cleocin phosphate 450 mg IV q6 h. Cleocin 150 mg/mL is available. How many milliliters will the nurse administer?

    a. 150 mg : 1 mL ::

    b. 150 mg : 1 mL :: _____ mg : _____ mL

       150 mg : 1 mL :: 450 mg : x mL

    c. 150 : 1 :: 450 : x

    d. $150x = 450$

$$x = \frac{450}{150}$$

$$x = 3$$

    e. Label your answer as determined by the abbreviation placed next to x in the original proportion.

$$x = 3 \text{ mL}$$

The nurse would measure 3 mL to administer 450 mg of Cleocin.

Parenteral Drug Dosage Calculation: Alternative Formula Method

In Chapter 13, the alternative formula was introduced as another method of calculating drug dosages. This formula also may be used when parenteral drug dosages are calculated.

Remember, the formula is

$$\frac{D}{A} \times Q = x$$

or

$$\frac{\text{Desired}}{\text{Available}} \times \text{Quantity available} = x \ (\text{unknown})$$

Example 1: The physician orders Amikin 150 mg IM q8 h. Amikin 500 mg/2 mL is available. How many milliliters will the nurse administer?

```
NDC 0015-3020-20        2 mL
EQUIVALENT TO           vial
500 mg AMIKACIN per 2 mL
AMIKIN®
Amikacin Sulfate
Injection, USP
FOR I.M. OR I.V. USE
CAUTION: Federal law prohibits
dispensing without prescription.
```
0.66% sodium bisulfite added as an antioxidant; buffered with 2.5% sodium citrate, adjusted to pH 4.5 with H₂SO₄. • Store at controlled room temperature 15°-30°C (59°-86° F). READ CIRCULAR
APOTHECON®
A Bristol-Myers Squibb Company
Princeton, NJ 08540 USA
3020200RL-3
Cont:
Exp. Date:

a. The desired amount of Amikin is 150 mg.

$$150 \text{ mg}$$

b. The available amount of Amikin is 500 mg.

$$\frac{150 \text{ mg}}{500 \text{ mg}}$$

c. The quantity of the medication for 500 mg is 2 mL.

$$\frac{150 \text{ mg}}{500 \text{ mg}} \times \frac{2 \text{ mL}}{1} = x$$

d. We can now solve for x.

$$x = \frac{150 \text{ mg}}{500 \text{ mg}} \times \frac{2 \text{ mL}}{1}$$

$$x = \frac{150 \text{ mg}}{500 \text{ mg}} \times \frac{\overset{1}{\cancel{2}} \text{ mL}}{1} = \frac{150}{250}$$

$$x = \frac{150}{250}$$

$$x = \frac{3}{5} \text{ or } 0.6$$

e. Label your answer as determined by the quantity.

$$150 \text{ mg} = 0.6 \text{ mL of Amikin}$$

If the physician's order is in one system of measurement and the drug is supplied in another system of measurement, one of the measurements must be converted so they are both expressed in the same system. After this is done, the formula may be used to calculate the amount of medication to be administered.

Example 2: Mr. Davis is to receive atropine gr $\frac{1}{150}$ IM stat. Atropine 0.4 mg/mL is available. How many milliliters will the nurse administer?

The physician's order is expressed in grains and the drug is supplied in milligrams. Convert the order to milligrams as outlined in Chapter 8.

$$60 \text{ mg} : 1 \text{ gr} :: x \text{ mg} : \frac{1}{150} \text{ gr}$$

$$60 : 1 :: x : \frac{1}{150}$$

$$x = \frac{60}{1} \times \frac{1}{150}$$

$$x = \frac{\overset{2}{\cancel{60}} \times 1}{1 \times \underset{5}{\cancel{150}}}$$

$$x = \frac{2}{5} \text{ or } 0.4$$

$$x = 0.4 \text{ mg}$$

$$\frac{1}{150} \text{ gr} = 0.4 \text{ mg of atropine}$$

Now the numbers may be filled into the formula.

    a. The desired amount is 0.4 mg.

$$\underline{0.4 \text{ mg}}$$

    b. The available amount or strength of atropine is 0.4 mg.

$$\frac{0.4 \text{ mg}}{0.4 \text{ mg}}$$

    c. The quantity available is in 1 mL.

$$\frac{0.4 \cancel{\text{ mg}}}{0.4 \cancel{\text{ mg}}} \times \frac{1 \text{ mL}}{1}$$

    d. Solve for x

$$x = \frac{0.4 \times 1}{0.4 \times 1}$$

$$x = 1$$

    e. Label your answer as determined by the quantity.

$$0.4 \text{ mg} = 1 \text{ mL of atropine}$$

Example 3: Mr. Lewis's physician has ordered 200 mg of Tigan IM for treatment of nausea. Tigan 100 mg/mL is available. How many milliliters will the nurse administer?

NDC 61570-541-20
100mg/mL
Tigan®
(trimethobenzamide HCl)   ℞ Only
Injection
20mL Multi-Dose Vial
Monarch
Pharmaceuticals®

NOT FOR USE IN CHILDREN.
For IM USE ONLY.
Store from 15° to 30° C (59° to 86°F).
Each mL of solution contains 100 mg trimetho-
benzamide hydrochloride compounded with 0.45%
phenol as preservative, 0.5 mg sodium citrate and
0.2 mg citric acid as buffers, and sodium hydroxide
to adjust pH to approximately 5.0.
Dosage: See accompanying prescribing
information. For IM use only (preferably by deep
IM Injection).
Distributed by:
Monarch Pharmaceuticals, Inc., Bristol, TN 37620
Manufactured by:
King Pharmaceuticals, Inc., Bristol, TN 37620
0934063 Rev. 11/99

a. The desired amount of Tigan is 200 mg.

$$200 \text{ mg}$$

b. The available amount or strength is 100 mg.

$$\frac{200 \text{ mg}}{100 \text{ mg}}$$

c. The quantity available is 1 mL.

$$\frac{200 \text{ mg}}{100 \text{ mg}} \times 1 \text{ mL}$$

d. Solve for x.

$$x = \frac{200 \text{ mg}}{100 \text{ mg}} \times \frac{1 \text{ mL}}{1}$$

$$x = \frac{200 \text{ mg} \times 1 \text{ mL}}{100 \text{ mg} \times 1}$$

$$x = \frac{200}{100}$$

$$x = 2$$

e. Label your answer as determined by the quantity.

$$200 \text{ mg} = 2 \text{ mL of Tigan}$$

Complete the following work sheet, which provides for extensive practice in the calculation of parenteral drug dosages. Check your answers. If you have difficulties, go back and review the necessary material. When you feel ready to evaluate your learning, take the first posttest. Check your answers. An acceptable score as indicated on the posttest signifies that you have successfully completed this chapter. An unacceptable score signifies a need for further study before taking the second posttest.

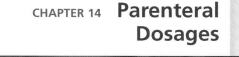

WORK SHEET

Directions: The medication order is listed at the beginning of each problem. Calculate the parenteral doses. Show your work. Shade the syringe when provided to indicate the correct dose.

1. The physician orders streptomycin 500 mg IM q12 h for your patient with an infection. How many milliliters will you administer? _____

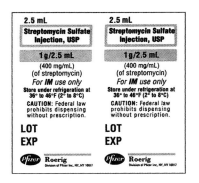

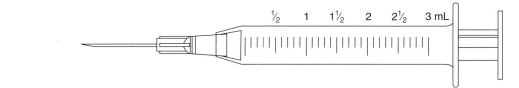

2. Your patient with an atrial valve repair has Lanoxin 110 mcg IV q12 h ordered. How many milliliters will you prepare? _____

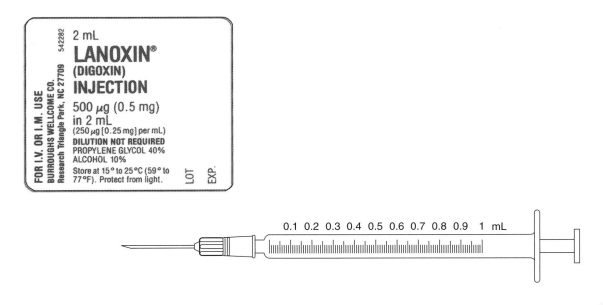

3. The physician orders atropine gr ¹⁄₂₀₀ IM at 0615. How many milliliters will the nurse administer? _____

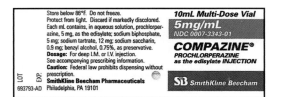

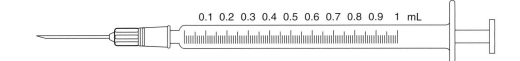

4. Your patient who has undergone pacemaker placement complains of nausea and has Compazine 10 mg IM q6 h ordered. How many milliliters will you administer? _____

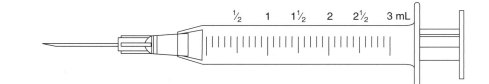

5. The physician orders ranitidine hydrochloride 50 mg IM q6 h. How many milliliters will the nurse administer? _____

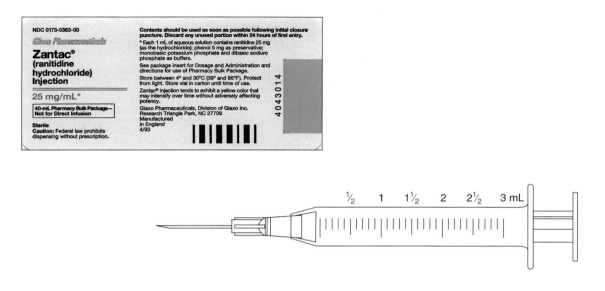

6. The physician orders piperacillin 3 g IV q8 h for your patient with sepsis. You have piperacillin 1 g/2.5 mL available. How many milliliters will you prepare? _____

7. The physician orders morphine 5 mg subcutaneous q4 h. How many milliliters will the nurse administer? _____

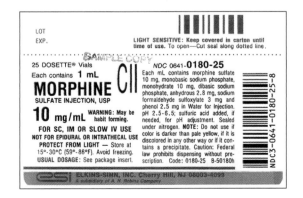

8. The physician orders vancomycin 0.5 g IV q12 h for your patient with a right-hand amputation. How many milliliters will you prepare? _____

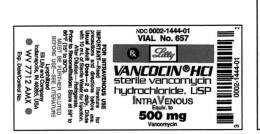

PREPARATION AND STABILITY

At the time of use, reconstitute by adding either 10 mL of Sterile Water for Injection to the 500-mg vial or 20 mL of Sterile Water for Injection to the 1-g vial of dry, sterile vancomycin powder. Vials reconstituted in this manner will give a solution of 50 mg/mL. **FURTHER DILUTION IS REQUIRED.**

After reconstitution, the vials may be stored in a refrigerator for 14 days without significant loss of potency. Reconstituted solutions containing 500 mg of vancomycin must be diluted with at least 100 mL of diluent. Reconstituted solutions containing 1 g of vancomycin must be diluted with at least 200 mL of diluent. The desired dose, diluted in this manner, should be administered by intermittent intravenous infusion over a period of at least 60 minutes.

9. Your patient with congestive heart failure requires furosemide 30 mg IV stat. How many milliliters will you administer? _____

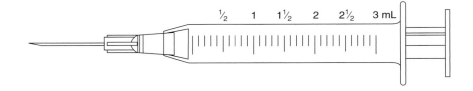

10. Your postoperative patient has Toradol 15 mg IM q6 h for 3 days ordered. You have 30 mg/mL prefilled syringes. How many milliliters will you administer? _____

11. The physician orders D$_5$W 1000 mL plus sodium bicarbonate (NaHCO$_3$) 25.8 mEq at 12 mL/h IV. NaHCO$_3$ is supplied in a 50-mL ampule containing 44.6 mEq. How many milliliters of NaHCO$_3$ will be added to the 1000 mL of D$_5$W? _____

12. Your patient with asthma requires aminophylline 100 mg IV q6 h. How many milliliters will you prepare? _____

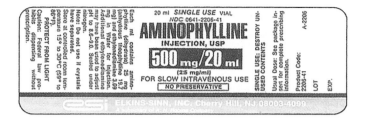

13. The physician orders amphotericin B 350 mg IV every day. You have a 100-mg/20-mL vial. How many milliliters will you prepare? _____

14. The physician orders Cipro 300 mg q12 h IV. How many milliliters will you prepare? _____

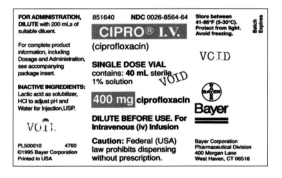

15. The physician orders Solu-Cortef 0.05 g IM q6 h for your patient with scleroderma. How many milliliters will you administer? _____

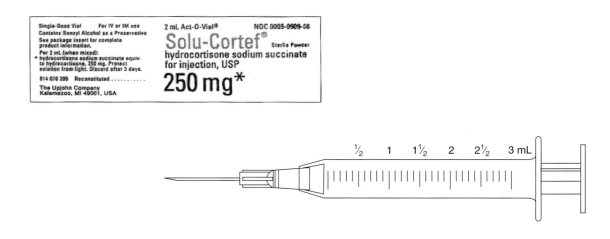

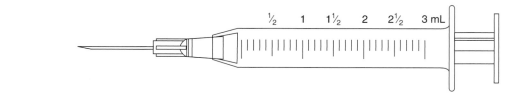

16. The physician orders naloxone 0.6 mg IV stat. How many milliliters will you administer? _____

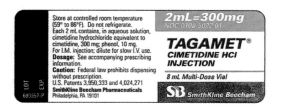

17. The physician orders Tagamet 300 mg IV q6 h. How many milliliters will the nurse prepare? _____

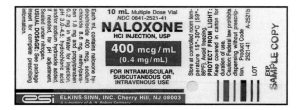

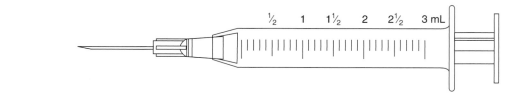

18. Mrs. Andis requires Duramorph 6 mg IV q4 h for pain. How many milliliters will the nurse administer? _____

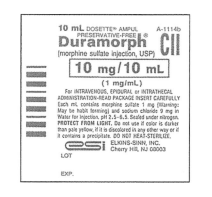

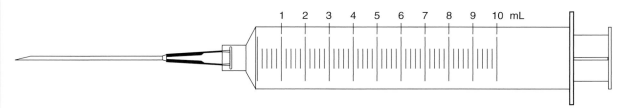

19. Loxapine 25 mg IM now is ordered for Mrs. Switzer who has been diagnosed with a psychotic disorder. Loxapine 50 mg/mL is available. How many milliliters will the nurse administer? _____

20. Mr. Lewis requires Ativan 1 mg IM stat for severe agitation. How many milliliters will the nurse administer? _____

21. Mrs. Carroll requires Apresoline 10 mg IM q6 h for high blood pressure. Apresoline is supplied in 1-mL ampules containing 20 mg. How many milliliters will the nurse prepare? _____

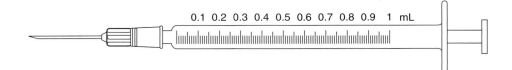

22. Mr. Fry has amikacin sulfate 400 mg IV q8 h ordered. You have amikacin sulfate for injection 500 mg/2 mL. How many milliliters will you administer? _____

NDC 0015-3020-20   2 mL vial
EQUIVALENT TO
500 mg AMIKACIN per 2 mL
AMIKIN®
Amikacin Sulfate Injection, USP
FOR I.M. OR I.V. USE
CAUTION: Federal law prohibits dispensing without prescription.

0.66% sodium bisulfite added as an antioxidant; buffered with 2.5% sodium citrate, adjusted to pH 4.5 with H₂SO₄. • Store at controlled room temperature 15°-30°C (59°-86°F). READ CIRCULAR
APOTHECON®
A Bristol-Myers Squibb Company
Princeton, NJ 08540 USA
3020200RL-3

Cont:

Exp. Date:

23. The physician orders diazepam 10 mg IM q6 h for your anxious patient. How many milliliters will you administer? _____

10 mL Multiple Dose Vial
NDC 0641-2289-41
6505-01-240-6894
DIAZEPAM CIV
INJECTION, USP
5 mg/mL
FOR INTRAMUSCULAR or INTRAVENOUS USE
ELKINS-SINN, INC. Cherry Hill, NJ 08003
A subsidiary of A. H. Robins Company

Each mL contains diazepam 5 mg, propylene glycol 0.4 mL, alcohol 0.1 mL, benzyl alcohol 0.015 mL and sodium benzoate/benzoic acid, a total of 50 mg in Water for Injection, pH 6.2-6.9. Seal under nitrogen.
USUAL DOSAGE: See package insert for complete prescribing information.
FOR INVENTORY ONLY

NOTE: Solution may appear colorless to light yellow.
Store at controlled room temperature 15°-30°C (59°-86°F).
Caution: Federal law prohibits dispensing without prescription.
Product Code 2289-41   A-2268c

LOT
EXP.

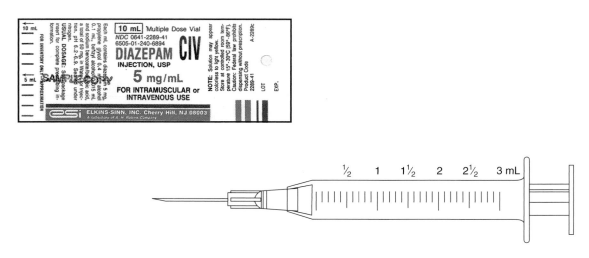

24. Mr. Keesling is diagnosed with an acoustic neuroma and complains of pain. He has codeine gr ¼ IM q3 h prn ordered. How many milliliters will the nurse administer? _____

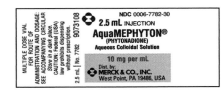

25. The physician orders AquaMEPHYTON 0.01 g IM every morning. How many milliliters will the nurse administer? _____

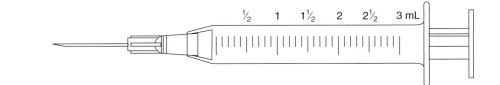

26. The physician orders Cipro 0.3 g IV q12 h. How many milliliters will the nurse prepare? _____

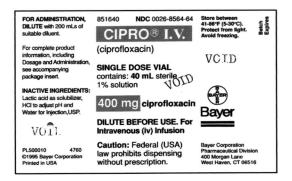

27. Mrs. Ring, who has undergone a hysterectomy, has morphine 6 mg IV q4 h prn ordered for pain relief. How many milliliters will the nurse administer? _____

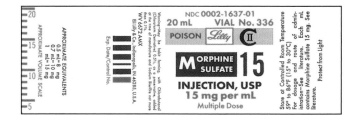

28. The physician orders Benadryl 100 mg IM four times a day. How many milliliters will the nurse administer? _____

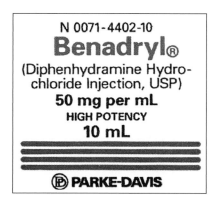

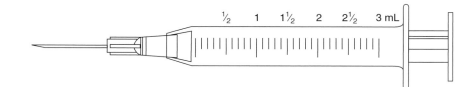

29. Mr. Fields requires digoxin 100 mcg IM daily for his cardiac dysrhythmia. How many milliliters will the nurse administer? _____

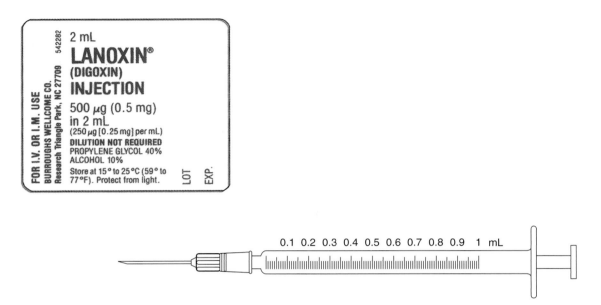

30. The physician orders Kefzol 500 mg IV q6 h × 4 days. How many milliliters will the nurse prepare? _____

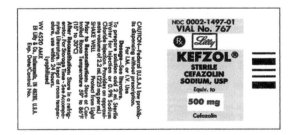

31. The physician orders Stadol 1.5 mg IV q4 h for pain. How many milliliters will the nurse administer? _____

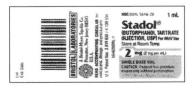

32. The physician orders Solu-Cortef 100 mg IV q8 h for your patient with severe contact dermatitis. How many milliliters will you administer? _____

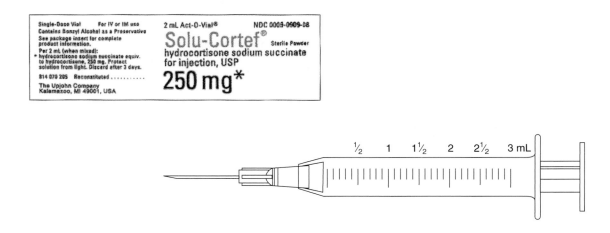

33. The physician orders D₅W 250 mL plus NaCl 7.5 mEq at 2 mL IV per hour. NaCl is supplied in a 40-mL vial containing 2.5 mEq/mL. How many milliliters of NaCl will be added to the 250 mL of D₅W? _____

34. Your patient with a lumbar laminectomy receives Vistaril 25 mg IM three times a day. How many milliliters does this patient receive in each dose? _____

35. The physician orders atropine gr ¹/₁₀₀ IM stat for your preoperative patient. How many milliliters will you administer? _____

36. Your patient admitted with neuroleptic disorder has Valproate 150 mg IM at bedtime prn ordered. The drug is available for injection at 100 mg/mL. How many milliliters will you administer? _____

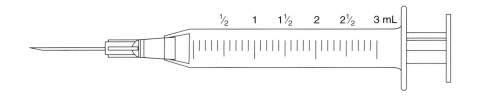

37. Ms. Barry has bumetanide 0.5 mg IV q3 h for edema caused by congestive heart failure ordered. Bumetanide 0.25 mg/mL is available. How many milliliters will the nurse administer? _____

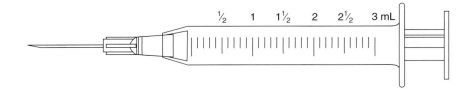

38. Your patient with chronic obstructive pulmonary disease receives aminophylline 75 mg IV q6 h. How many milliliters will you prepare? _____

39. The physician orders naloxone 0.6 mg IM stat. How many milliliters will the nurse prepare? _____

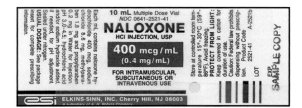

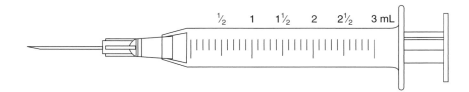

40. The physician orders diazepam 10 mg IV stat. How many milliliters will the nurse prepare? _____

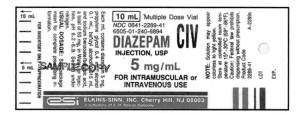

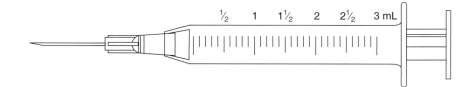

41. Mr. Ortiz has psoriasis and requires hydrocortisone 25 mg IM daily. The drug is available at a concentration of 100 mg/2 mL. How many milliliters will the nurse administer? _____

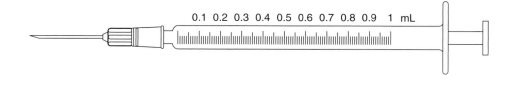

42. Mrs. Kite has ciprofloxacin 200 mg IV q12 h ordered for a urinary tract infection. Ciprofloxacin 400 mg/40 mL is available. How many milliliters will the nurse administer? _____

43. The physician orders ascorbic acid 0.25 g IM daily for your patient admitted with an alcohol abuse problem. You have ascorbic acid 500 mg/mL. How many milliliters will you administer? _____

44. The physician orders D_5W 250 mL plus calcium chloride ($CaCl_2$) 5 mEq at 2 mL/h IV. $CaCl_2$ is supplied in a 10-mL ampule containing 13.6 mEq. How many milliliters of $CaCl_2$ will be added to the 250 mL of D_5W? _____

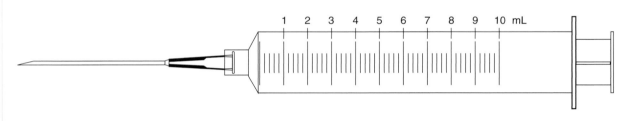

45. The physician orders phenobarbital 70 mg IV q8 h for your patient with epilepsy. The drug is supplied in a 1-mL ampule containing 130 mg. How many milliliters will you administer? _____

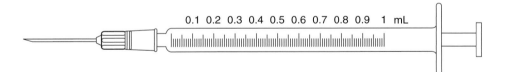

46. The physician orders Vibramycin 200 mg IV daily. You have Vibramycin 10 mg/mL after reconstitution. How many milliliters will you prepare? _____

47. The physician orders Dilaudid 2 mg IV q4 h prn for pain. How many milliliters will the nurse administer? _____

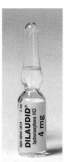

48. Your patient with atrial fibrillation has digoxin 0.2 mg IM daily ordered. How many milliliters will you administer? _____

LANOXIN®   **2mL**
(digoxin) Injection
500 µg (0.5 mg) in 2 mL
(250 µg [0.25 mg] per mL)
Store at 15° to 25°C (59° to 77°F).
PROTECT FROM LIGHT.
Glaxo Wellcome Inc.
Research Triangle Park, NC 27709
Rev. 1/96

542308

LOT
EXP

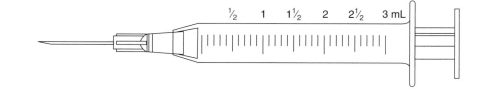

49. The physician orders morphine gr ⅙ subcutaneous q3 h. How many milliliters will the nurse administer? _____

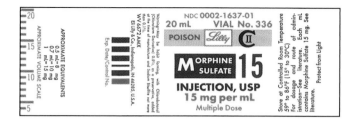

50. Mr. Lee is receiving Benadryl 25 mg IV q6 h for severe itching. Benadryl 50 mg/mL is available. How many milliliters will the nurse administer? _____

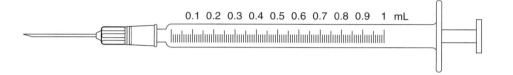

51. The physician orders Cefadyl 600 mg IM q6 h. How many milliliters will the nurse administer? _____

52. Your preoperative patient needs atropine 0.9 mg IM at 0615. How many milliliters will you administer? _____

53. The physician orders codeine gr ss subcutaneous q4 h for your patient after a lumbar laminectomy for pain relief. How many milliliters will you administer? _____

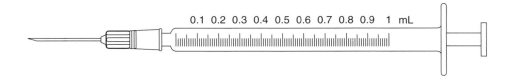

54. Mrs. Das has Ativan 3 mg IM now ordered for anxiety. Ativan 4 mg/mL is available. How many milliliters will the nurse administer? _____

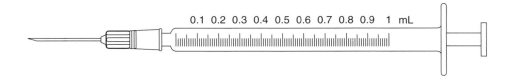

55. The physician orders D_5W 500 mL plus 6 mEq of $NaHCO_3$ at 42 mL/h IV. $NaHCO_3$ is available in a 10-mL ampule containing 0.89 mEq/mL. How many milliliters of $NaHCO_3$ will be added to the 500 mL of D_5W? _____

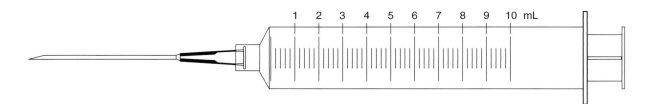

56. Mrs. Luther has Decadron 10 mg IV now for cerebral edema. Decadron 20 mg/mL is available. How many milliliters will the nurse administer? _____

57. Mr. Ali receives Thorazine 5 mg q4 h for severe hiccups. How many milliliters does Mr. Ali receive in each dose? _____

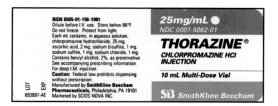

58. Your patient with sinusitis receives ampicillin 500 mg IV q12 h. You have ampicillin 125 mg/mL. How many milliliters will you prepare? _____

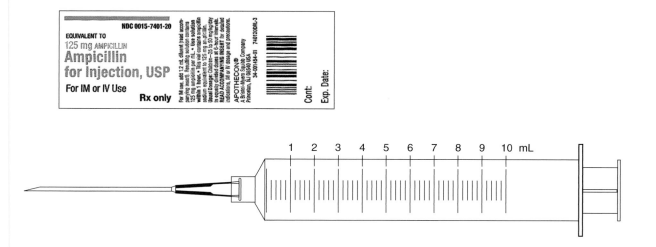

59. Mrs. Calhoun has ergonovine 0.2 mg IM now. Ergonovine 0.25 mg/mL is available. How many milliliters will the nurse administer? _____

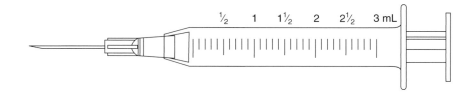

60. The physician orders Ativan 0.5 mg IM stat for your patient with severe anxiety. The drug is supplied in a 1-mL vial containing 2 mg/mL. How many milliliters will you administer?

_____

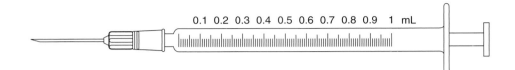

61. Aminophylline 0.2 g IV three times a day is ordered. Aminophylline is supplied in a 20-mL single-use vial containing 500 mg/20 mL. How many milliliters will the nurse prepare?

_____

62. Codeine 15 mg IM q4 h is ordered. Codeine is available in a vial containing gr ss/mL. How many milliliters will the nurse administer? _____

63. Mr. Ciele, who has undergone partial craniotomy, receives Dilantin 100 mg IV q8 h. You have available Dilantin 50 mg/mL. How many milliliters will you prepare? _____

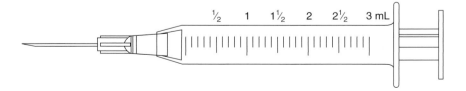

64. The physician orders digoxin 0.25 mg IV daily for your patient with atrial flutter. Digoxin is supplied in a 2-mL ampule containing 0.5 mg. How many milliliters will you prepare? _____

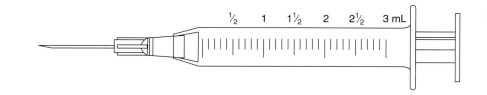

65. Mrs. Snow has Kytril 500 mcg IV ordered 30 minutes before beginning her chemotherapy. Kytril is available in 1 mg/mL. How many milliliters will the nurse administer? _____

66. The physician orders D_5W 250 mL plus calcium gluconate 5 mEq at 2 mL IV per hour. Calcium gluconate is supplied in a 10-mL ampule containing 4.8 mEq. How many milliliters of calcium gluconate will be added to the 250 mL of D_5W? _____

67. Mr. Thompson, admitted with erythrasma, receives Cleocin 50 mg IV q8 h. How many milliliters will the nurse prepare? _____

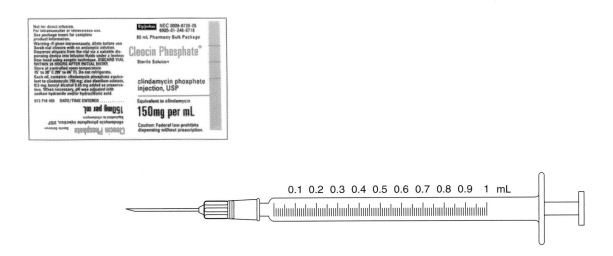

68. Atropine 0.2 mg IM at 0730 is ordered. How many milliliters will the nurse administer? _____

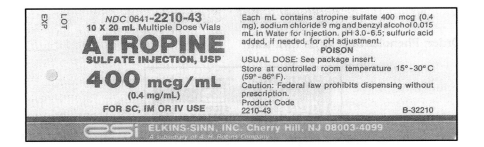

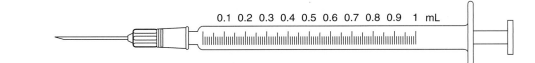

69. Mr. Riley receives tobramycin 55 mg IV q8 h for sepsis. How many milliliters will the nurse prepare? _____

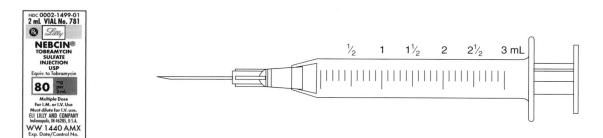

70. Mr. Russo has amikacin sulfate 600 mg IV q8 h ordered. You have amikacin sulfate for injection 500 mg/2 mL. How many milliliters will you administer? _____

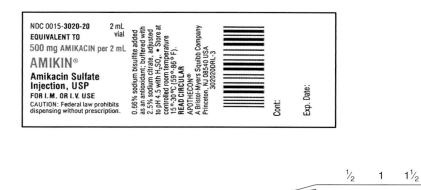

71. Your patient needs morphine gr ⅙ subcutaneous stat for myocardial infarction. How many milliliters will you administer? _____

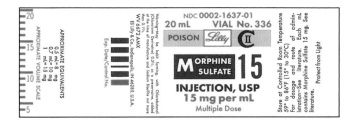

72. The physician orders vitamin B_{12} 1000 mcg IM every Monday. How many milliliters will the nurse administer? _____

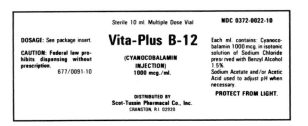

73. The physician orders Monocid 800 mg IM daily. How many milliliters will the nurse administer? _____

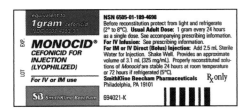

74. Mr. Paley receives promethazine 30 mg IM at 0930 for relief of nausea after a colonoscopy. How many milliliters will the nurse administer? _____

25 DOSETTE® AMPULS   Each co

NDC 0641-**1496-35**

PROMETHAZINE

HCI INJECTION, USP

50 mg / mL

FOR DEEP INTRAMUSCULAR USE ONLY

Each mL contains promethazine hydrochloride 50 mg, ede-
tate disodium 0.1 mg, calcium chloride 0.04 mg, sodium
metabisulfite 0.25 mg and phenol 5 mg in Water for Injec-
tion. pH 4.0-5.5; buffered with acetic acid-sodium acetate.
Sealed under nitrogen. **USUAL DOSAGE:** See package insert.
PROTECT FROM LIGHT: Keep covered in carton until time
of use. Store at 15°-30°C (59°-86°F).
**DO NOT USE IF SOLUTION HAS DEVELOPED COLOR OR
CONTAINS A PRECIPITATE.**
To open ampuls, ignore color line; break at constriction.
Caution: Federal law prohibits dispensing without prescription.
Product Code: 1496-35   B-51496d

ELKINS-SINN, INC. Cherry Hill, N
A subsidiary of A. H. Robins Company

0.1 0.2 0.3 0.4 0.5 0.6 0.7 0.8 0.9 1 mL

75. Your patient receives Robinul 0.28 mg IM at 0600. How many milliliters will you administer? _____

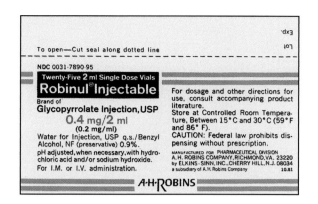

76. Mrs. Lopez has Ativan 3 mg IM ordered at bedtime for insomnia. Ativan is supplied in a 4 mg/mL prefilled syringe. How many milliliters will the nurse administer? _____

77. The physician orders D$_5$W 1000 mL plus NaCl 15 mEq at 30 mL IV per hour. NaCl is supplied in a 40-mL vial containing 100 mEq. How many milliliters of NaCl will be added to the 1000 mL of D$_5$W? _____

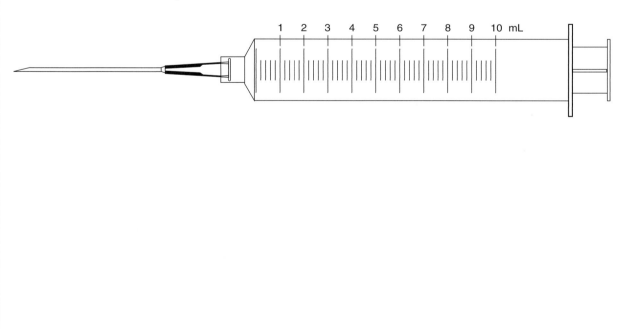

78. Mr. Neal receives Kefzol 250 mg IV q6 h for 12 doses after an ethmoidectomy. How many milliliters will the nurse prepare? _____

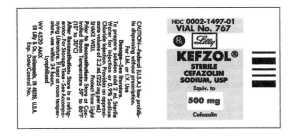

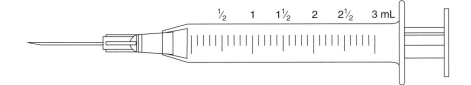

79. Your patient receives the antibiotic Cleocin phosphate 300 mg IV q6 h for treatment of diphtheria. How many milliliters will you prepare? _____

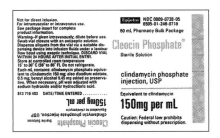

80. The physician orders lidocaine 75 mg IV stat. Lidocaine is available in a 5-mL vial containing 100 mg/5 mL. How many milliliters will the nurse prepare? _____

81. The physician orders Ticar 0.8 g IM q6 h. How many milliliters will the nurse prepare? _____

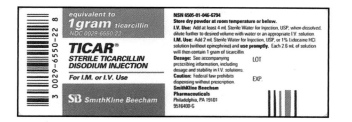

82. The physician orders Solu-Medrol 100 mg IV stat. How many milliliters will the nurse prepare? _____

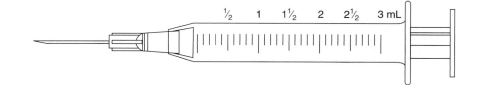

83. Mr. Scott takes Cerebyx 300 mg IV stat for grand mal seizure. Cerebyx 75 mg/mL in a 10-mL vial is available. How many milliliters will the patient receive? _____

84. The physician orders scopolamine gr ¹⁄₁₅₀ subcutaneous at 0700. How many milliliters will the nurse administer? _____

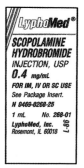

85. The physician orders for your patient promethazine 10 mg IM stat for relief of nausea and vomiting. How many milligrams will the patient receive? _____

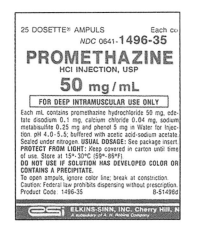

86. The physician orders Dilaudid gr ⅟₆₀ IV q4 h prn. How many milliliters will the nurse administer? _____

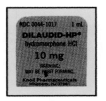

87. Your patient requires Vistaril 50 mg IM q4 h prn for severe agitation. How many milliliters will you administer? _____

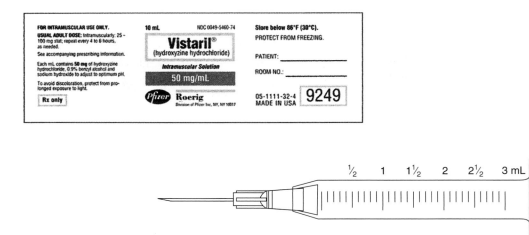

88. Ms. Jones has fentanyl citrate 60 mcg IM ordered q2 h prn for pain. How many milliliters will the nurse administer? _____

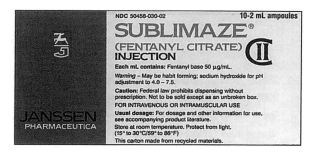

89. Atropine gr ¹⁄₁₂₀ IM stat is ordered. How many milliliters will the nurse administer? _____

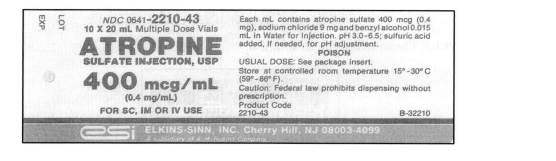

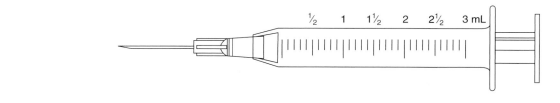

90. Your patient has Thorazine 15 mg IM q6 h ordered for severe agitation. How many milliliters will you administer? _____

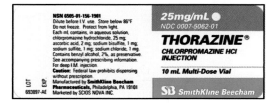

91. The physician orders Vancocin 500 mg IV q12 h. Vancocin 250 mg/5 mL is available after reconstitution. How many milliliters will the nurse prepare? _____

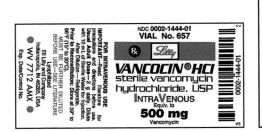

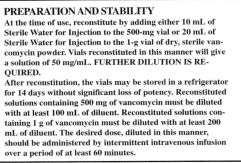

PREPARATION AND STABILITY

At the time of use, reconstitute by adding either 10 mL of Sterile Water for Injection to the 500-mg vial or 20 mL of Sterile Water for Injection to the 1-g vial of dry, sterile van-comycin powder. Vials reconstituted in this manner will give a solution of 50 mg/mL. FURTHER DILUTION IS RE-QUIRED.

After reconstitution, the vials may be stored in a refrigerator for 14 days without significant loss of potency. Reconstituted solutions containing 500 mg of vancomycin must be diluted with at least 100 mL of diluent. Reconstituted solutions con-taining 1 g of vancomycin must be diluted with at least 200 mL of diluent. The desired dose, diluted in this manner, should be administered by intermittent intravenous infusion over a period of at least 60 minutes.

92. Mr. Garcia has Robinul 75 mcg IM ordered 39 minutes before surgery. Robinul 0.2 mg/mL is available. How many milliliters will the nurse administer? _____

93. Your patient with delirium tremens receives diazepam 2 mg IM q6 h. How many milliliters will you administer? _____

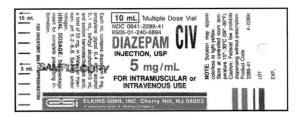

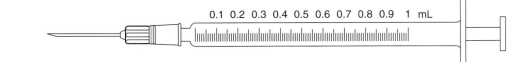

0.1 0.2 0.3 0.4 0.5 0.6 0.7 0.8 0.9 1 mL

94. The physician orders Flagyl 500 mg IV q6 h to treat Ms. King's yeast infection. After reconstitution you have Flagyl 100 mg/mL. How many milliliters will you prepare? _____

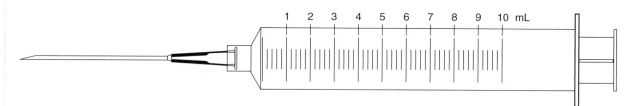

95. The physician orders streptomycin 0.64 g IM daily. After reconstitution you have streptomycin 400 mg/mL. How many milliliters will you administer? _____

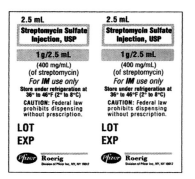

96. Your patient receives nafcillin 500 mg IM q6 h for treatment of a *Staphylococcus aureus* infection. You have nafcillin 250 mg/mL. How many milliliters will you administer? _____

NDC 0015-7226-20
EQUIVALENT TO
2 gram NAFCILLIN
NAFCILLIN SODIUM
FOR INJECTION, USP
Buffered-For IM or IV Use
CAUTION: Federal law prohibits
dispensing without prescription.
APOTHECON

97. The physician orders Stadol 1.5 mg IV q4 h for pain. How many milliliters will the nurse administer? _____

NDC 0015-5646-20   1 mL
Stadol®
(BUTORPHANOL TARTRATE
INJECTION, USP) For IM/IV Use
Store at Room Temp
2 mg (2 mg per mL)
SINGLE DOSE VIAL

98. The physician orders Imferon 100 mg IM every other day for your patient with pernicious anemia. The drug is supplied in ampules containing 25 mg/0.5 mL. How many milliliters will you administer? _____

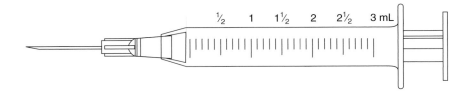

99. Your patient with arthritis receives Solganal 10 mg IM. Solganal is supplied 50 mg/mL. How many milliliters will you administer? _____

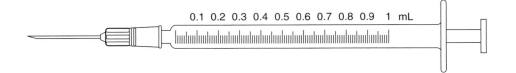

100. Mrs. Sutter has Versed 3.5 mg IM ordered 1 hour before her surgery. You have Versed 5 mg/mL supplied in a 2-mL vial. How many milliliters will you administer? _____

Answers on pp. 517–536.

Name _____

Date _____

ACCEPTABLE SCORE ___19___

YOUR SCORE _____

POSTTEST 1

Directions: The medication order is listed at the beginning of each problem. Calculate the parenteral doses. Show your work. Shade the syringe when provided to indicate the correct dose.

1. The physician orders Vistaril 25 mg IM three times a day q6 h prn to enhance the effects of pain medication for your patient with a thyroidectomy. How many milliliters will you administer? _____

FOR INTRAMUSCULAR USE ONLY.

USUAL ADULT DOSE: Intramuscularly: 25-100 mg stat; repeat every 4 to 6 hours, as needed.

See accompanying prescribing information.

Each mL contains **50 mg** of hydroxyzine hydrochloride, 0.9% benzyl alcohol and sodium hydroxide to adjust to optimum pH.

To avoid discoloration, protect from prolonged exposure to light.

Rx only

10 mL   NDC 0049-5460-74

Vistaril®
(hydroxyzine hydrochloride)

Intramuscular Solution

50 mg/mL

Pfizer **Roerig**
Division of Pfizer Inc, NY, NY 10017

Store below 86°F (30°C).

PROTECT FROM FREEZING.

PATIENT: _____

ROOM NO.: _____

05-1111-32-4   **9249**
MADE IN USA

2. Your patient with a septoplasty complains of nausea and has promethazine 25 mg IM four times a day ordered. How many milliliters will you administer? _____

25 DOSETTE® AMPULS   Each co

*NDC 0641-***1496-35**

PROMETHAZINE
HCl INJECTION, USP

50 mg/mL

FOR DEEP INTRAMUSCULAR USE ONLY

Each mL contains promethazine hydrochloride 50 mg, edetate disodium 0.1 mg, calcium chloride 0.04 mg, sodium metabisulfite 0.25 mg and phenol 5 mg in Water for Injection. pH 4.0-5.5; buffered with acetic acid-sodium acetate. Sealed under nitrogen. USUAL DOSAGE: See package insert. PROTECT FROM LIGHT: Keep covered in carton until time of use. Store at 15°-30°C (59°-86°F). DO NOT USE IF SOLUTION HAS DEVELOPED COLOR OR CONTAINS A PRECIPITATE.

To open ampuls, ignore color line; break at constriction. Caution: Federal law prohibits dispensing without prescription.

Product Code: 1496-35   8-51496d

esi ELKINS-SINN, INC. Cherry Hill, N
A subsidiary of A. H. Robins Company

0.1 0.2 0.3 0.4 0.5 0.6 0.7 0.8 0.9   1 mL

3. Your patient who has undergone tympanomastoidectomy complains of pain and has codeine 30 mg IM q2 h prn ordered. Codeine is supplied in a 1-mL ampule containing gr ¼. How many milliliters will you administer? _____

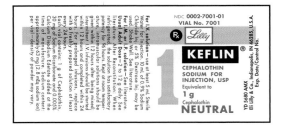

4. The physician orders Keflin 500 mg IM q6 h for your patient with a *Klebsiella* infection. Keflin 1 g/10 mL is available. How many milliliters will you administer? _____

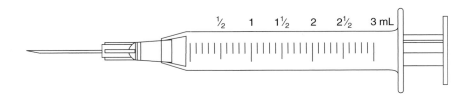

5. Your patient, who has undergone medullary carcinoma excision, has hydrocortisone 50 mg IM twice a day ordered. You have hydrocortisone 100 mg/2 mL available. How many milliliters will you administer? _____

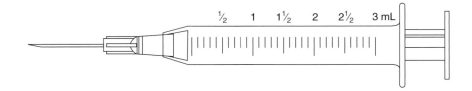

6. The physician orders Dilaudid 0.5 mg IM q4 h prn. How many milliliters will the nurse administer? _____

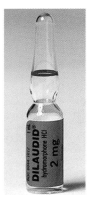

7. Mr. Harrison has Toradol 15 mg IM ordered q6 h for pain after a hip replacement. A prefilled syringe with Toradol 30 mg/mL is available. How many milliliters will the nurse administer? _____

8. The physician orders scopolamine gr ⅟₃₀₀ IM at 0600 before surgery. How many milliliters will the nurse administer? _____

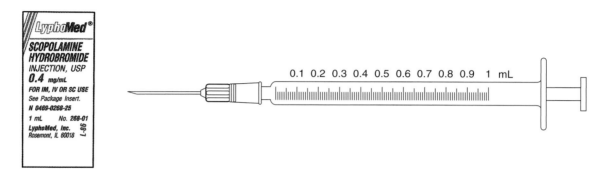

9. The physician orders Thorazine 100 mg IM stat. Thorazine is supplied in a 10-mL vial containing 25 mg/mL. How many milliliters will the nurse administer? _____

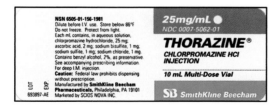

10. Your severely agitated patient has diazepam 2 mg IM q6 h prn ordered. How many milliliters will you administer? _____

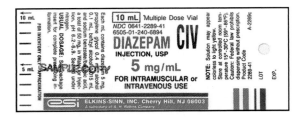

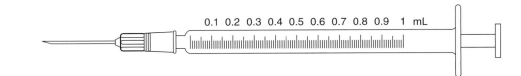

11. Atropine 0.7 mg IM stat is ordered for your patient before surgery. You have atropine gr ¹⁄₁₂₀/mL. How many milliliters will you administer? _____

12. Your patient with a medication reaction complains of pruritus and has Benadryl 25 mg IM prn ordered. You have Benadryl 50 mg/mL available. How many milliliters will you administer? _____

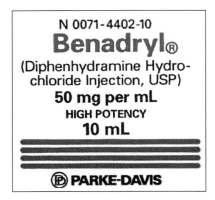

13. The physician orders Depo-Medrol 50 mg IM twice a day. How many milliliters will the nurse administer? _____

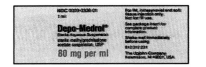

14. The physician orders ampicillin 500 mg IM q4 h for a patient who has undergone lumbar laminectomy. How many milliliters will the nurse administer? _____

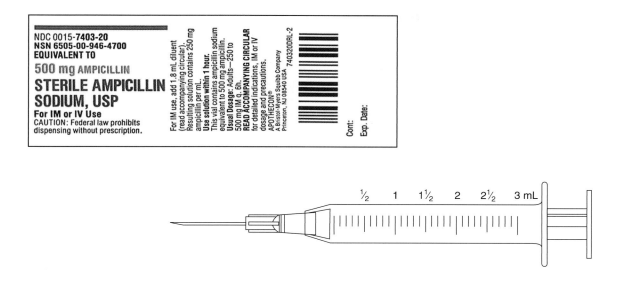

15. The physician orders Ancef 300 mg IV q8 h. You have Ancef 1 g/50 mL vial available. How many milliliters will you administer? _____

16. The physician orders morphine 6 mg IM q3 h prn. How many milliliters will the nurse administer? _____

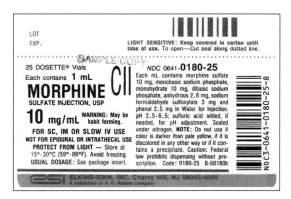

17. The physician orders dexamethasone 6 mg IM stat. You have dexamethasone 10 mg/mL. How many milliliters will you administer? _____

18. Your patient with congestive heart failure has furosemide 20 mg IV daily ordered. How many milliliters will you administer? _____

FUROSEMIDE
INJECTION, USP
40 mg/4 mL
(10 mg/mL)
For IM or IV Use
4 mL Single Dose Vial

N 63323-280-04   Sterile, Nonpyrogenic   28004

Preservative Free
Discard unused portion.
Each mL contains: Furosemide
10 mg, Water for Injection q.s.
Sodium chloride to adjust
isotonicity, pH adjusted with
sodium hydroxide and if
necessary hydrochloric acid.
Usual Dosage: See insert.
PROTECT FROM LIGHT. Do not
use if discolored. Use only if
solution is clear and seal intact.
Store at controlled room
temperature 15°-30°C
(59°-86°F).
Rx only

American
Pharmaceutical
Partners, Inc.
Los Angeles, CA 90024

401736

LOT
EXP

19. The physician orders digoxin 0.3 mg IM now. How many milliliters will the nurse administer? _____

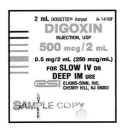

2 mL DOSETTE® Ampul   A-1410F
DIGOXIN
INJECTION, USP
500 mcg / 2 mL
0.5 mg/2 mL (250 mcg/mL)
FOR SLOW IV OR
DEEP IM USE
GSI ELKINS-SINN, INC.
CHERRY HILL, NJ 08003

SAMPLE COPY

20. Mrs. Joyce has verapamil 5 mg IV bolus ordered to be given over 2 minutes now for dysrhythmia. Verapmil 2.5 mg/mL is supplied. How many milliliters will Mrs. Joyce receive? _____

Answers on pp. 536–539.

Name _____

Date _____

ACCEPTABLE SCORE ___19___

YOUR SCORE _____

POSTTEST 2

Directions: The medication order is listed at the beginning of each problem. Calculate the parenteral doses. Show your work. Shade the syringe when provided to indicate the correct dose.

1. Your patient who was involved in a motor vehicle accident complains of pain and has Dilaudid 2 mg IM q3 h prn ordered. How many milliliters will you administer? _____

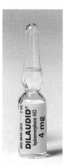

2. Your preoperative patient complains of anxiety and has Ativan 2 mg IM q6 h ordered. Ativan is supplied 4 mg/mL. How many milliliters will you administer? _____

3. The physician orders erythromycin 0.4 g IV today. The drug is supplied in vials containing 500 mg/10 mL. How many milliliters will the nurse prepare? _____

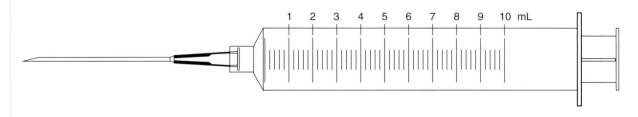

4. Mrs. Jesse has Cardizem 20 mg IV ordered stat for hypertension. How many milliliters will the nurse administer? _____

NDC 0088-1790-32
CARDIZEM® Injectable
(diltiazem HCl Injection)
FOR DIRECT INTRAVENOUS BOLUS INJECTION AND CONTINUOUS INTRAVENOUS INFUSION
25 mg (5 mg/mL)
Sterile 5-mL Vial
SINGLE-USE CONTAINER. DISCARD UNUSED PORTION. Mfd. for
Date Removed From Refrigeration _____ Hoechst Marion Roussel, Inc.
Date To Be Discarded _____ Kansas City, MO 64137 USA
50007742   06

5. Your patient who has had a lumpectomy has codeine 60 mg IM q3 h ordered. How many milliliters will you administer? _____

NDC 0002-1636-01
20 ml VIAL No. 335
POISON
CODEINE PHOSPHATE 30
INJECTION, USP
30 mg
(1/2 gr) per ml
Multiple Dose

APPROXIMATE VOLUME SCALE
APPROXIMATE EQUIVALENTS
0.5 ml=15 mg (1/4 gr)
1 ml=30 mg (1/2 gr)
2 ml=60 mg (1 gr)
Eli Lilly & Co., Indianapolis, IN 46285, U.S.A.
YA 9275 AMX

6. Mr. Ryan has Tigan 200 mg IM ordered three times a day for nausea and vomiting. How many milliliters will you administer? _____

NDC 61570-541-20
100mg/mL
Tigan®
(trimethobenzamide HCl)
Injection   **℞ Only**
20mL Multi-Dose Vial
Monarch Pharmaceuticals

NOT FOR USE IN CHILDREN.
FOR IM USE ONLY.
Store from 15° to 30° C (59° to 86°F).
Each mL of solution contains 100 mg trimetho-benzamide hydrochloride compounded with 0.45% phenol as preservative, 0.5 mg sodium citrate and 0.2 mg citric acid as buffers, and sodium hydroxide to adjust pH to approximately 5.0.
Dosage: See accompanying prescribing information. For IM use only (preferably by deep IM Injection).
Distributed by:
Monarch Pharmaceuticals, Inc., Bristol, TN 37620
Manufactured by:
King Pharmaceuticals, Inc., Bristol, TN 37620
0934063 Rev. 11/99

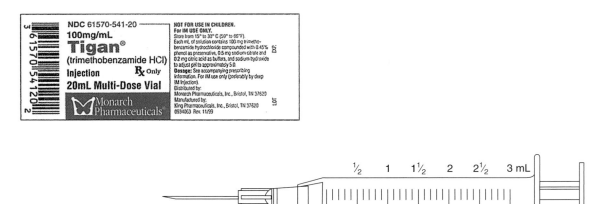

7. The physician orders atropine gr ¹⁄₂₀₀ IM at 0600. How many milliliters will the nurse administer? _____

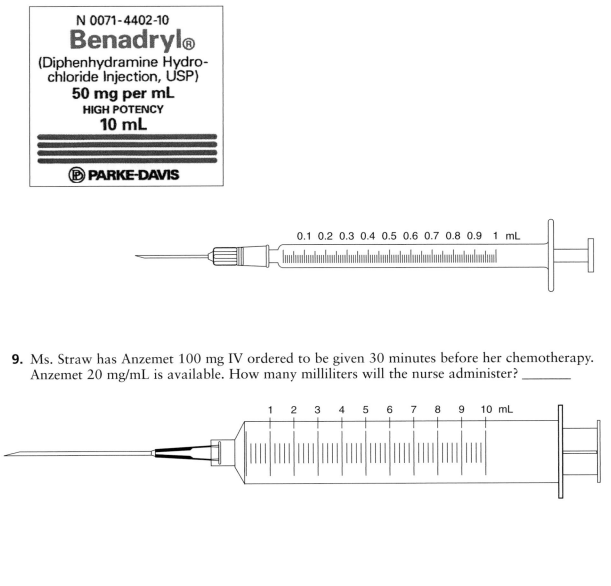

8. The physician orders Benadryl 25 mg IV now for your patient with a mild medication reaction. How many milliliters will you prepare? _____

N 0071-4402-10

Benadryl®

(Diphenhydramine Hydro-chloride Injection, USP)

50 mg per mL

HIGH POTENCY

10 mL

℗ **PARKE-DAVIS**

0.1 0.2 0.3 0.4 0.5 0.6 0.7 0.8 0.9 1 mL

9. Ms. Straw has Anzemet 100 mg IV ordered to be given 30 minutes before her chemotherapy. Anzemet 20 mg/mL is available. How many milliliters will the nurse administer? _____

1   2   3   4   5   6   7   8   9   10 mL

10. Mr. Trent has hydroxyzine 75 mg IM now ordered for severe motion sickness. You have hydroxyzine 50 mg/mL. How many milliliters will you administer? _____

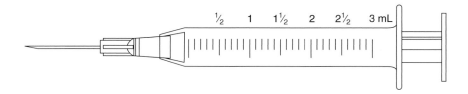

11. Your patient who has undergone parathyroidectomy receives ampicillin 200 mg IV q6 h. Ampicillin 125 mg/mL is available. How many milliliters will you prepare? _____

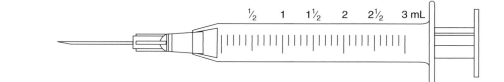

12. The physician orders scopolamine gr ¹⁄₁₅₀ IM at 0700. Scopolamine gr ¹⁄₂₀₀/mL is available. How many milliliters will the nurse administer? _____

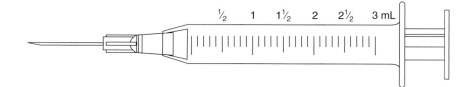

13. The physician orders piperacillin 2 g IV q8 h for your patient with sepsis. Piperacillin 1 g/2.5 mL is available. How many milliliters will you prepare? _____

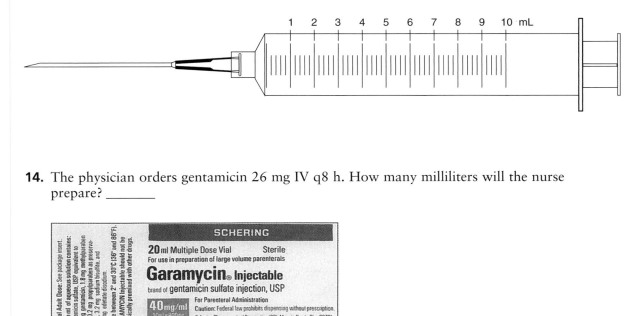

14. The physician orders gentamicin 26 mg IV q8 h. How many milliliters will the nurse prepare? _____

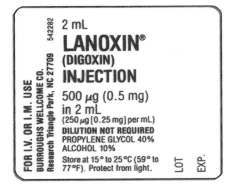

15. The physician orders Lovenox 85 mg subcutaneous q12 h. The drug is available 100 mg/mL. How many milliliters will the nurse administer? _____

16. Your patient, who has undergone tricuspid valve repair, has Lanoxin 80 mcg IM twice a day ordered. How many milliliters will you administer? _____

17. The physician orders morphine 4 mg subcutaneous q4 h prn. Morphine is supplied in a 1-mL ampule containing gr ⅛. How many milliliters will the nurse administer? _____

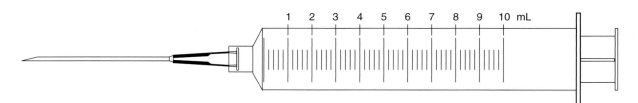

18. Your patient with a history of seizures has Dilantin 100 mg IV q8 h ordered. Dilantin 50 mg/2 mL is available. How many milliliters will you prepare? _____

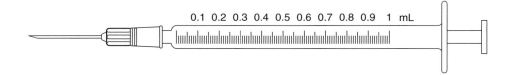

19. Mr. Richards has Floxin 300 mg IV q12 h ordered to treat his prostatitis. Floxin 400 mg/100 mL is available. How many milliliters will the nurse administer? _____

20. The physician orders D_5W 500 mL plus calcium chloride ($CaCl_2$) 10 mEq at 10 mL per hour IV. $CaCl_2$ is supplied in a 10-mL ampule containing 13.6 mEq. How many milliliters of $CaCl_2$ will be added to the 500 mL of D_5W? _____

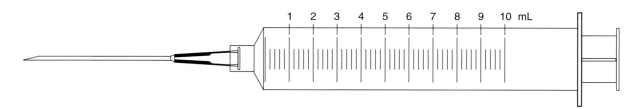

Answers on pp. 540–543.

Refer to Basic Calculations: Parenteral Dosages and Reconstitution of Powdered Drugs on the enclosed CD for additional help and practice problems.

Dosages Measured in Units

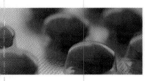

LEARNING OBJECTIVES

On completion of the materials provided in this chapter, you will be able to perform computations accurately by mastering the following mathematical concepts:

1 Calculating drug dosage problems that first require reconstitution of a powdered drug into a liquid form

2 Using a proportion to solve problems involving drugs measured in unit dosages

3 Drawing a line through an insulin syringe to indicate the number of units desired

A unit is the amount of a drug needed to produce a given result. Various drugs are measured in units; the examples used in this chapter are among the more common drugs prescribed.

Drugs used in this chapter include:

Epogen—A drug that increases the production of red blood cells

Fragmin—An anticoagulant that prevents the clotting of blood

Penicillin—An antibiotic that reduces organisms within the body that cause infection

Heparin—An anticoagulant that inhibits clotting of the blood

Insulin—A hormone secreted by the pancreas that lowers blood glucose

Epogen is a drug that helps to combat the effects of anemia caused by chemotherapy or chronic renal failure. After administering the medicine, the nurse should monitor the patient's blood pressure and laboratory results on a routine basis.

Fragmin is used in the prevention of deep vein thrombosis after abdominal surgery, hip replacements, and unstable angina/non–Q wave myocardial infarction. It may also be used with patients who have restricted mobility during an acute illness. Fragmin may only be given by subcutaneous injections—never intramuscularly or intravenously. The patient's blood studies must be monitored on a routine basis during treatment with Fragmin.

Penicillin can be administered orally or parenterally, but heparin, insulin, and epogen must be given subcutaneously or intravenously.

Before administering penicillin, the nurse must confer with the patient regarding previous allergies to the drug. After administering the drug, the nurse must still observe the patient for signs of an allergic reaction.

Because heparin prolongs the time blood takes to clot, the dosage must be accurate. A larger dose may cause hemorrhage, and an insufficient dose may not have the desired result. After administering the drug, the nurse should observe the patient for signs of hemorrhage.

Insulin is used in the treatment of diabetes mellitus. Accuracy is important in the preparation of insulin. A higher dosage than needed may cause insulin shock. An insufficient amount of insulin may result in diabetic coma. Both conditions are extremely serious, and the nurse must be able to recognize the symptoms of each condition so that immediate treatment can be initiated to stabilize the patient. In many institutions, both insulin and heparin dosages are checked for accuracy by another nurse before the drug is administered to the patient.

A U-100 insulin syringe and U-100 insulin are necessary to ensure an accurate insulin dosage. U-100 insulin means that 100 units of insulin is contained in 1 mL of liquid. U-100 insulin is a universal insulin preparation that all persons requiring insulin can use. Another type of U-100 syringe is the U-100 Lo-Dose syringe, which measures 50 units; however, for accuracy, no more than 40 units should be measured in the U-100 Lo-Dose syringe. Because the doses are minute, the U-100 syringe provides the most accurate measurement of insulin dosages. The 30-unit U-100 syringe is used for insulin doses that equal less than 30 units.

IMPORTANT NOTE: Only insulin is measured and given in the syringes that are marked in units.* Heparin, penicillin, and other medication measured in units can be measured and given only in syringes marked in milliliters.

Powder Reconstitution

A drug in powdered form is necessary when a medication is unstable as a liquid form for a long period. This powdered drug must be reconstituted—dissolved with a sterile diluent—before administration. The diluents commonly used include sterile water, sterile normal saline solution, 5% dextrose solution (D_5W), and bacteriostatic normal saline.

Before reconstituting the medication, the nurse must follow several principles:
1. Carefully read the information and directions on the vial or package insert for reconstitution of the medication.
2. If no directions are available with the medication, consult the *Physicians' Desk Reference*, hospital drug formulary, pharmacology text, or hospital pharmacy.
3. Identify the type and amount of diluent and the route of administration.
4. Note the drug strength or concentration after reconstitution and circle or place this on the label, if not already written, when you use a multidose vial.
5. Note the length of time for which the medication is good once reconstituted and the directions for storage.
6. Be aware that the total reconstitution amount may be greater than the amount of diluent.
7. After reconstitution of a multidose vial, place your initials, date of preparation, time of preparation, date of expiration, and time of expiration on the label.

---

*Only regular insulin can be given intravenously.

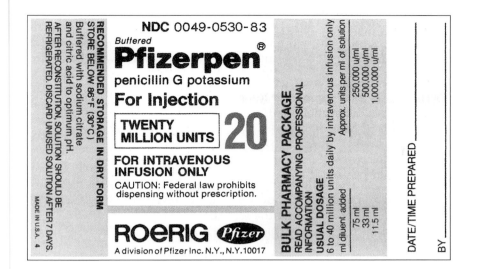

NDC 0049-0530-83

Buffered

Pfizerpen®

penicillin G potassium

For Injection

TWENTY
MILLION UNITS **20**

**FOR INTRAVENOUS
INFUSION ONLY**

CAUTION: Federal law prohibits
dispensing without prescription.

ROERIG *Pfizer*

A division of Pfizer Inc. N.Y., N.Y. 10017

RECOMMENDED STORAGE IN DRY FORM
STORE BELOW 86°F (30°C)
Buffered with sodium citrate
and citric acid to optimum pH.
AFTER RECONSTITUTION, SOLUTION SHOULD BE
REFRIGERATED. DISCARD UNUSED SOLUTION AFTER 7 DAYS.

MADE IN U.S.A. 4

BULK PHARMACY PACKAGE
READ ACCOMPANYING PROFESSIONAL
INFORMATION
USUAL DOSAGE
6 to 40 million units daily by intravenous infusion only

Approx. units per ml of solution

ml diluent added		
75 ml	33 ml	11.5 ml
250,000 u/ml	500,000 u/ml	1,000,000 u/ml

DATE/TIME PREPARED _____

BY _____

Example:

a. What is the route of administration?   IV
b. What type of diluent can be used?   Check insert
c. How much diluent must be added?   75 mL
d. What is the medication concentration?   250,000 units/mL
e. How long will the medication maintain
   its potency at room temperature?   7 days
f. The physician orders 2,000,000 units IV
   q4 h. How many milliliters will you give?
   Shade the syringe.   8 mL

   a. 250,000 units : 1 mL ::
   b. 250,000 units : 1 mL :: _____ units : _____ mL
   c. 250,000 units : 1 mL :: 2,000,000 units : x mL
   d. $250,000x = 2,000,000$

   $$x = \frac{2,000,000}{250,000}$$

   $x = 8$
   e. $x = 8$ mL

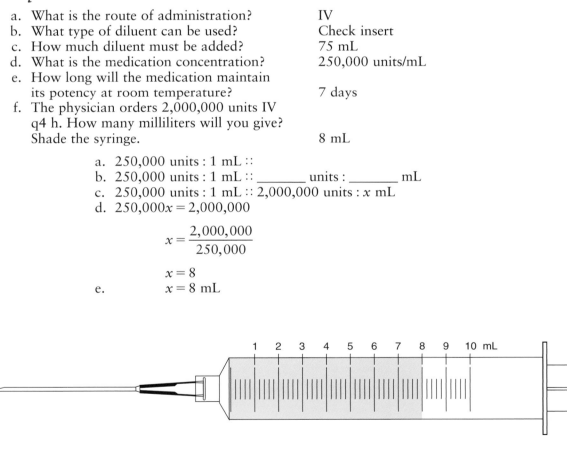

Dosages Measured in Units Involving Oral Medications

Example: The physician orders mycostatin 400,000 units po four times a day. The drug is supplied 100,000 units/mL after reconstitution. How many milliliters will the nurse administer?

    a. On the left side of the proportion, place what you know or have available. In this example, each milliliter contains 100,000 units. So the left side of the proportion would be

$$100{,}000 \text{ units} : 1 \text{ mL} ::$$

    b. The right side of the proportion is determined by the physician's order and the abbreviations on the left side of the proportion. Only *two* different abbreviations may be used in a single proportion. The abbreviations must be in the same position on the right side as on the left side.

$$100{,}000 \text{ units} : 1 \text{ mL} :: 400{,}000 \text{ units} : \underline{\hspace{1cm}} \text{ mL}$$

We need to find the number of milliliters to be administered, so we use the symbol x to represent the unknown.

$$100{,}000 \text{ units} : 1 \text{ mL} :: 400{,}000 \text{ units} : x \text{ mL}$$

    c. Rewrite the proportion without the abbreviations.

$$100{,}000 : 1 :: 400{,}000 : x$$

    d. Solve for x.

$$100{,}000 : 1 :: 400{,}000 : x$$
$$100{,}000x = 400{,}000$$
$$x = \frac{400{,}000}{100{,}000}$$
$$x = 4$$

    e. Label your answer as determined by the abbreviation placed next to x in the original proportion.

$$x = 4 \text{ mL}$$

The nurse would measure 4 mL to administer 400,000 units of mycostatin.

Dosages Measured in Units Involving Parenteral Medications

Example: The physician orders heparin 4000 units subcutaneous q8 h. How many milliliters will the nurse administer?

    a. $5000 \text{ units} : 1 \text{ mL} ::$
    b. $5000 \text{ units} : 1 \text{ mL} :: \underline{\hspace{1cm}} \text{ units} : \underline{\hspace{1cm}} \text{ mL}$

```
N 0469-1262-15    926201
HEPARIN SODIUM
INJECTION, USP
5,000 USP Units/mL
(Derived from Porcine
Intestinal Mucosa)
For IV or SC Use
1 mL Multiple Dose Vial
Usual Dosage: See insert.
Fujisawa USA, Inc.
Deerfield, IL 60015-2548

        40213F

LOT
EXP
```

$$5000 \text{ units} : 1 \text{ mL} :: 4000 \text{ units} : x \text{ mL}$$

c. $5000 : 1 :: 4000 : x$

d. $5000x = 4000$

$$5000x = 4000$$

$$x = \frac{4000}{5000}$$

$$x = 0.8$$

e. $x = 0.8 \text{ mL}$

Therefore 0.8 mL of heparin would be the amount of each individual dose of heparin given q8 h.

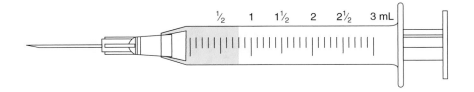

Insulin Given with a Lo-Dose Insulin Syringe

Example: The physician orders Humulin Lente U-100 insulin 36 units subcutaneous injection in AM. A U-100 Lo-Dose syringe is available. Shade the syringe to indicate the correct dose.

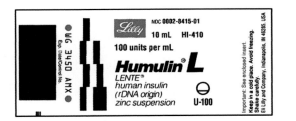

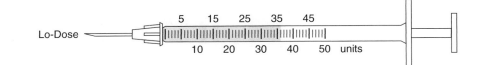

With a Lo-Dose insulin syringe, 36 units of U-100 insulin would be measured as indicated.

Mixed Insulin Administration*

The physician may prescribe two types of insulin to be administered at the same time. As long as they are compatible, these insulins will be drawn up in the same syringe to avoid injecting the patient twice.

---

*NOTE: Some insulins such as Lantus should never be mixed. Be sure to always check if an insulin can be mixed with another insulin.

Several guidelines apply to this type of administration:
1. Air equal to the amount of insulin being withdrawn should be injected into each vial. Do *not* touch the solution with the tip of the needle.
2. Using the same syringe, draw up the desired amount of insulin from the **regular** insulin bottle first.
3. Remove the syringe from the regular insulin bottle. Check the syringe for any air bubbles and remove them.
4. Using the same syringe, draw up the amount of cloudy insulin to the desired dose.
5. Hospitals usually require that you check your insulin dosages with another nurse before administration. Consult your hospital policy and procedures.

Example 1: The physician orders Humulin Regular U-100 10 units plus Humulin NPH U-100 20 units subcutaneous now.

The total amount of insulin is 30 units (10 units + 20 units = 30 units).

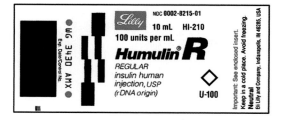

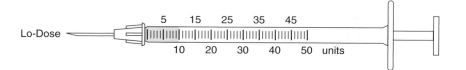

10 units of regular insulin is drawn up first, then 20 units of NPH insulin is drawn up.

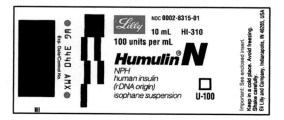

10 units of regular insulin + 20 units of NPH insulin = 30 units of insulin

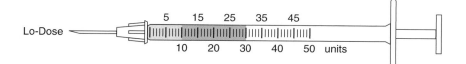

Example 2: The physician orders Humulin Lente U-100 46 units subcutaneous daily, plus regular Humulin U-100 20 units. A U-100 insulin syringe is available. Shade the syringe to indicate the amount of Lente Humulin insulin to be given, and in a different color to indicate the total dose.

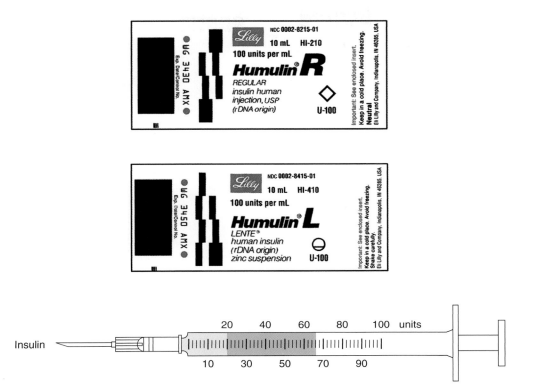

Complete the following work sheet, which provides for extensive practice in the calculation of dosages measured in units. Check your answers. If you have difficulties, go back and review the necessary material. When you feel ready to evaluate your learning, take the first posttest. Check your answers. An acceptable score as indicated on the posttest signifies that you have successfully completed this chapter. An unacceptable score signifies a need for further study before taking the second posttest.

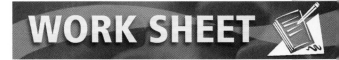

WORK SHEET

Directions: The medication order is listed at the beginning of each problem. Calculate the doses. Show your work. Mark the syringe when provided to indicate the correct dose.

1. Your patient with pneumonia receives penicillin V 200,000 units po four times a day. You have penicillin V oral solution 400,000 units/5 mL available. Draw a vertical line through the syringe to indicate the number of milliliters to be given.

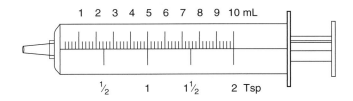

2. Mr. Curtis has Epogen 12,000 units subcutaneous injection three times a week to treat anemia related to chemotherapy. How many milliliters will you administer? _____

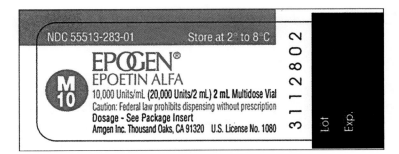

3. The physician orders NPH U-100 insulin 20 units subcutaneous daily at 0800. Draw a vertical line through the syringe to indicate the amount of NPH insulin to be given.

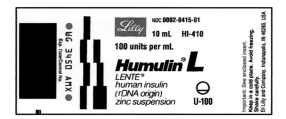

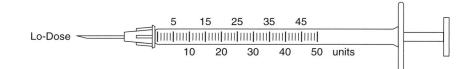

Lo-Dose

4. A patient with a temporal bone infection receives penicillin G 500,000 units IM q6 h. How much diluent should be added? _____ What is the medication concentration? _____ How many milliliters will you administer? _____ What would you circle on the label to indicate concentration? _____

PENICILLIN G
POTASSIUM
FOR INJECTION
USP
(BUFFERED)
1,000,000 Units

NDC 0002-1406-01
VIAL No. 526

Add diluent	Conc. of Solution
9.6 ml	100,000 Units/ml
4.6 ml	200,000 Units/ml
1.6 ml	500,000 Units/ml

5. Mr. Stephens, following his right total hip replacement, has Fragmin 5000 international units subcutaneous injections daily ordered. How many milliliters will the nurse administer? _____

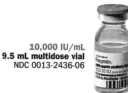

10,000 IU/mL
9.5 mL multidose vial
NDC 0013-2436-06

Reproduced with permission from Pfizer, Inc. All rights reserved.

6. The physician orders regular Humulin insulin 2 units subcutaneous daily at 1900. Draw a vertical line through the syringe to indicate the dose.

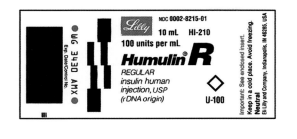

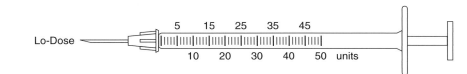

7. Your postoperative patient receives heparin 3000 units subcutaneous q8 h to prevent deep vein thrombosis. How many milliliters will you administer? _____

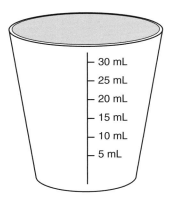

8. The physician orders V-Cillin K suspension 400,000 units po q6 h. V-Cillin K suspension is supplied 200,000 units/5 mL. How many milliliters will the nurse administer? _____

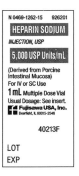

9. The physician orders Lente insulin 14 units, regular insulin 6 units subcutaneous every morning. Lente insulin U-100, regular insulin U-100, and a U-100 Lo-Dose syringe are supplied. Draw a vertical line through the syringe to indicate the amount of regular insulin to be given and a second line to indicate the total dose.

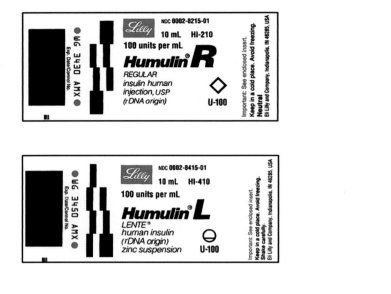

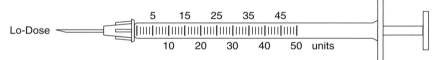

10. Your patient with an appendectomy has penicillin V 300,000 units po four times a day ordered. You have penicillin V oral solution 400,000 units/5 mL available. How many milliliters will you administer? _____ Draw a vertical line through the syringe to indicate the dose.

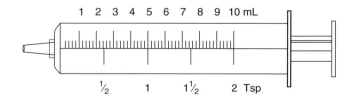

11. Mrs. Alvarez has Epogen 4500 units subcutaneous injection three times a week for anemia caused by chronic renal failure. How many milliliters will you administer? _____

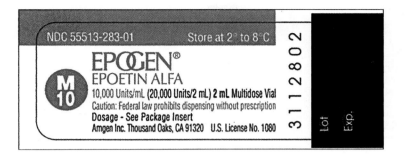

12. The physician orders Humulin regular insulin 18 units subcutaneous at 0700 daily. Draw a vertical line through the syringe to indicate the dose.

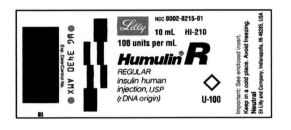

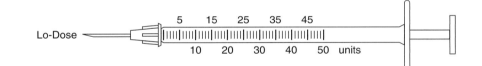

13. The physician orders Humulin 70/30 insulin 32 units subcutaneous tomorrow at 0745. Draw a vertical line through the syringe to indicate the dose.

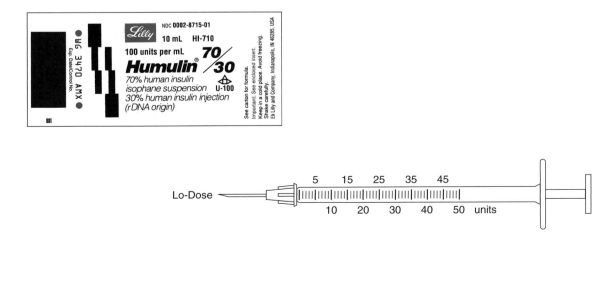

14. Your patient with a thoracotomy receives penicillin G 600,000 units IM twice a day. How much diluent should be added? _____ What is the medication concentration? _____ How many milliliters will you administer? _____

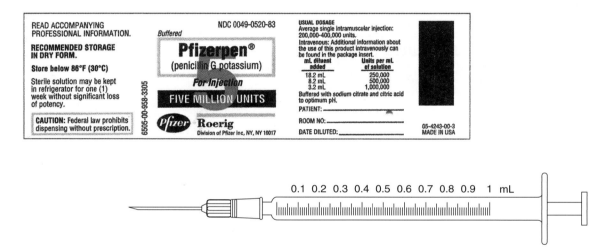

15. Mr. Rose has Pfizerpen 250,000 units IM now ordered. How much diluent will be added? _____ How many milliliters will the nurse administer? _____

0.1 0.2 0.3 0.4 0.5 0.6 0.7 0.8 0.9 1 mL

16. Mrs. Garden has penicillin G potassium 175,000 units IM now ordered. If 18.2 mL of diluent are added, how many milliliters will the nurse administer? _____

17. Your patient with a stapedectomy receives penicillin V 300,000 units po four times a day. The drug is supplied in oral solution 200,000 units/5 mL. How many milliliters will you administer? _____

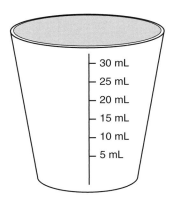

18. Your patient with insulin-dependent diabetes receives Humulin U Insulin 24 units subcutaneous every morning. Draw a vertical line through the syringe to indicate the dose.

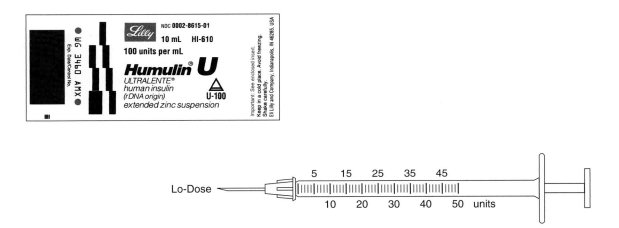

19. Your postoperative patient receives heparin 2500 units subcutaneous injection now. Draw a vertical line through the syringe to indicate the dose.

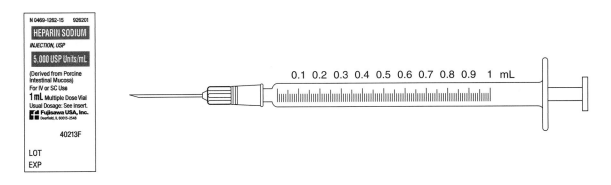

20. Your patient with a gastric pull-up receives penicillin G 200,000 units IM q6 h. You have penicillin G 250,000 units/mL available. How many milliliters will you administer? _____ Draw a vertical line through the syringe to indicate the dose.

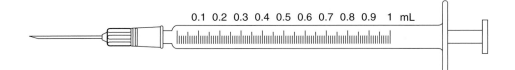

21. Mrs. Schroeder has Fragmin 5500 international units by subcutaneous injection twice a day for system anticoagulation. You have Fragmin 10,000 international units/mL. How many milliliters will you administer? _____

22. The physician orders Humulin regular insulin 40 units and Humulin NPH 35 units every morning before breakfast. Draw a vertical line through the syringe to indicate the dosage for regular Humulin first, and then with the Humulin NPH dosage.

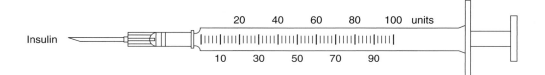

23. The physician orders heparin 2500 units subcutaneous q12 h for your patient with a jejunostomy. How many milliliters will you administer? _____ Draw a vertical line through the syringe to indicate the dose.

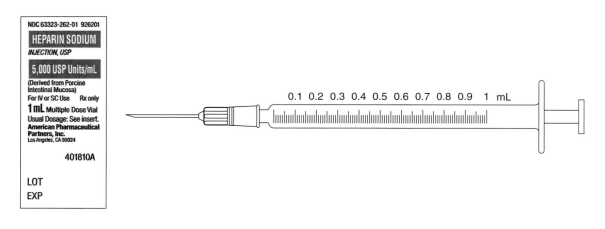

24. The physician orders 24 units Humulin U subcutaneous injection now. Draw a vertical line through the syringe to indicate the dose.

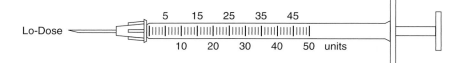

25. The physician orders Humulin 50/50 70 units subcutaneous injection. Draw a vertical line through the syringe to indicate the dose.

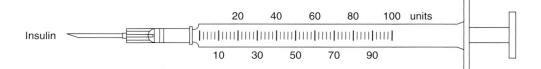

Answers on pp. 544–548.

Name _____

Date _____

ACCEPTABLE SCORE ___14___

YOUR SCORE _____

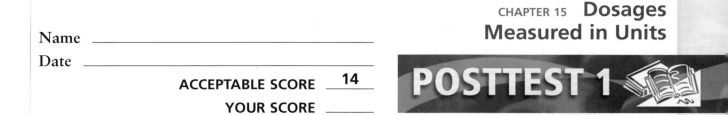

POSTTEST 1

Directions: The medication order is listed at the beginning of each problem. Calculate the doses. Show your work. Mark the syringe when provided to indicate the correct dose.

1. The physician orders penicillin V 500,000 units po four times a day for your patient with a hysterectomy. Penicillin V pediatric suspension 400,000 units/5 mL is supplied. How many milliliters will you administer? _____ Draw a vertical line through the syringe to indicate the dose.

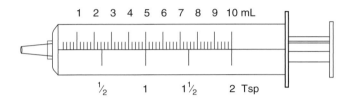

2. The physician orders Lente insulin 40 units subcutaneous daily. Draw a vertical line through the syringe to indicate the dose.

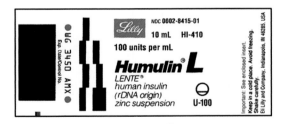

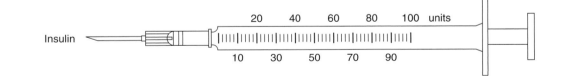

3. In preparation for his upcoming hip replacement surgery, Mr. Stone has Epogen 36,000 units subcutaneous injection once 3 weeks before his surgery. Epogen 40,000 units/mL is available. How many milliliters will the nurse administer? _____

4. The physician orders Humulin 50/50 insulin 6 units subcutaneous now. Draw a vertical line through the syringe to indicate the dose.

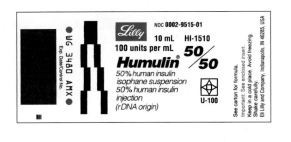

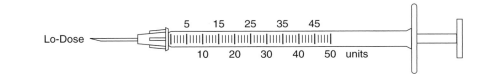

5. The physician orders penicillin G potassium 3,000,000 units IM q6 h for your patient with an ethmoidectomy. What is the best amount of diluent to add? _____ What is the medication concentration? _____ How many milliliters will you administer? _____

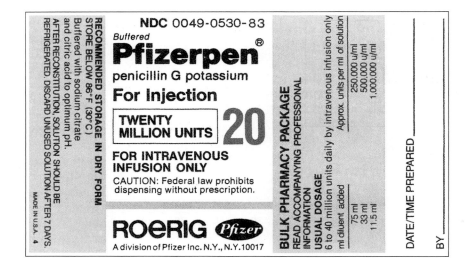

6. Your patient with insulin-dependent diabetes has Humalog insulin 60 units subcutaneous four times a day. You have Humalog insulin U-100 and a U-100 syringe. Draw a vertical line through the syringe to indicate the dose.

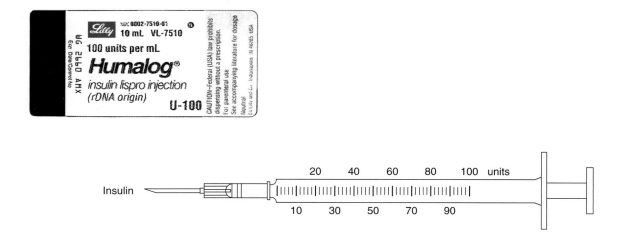

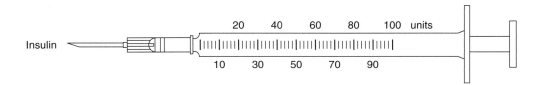

7. Mr. Cory has Pfizerpen 600,000 units IM q6 h for a serious pneumococcal infection. Select the most appropriate dilution. How many milliliters of diluent will you add? _____ How many milliliters will you administer? _____

8. The physician orders Lente insulin 38 units, regular insulin 18 units subcutaneous daily. Lente U-100, regular insulin U-100, and a U-100 syringe are supplied. Draw a vertical line through the syringe to indicate the amount of regular insulin to be given and a second line to indicate the total dose.

9. The physician orders penicillin V 300,000 units po four times a day for your patient with chronic otitis. The drug is supplied in oral solution 200,000 units/5 mL. How many milliliters will you administer? _____

10. The physician orders Pfizerpen 1.2 million units IM in a single dose today. How much diluent should be added? _____ What is the medication concentration? _____ How many milliliters will the nurse administer? _____

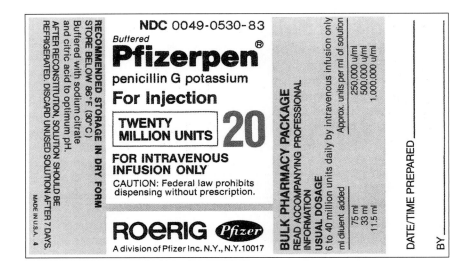

11. Your patient with a sacral decubitus receives penicillin V 200,000 units po four times a day. You have penicillin V oral solution 400,000 units/5 mL. How many milliliters will you administer? _____

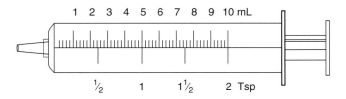

12. Your postoperative patient receives heparin 5000 units subcutaneous q12 h. Heparin 2500 units/mL is available. How many milliliters will you administer? _____

13. Mrs. Tanaka has been admitted with unstable angina. The physician orders Fragmin 8700 international units subcutaneous injection q12 h. How many milliliters will be administered? _____

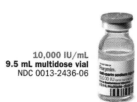

10,000 IU/mL
9.5 mL multidose vial
NDC 0013-2436-06

Reproduced with permission from Pfizer, Inc. All rights reserved.

14. Mrs. Daisy receives nystatin oral suspension 600,000 units po four times a day. How many milliliters will the nurse administer? _____

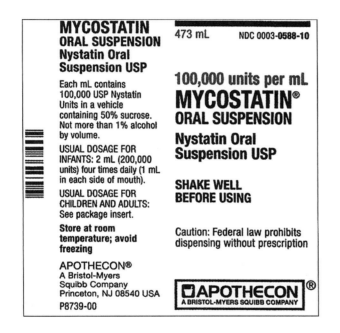

MYCOSTATIN
ORAL SUSPENSION
Nystatin Oral
Suspension USP

Each mL contains
100,000 USP Nystatin
Units in a vehicle
containing 50% sucrose.
Not more than 1% alcohol
by volume.

USUAL DOSAGE FOR
INFANTS: 2 mL (200,000
units) four times daily (1 mL
in each side of mouth).

USUAL DOSAGE FOR
CHILDREN AND ADULTS:
See package insert.

**Store at room
temperature; avoid
freezing**

APOTHECON®
A Bristol-Myers
Squibb Company
Princeton, NJ 08540 USA

P8739-00

473 mL   NDC 0003-0588-10

100,000 units per mL
MYCOSTATIN®
ORAL SUSPENSION
Nystatin Oral
Suspension USP

SHAKE WELL
BEFORE USING

Caution: Federal law prohibits
dispensing without prescription

☐APOTHECON®
A BRISTOL-MYERS SQUIBB COMPANY

15. Ms. Sanders has Epogen 2200 units subcutaneous injection three times a week ordered for the anemia caused by chronic renal failure. Epogen 3000 units/mL is available. How many milliliters will the patient receive for each dose? _____

Answers on pp. 549–551.

Name _____

Date _____

ACCEPTABLE SCORE ___14___

YOUR SCORE _____

POSTTEST 2

Directions: The medication order is listed at the beginning of each problem. Calculate the doses. Show your work. Mark the syringe when provided to indicate the correct dose.

1. The physician orders regular insulin 10 units subcutaneous. Regular insulin U-100 and a U-100 Lo-Dose syringe are supplied. Draw a vertical line through the syringe to indicate the dose.

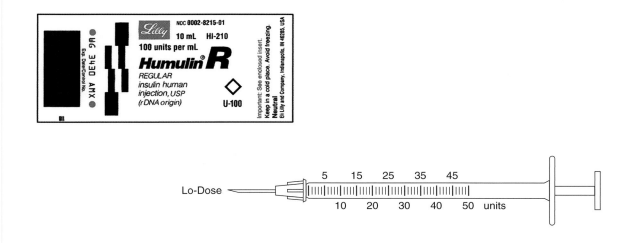

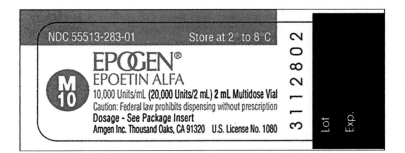

2. Mr. Blackwell has 14,000 units Epogen subcutaneous injection ordered three times a week for anemia related to his chemotherapy. How many milliliters will he receive each time? _____

3. Your patient with a septoplasty receives V-Cillin K 500,000 units po q6 h. You have 200,000 units/5 mL available. How many milliliters will you administer? _____

4. The physician orders Novolin L insulin 28 units subcutaneous at 0745. Draw a vertical line through the syringe to indicate the dose of NPH insulin to be given.

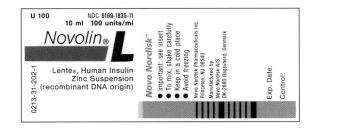

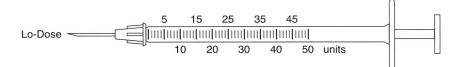

5. Mr. Noah has Fragmin 2500 international units subcutaneous 2 hours before surgery for a total hip replacement. How many milliliters will he receive? _____

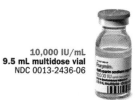

Reproduced with permission from Pfizer, Inc. All rights reserved.

6. The physician orders penicillin G potassium 1.2 million units IV q4 h for your patient after dental extraction. You have a vial containing 1,000,000 units/mL. How many milliliters will you prepare? _____

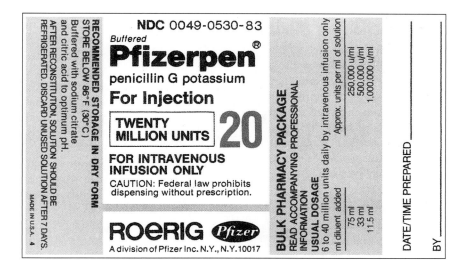

7. The physician orders Humulin L Lente insulin 54 units subcutaneous. You have Lente insulin U-100 and a U-100 syringe. Draw a vertical line through the syringe to indicate the amount of Lente insulin to be given.

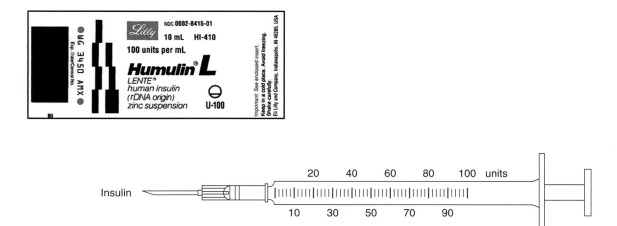

Insulin

8. The physician orders NPH insulin 16 units and regular insulin 8 units subcutaneous daily at 0800. You have NPH insulin U-100, regular insulin U-100, and a U-100 Lo-Dose syringe. Draw a vertical line through the syringe to indicate the amount of regular insulin to be given and a second line to indicate the total dose.

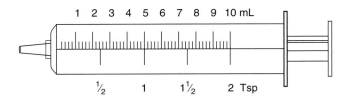

9. Your patient with chronic sinusitis receives penicillin V 300,000 units po four times a day. You have penicillin V oral solution 400,000 units/5 mL. How many milliliters will you administer? _____

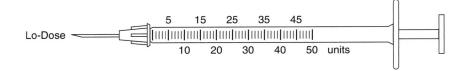

10. Ms. Martinez has 2 million units IV Pfizerpen q4 h ordered for a severe pneumococcal infection. How much diluent will you add? _____ How many milliliters will you administer? _____

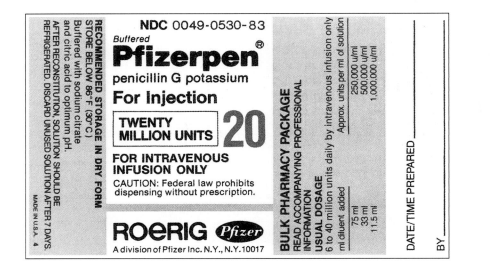

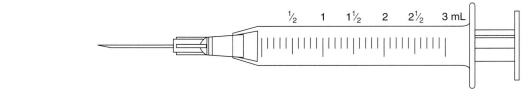

11. Your patient with osteomyelitis receives penicillin G 600,000 units IM twice daily. How much diluent should be added? _____ What is the medication concentration? _____ How many milliliters will you administer? _____

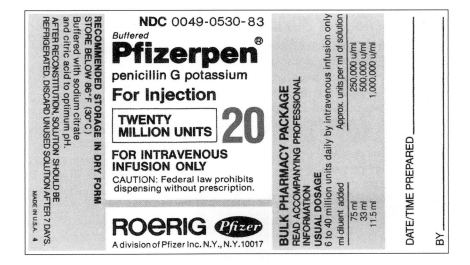

12. Miss Garrett has Pfizerpen 400,000 units IV q4 h ordered for a severe streptococcal infection. You add 75 mL of diluent. How many milliliters will you administer? _____

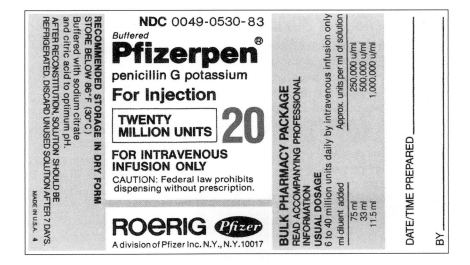

13. Your patient with insulin-dependent diabetes receives Lente insulin 25 units subcutaneous daily at 0800. Draw a vertical line through the syringe to indicate the amount of Lente insulin to be given.

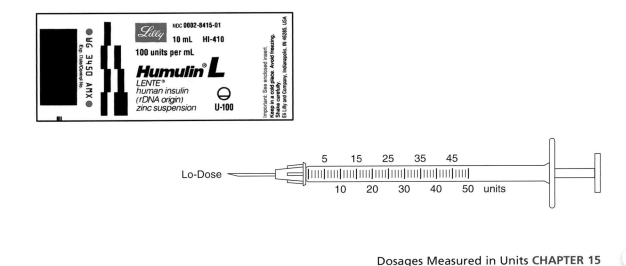

14. Mrs. Roy has Pfizerpen (penicillin G potassium) 300,000 units IM q4 h ordered for a serious streptococcal infection. How much diluent will you add? _____ How many milliliters will you administer? _____

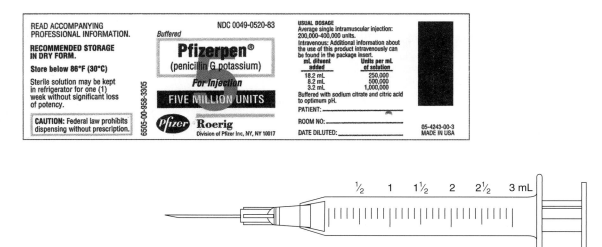

15. Mrs. Star has Epogen 16,000 units subcutaneous injection three times a week for anemia as a result of her chemotherapy. How many milliliters will you administer for each dose? _____

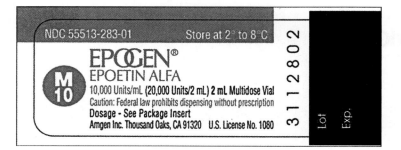

Answers on pp. 551–553.

Refer to Introducing Drug Measures: Measuring Dosages and Advanced Calculations: Insulin and Heparin on the enclosed CD for additional help and practice problems.

Intravenous Flow Rates

Linda K. Fluharty, MSN, RN

LEARNING OBJECTIVES

On completion of the materials provided in this chapter, you will be able to perform computations accurately by mastering the following mathematical concepts:

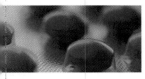

1 Calculating drops per minute (gtt/min) when given the total volume and time over which an IV solution or intravenous piggyback is to be infused

2 Calculating milliliters per hour (mL/h) when given the total volume and time over which an IV solution or intravenous piggyback is to be infused

It is sometimes necessary to deliver fluids and medications to a patient intravenously. Intravenous (IV) solutions and medications are placed directly into a vein. Infusions are injections of moderate to large quantities of fluids and nutrients into the patient's venous system. An IV medication or infusion may be prepared and administered by a physician, nurse, or technician as regulated by state law and the policies of the particular health care agency. Medications and electrolyte milliequivalents are commonly ordered as additives to IV fluids. Medications may also be diluted and given in conjunction with IV solutions.

IV fluids are administered via an IV infusion set. This set includes two parts: the sealed bottle or bag containing the fluids and the tubing. The tubing is made up of the following parts: a drip chamber connected to the bottle or bag by a small tube or spike, and tubing that leads from the drip chamber down to and connecting with the needle or catheter at the site of insertion into the patient (Figure 16-1). The flow rate is adjusted to the desired drops per minute by a clamp placed around the tubing. The nurse must be knowledgeable about the equipment being used and, in particular, about the flow rate, or drops per milliliter, that a particular set of tubing will deliver.

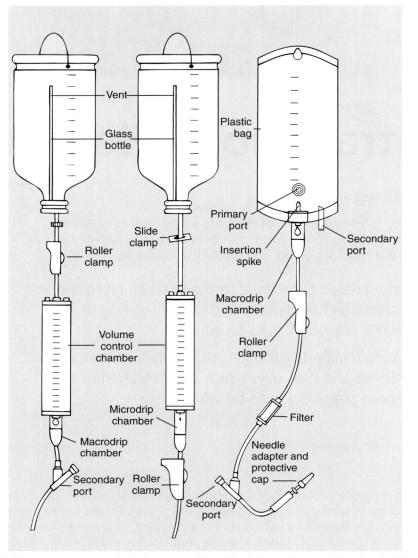

FIGURE 16-1 Intravenous infusion sets. (Modified from Clayton BD, Stock YN: *Basic pharmacology for nurses,* ed 13, St Louis, 2004, Mosby.)

Infusion sets come in a variety of sizes. The larger the diameter of the tubing where it enters the drip chamber, the bigger the drop will be. The **drop factor** of an infusion set is the number of drops contained in 1 mL. This equivalent may vary with different manufacturers. The most common drop factors are 10, 15, 20, and 60 drops/mL. Sets that deliver 10, 15, or 20 drops/mL are called *macrodrip sets*. A set that delivers 60 drops/mL is called *a microdrip set*. Macrodrip sets are larger than microdrip sets.

If large volumes of fluid must be administered (125 mL/h or more), a macrodrip set is required. Microdrip sets are unable to deliver large volumes per hour because their drop size is so small. When an IV solution is to run at a rate of 50 mL/h or less, a microdrip set should be used. Some hospitals may even require a microdrip set for rates of 60 to 80 mL/h, for accuracy of flow rate and to help maintain the patency of the line. The number of drops per milliliter for the IV administration set is written on the outside of the box. This information is essential for solving problems related to the regulation of IV flow rates (Figure 16-2).

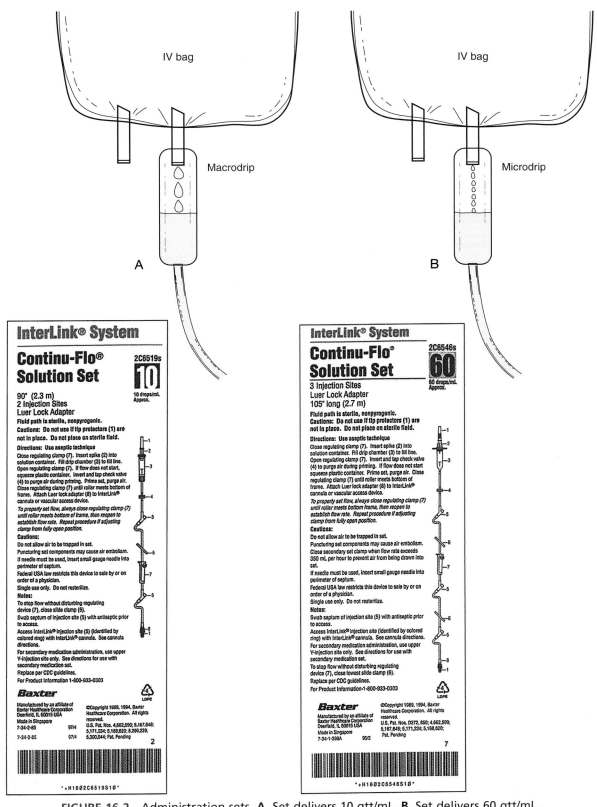

FIGURE 16-2 Administration sets. **A,** Set delivers 10 gtt/mL. **B,** Set delivers 60 gtt/mL. (Modified from Morris DG: *Calculate with confidence,* ed 4, St Louis, 2006, Mosby.)

The physician is responsible for writing the order for the type and amount of IV or hyperalimentation fluids. The number of hours the IV fluid will run or rate of infusion is also ordered by the physician. It is usually the nurse's responsibility to regulate and maintain the infusion flow rate. It is the nurse's goal to ensure that the IV flow is regular. If the rate is irregular, too much or too little fluid may be infused. This may lead to complications such as fluid overload, dehydration, or medication overdose. Sometimes the flow rate must be adjusted because of interruptions caused by needle placement, condition of the vein, or infiltration.

The nurse must be able to determine the number of drops per minute (gtt/min) the patient must receive for the infusion to be completed within the specified time.

When the volume, time or length of the infusion, and the constant drop factor are known, a simple formula can be used:

$$\frac{V \text{ (Volume)}}{T \text{ (Time)}} \times C \text{ (Constant drop factor)} = R \text{ (gtt/min)}$$

IV Administration of Fluids by Gravity

Example 1: Hespan 500 mL is ordered to be infused over 3 hours. The drop factor is 15 gtt/mL. How many drops per minute should be given to infuse the total amount of Hespan over 3 hours?

$$\text{The formula:} \frac{\text{Total volume to be infused}}{\text{Total amount of time in minutes}} \times \text{Drop factor} = x \text{ gtt/min}$$

a. Convert total hours to minutes.

1 h : 60 min :: 3 h : x min
$x = 180$

Therefore 3 hours equals 180 minutes.

b. Calculate gtt/min.

This calculation depends on the drop factor of the tubing being used. Remember, this information is found on the package. For the problems in this work text, the drop factor is indicated. The drop factor for this problem is 15.

$$\text{(Formula setup)} \quad \frac{500 \text{ mL}}{180 \text{ min}} \times \frac{15 \text{ gtt/mL}}{1} = x \text{ gtt/min}$$

$$\text{(Cancel)} \quad \frac{500 \cancel{\text{ mL}}}{\cancel{180} \text{ min}} \times \frac{\cancel{15} \text{ gtt/}\cancel{\text{mL}}}{1} = x \text{ gtt/min}$$
$$12$$

$$\text{(Calculate)} \quad \frac{500}{12 \text{ min}} \times \frac{1 \text{ gtt}}{1} = \frac{500}{12} = 41.6 \text{ or } 42 \text{ gtt/min}$$

Therefore the nurse will regulate the IV to drip at 42 drops/min, and the 500 mL of Hespan will be infused over 3 hours (Figure 16-3). Since the nurse cannot count a fraction of a drop, drops per minute are always rounded to a whole number.

Example 2: 1000 mL of dextrose 5% in water (D_5W) is ordered to be infused over 5 hours. The drop factor is 10 gtt/mL. How many drops per minute should be given to infuse the 1000 mL over 5 hours?

$$\text{The formula:} \frac{\text{Total volume to be infused}}{\text{Total amount of time in minutes}} \times \text{Drop factor} = x \text{ gtt/min}$$

$$\frac{V}{T} \times C = R$$

346 **CHAPTER 16** Intravenous Flow Rates

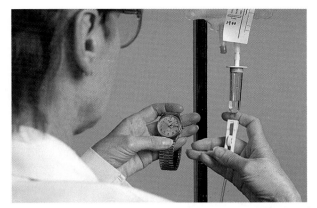

FIGURE 16-3 Count drops per minute by watching the drip chamber for 1 minute and adjusting the roller clamp as needed to deliver the desired number of drops per minute. (From Potter PA, Perry AG: *Fundamentals of nursing,* ed 6, St Louis, 2005, Mosby.)

    a. Convert the total hours to minutes.

$$1 \text{ h} : 60 \text{ min} :: 5 \text{ h} : x \text{ min}$$
$$x = 300$$

      Therefore 5 hours equals 300 minutes.

    b. Calculate gtt/min.

(Formula setup) $\dfrac{1000 \text{ mL}}{300 \text{ min}} \times \dfrac{10 \text{ gtt/mL}}{1} = x \text{ gtt/min}$

(Cancel) $\dfrac{1000 \cancel{\text{ mL}}}{\underset{30}{\cancel{300} \text{ min}}} \times \dfrac{\overset{1}{\cancel{10} \text{ gtt/}\cancel{\text{mL}}}}{} = x \text{ gtt/min}$

(Calculate) $\dfrac{1000}{30 \text{ min}} \times \dfrac{1 \text{ gtt}}{} = \dfrac{1000}{30} = 33.3 \text{ or } 33 \text{ gtt/min}$

The nurse will regulate the IV to drip at a rate of 33 gtt/min, and the 1000 mL of D_5W will be infused over 5 hours.

Infusion of IV Piggybacks by Gravity

Sometimes the physician will order medications to be administered in a small amount of IV fluid. This medication will need to be infused in addition to the regular IV fluids; it is called an *IV piggyback* (IVPB) because it is attached to the main IV tubing with shorter tubing of its own (Figure 16-4). The medication for the IVPB may be received premixed by the pharmacy or may need to be prepared by the nurse. The time frame for the IVPB infusion is usually 60 minutes or less.

If the physician does not include an infusion time or rate, it is the nurse's responsibility to follow the manufacturer's guidelines. The hospital pharmacy and drug books such as the *Hospital Formulary* and *A Handbook for Intravenous Medication* published by Mosby are known resources for fluid rates. The nurse should always refer to recommended fluid limits and rates before IVPB administration.

When the volume, time of infusion, and tubing drop factor are known, the same formula that was used for IV Administration of Fluids by Gravity is used to calculate the flow rate for the IVPB.

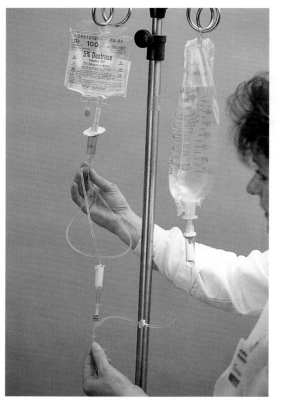

FIGURE 16-4   Tandem/intravenous piggyback (IVPB) administration setup. (From Potter PA, Perry AG: *Fundamentals of nursing,* ed 5, St Louis, 2001, Mosby.)

Example 1:   The physician orders cefuroxime 1 g in 50 mL of normal saline solution (NS) to be infused over 30 minutes. The tubing drop factor is 60 gtt/mL. How many drops per minute should be given to infuse the total amount of cefuroxime over 30 minutes?

$$\text{The formula:}\ \frac{\text{Total volume to be infused}}{\text{Total amount of time in minutes}} \times \text{Drop factor} = x\ \text{gtt/min}$$

Calculate gtt/min.

$$\text{(Formula setup)}\quad \frac{50\ \text{mL}}{30\ \text{min}} \times \frac{60\ \text{gtt/mL}}{} = x\ \text{gtt/min}$$

$$\text{(Cancel)}\quad \frac{50\ \cancel{\text{mL}}}{\cancel{30}\ \text{min}} \times \frac{\overset{2}{\cancel{60}}\ \text{gtt/}\cancel{\text{mL}}}{\underset{1}{}} = x\ \text{gtt/min}$$

$$\text{(Calculate)}\quad \frac{50}{1} \times 2 = 100\ \text{gtt/min}$$

Therefore the nurse will regulate the IVPB to drip at 100 gtt/min, and the cefuroxime will be infused over 30 minutes.

Example 2: The physician orders gentamicin 80 mg in 100 mL D$_5$W to be infused over 1 hour. The tubing drop factor is 60 gtt/mL. How many drops per minute should be given to infuse the gentamicin over 1 hour?

    a. Convert the total hours to minutes.

       1 h : 60 min

    b. Calculate the gtt/min.

$$\text{(Formula setup)} \qquad \frac{100 \text{ mL}}{60 \text{ min}} \times \frac{60 \text{ gtt/mL}}{} = x \text{ gtt/min}$$

$$\text{(Cancel)} \qquad \frac{100 \text{ mL}}{\underset{1}{\cancel{60}} \text{ min}} \times \frac{\overset{2}{\cancel{60}} \text{ gtt/}\cancel{\text{mL}}}{} = x \text{ gtt/min}$$

$$\text{(Calculate)} \qquad \frac{100}{1 \text{ min}} \times \frac{1 \text{ gtt}}{} = 100 \text{ gtt/min}$$

Therefore the nurse will regulate the IVPB to drip at 100 gtt/min, and the gentamicin will be infused over 1 hour.

NOTE: If the infusion time is 60 minutes and a microdrip set (drop factor of 60 gtt/mL) is used, the drops per minute will be the same as the number of milliliters per hour.

INFUSION OF IV BY PUMP

IV flow rates are often controlled by an electronic device or pump. The IV pumps are programmed to deliver a set amount of fluid per hour. Safety for the patient is an advantage of electronic IV pumps. The pumps are used for patients in regular medical-surgical units, critical care areas, pediatrics, the operating room, and ambulatory care settings.

Many electronic pumps are on the market today. These vary from simple one-channel models to four multichannel pumps. Many of the newer models actually calculate flow rates and automatically start infusions at a later time. Convenience, safety, accuracy, and time-saving options are driving forces in the innovations currently available.

Some examples of equipment are pictured in Figures 16-5 to 16-8; in Figure 16-6 the Medley Medication Safety System and the Medley pump module (attached to the programming module) are shown. In Figure 16-7 the Medley Medication Safety System is being used on a patient in a critical care setting. Each company offers tubing for use with its pumps.

Newer IV pumps, as pictured in Figures 16-6 and 16-8, contain software that allows each facility to program safeguard information for medications into the IV pump. If a health care professional programs a rate, dose, or duration that is considered to be unsafe, a visual or audible alert will sound. The safeguards are determined by the facility to prevent IV medication errors.

Intravenous Flow Rates **CHAPTER 16**   349

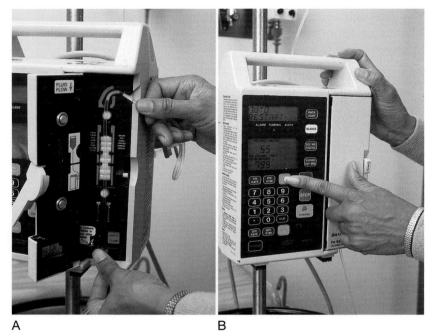

FIGURE 16-5 Single infusion pumps with decimal capability. **A,** Place infusing tubing within ridges of pump. **B,** Press start button to begin infusion. (From Potter PA, Perry AG: *Fundamentals of nursing,* ed 6, St Louis, 2005, Mosby.)

Infusion of IV Fluids with an IV Pump

In many facilities IV fluids are infused using an IV pump. IV pumps are programmed to infuse IV fluids by milliliters per hour (mL/h).

$$\text{The formula: } \frac{\text{Total volume in milliliters}}{\text{Total time in hours}} = x \text{ mL/h}$$

Example 1: Infuse 250 mL of 0.9% NS over 2 hours. How many milliliters per hour should the IV pump be programmed for to infuse 250 mL over 2 hours?

$$\text{The formula: } \frac{\text{Total volume in milliliters}}{\text{Time in hours}} = x \text{ mL/h}$$

Calculate mL/h.

$$(\text{Formula setup}) \quad \frac{250 \text{ mL}}{2 \text{ h}} = 125 \text{ mL/h}$$

Therefore the nurse will program the IV pump for 125 mL/h, and the 250 mL of NS will be infused over 2 hours.

Example 2: Infuse 1000 mL of lactated Ringer's solution (LR) over 12 hours. How many mL/h should the IV pump be programmed for?

Calculate mL/h.

$$(\text{Formula setup}) \quad \frac{1000 \text{ mL}}{12 \text{ h}} = 83.3 \text{ or } 83 \text{ mL/h}$$

Therefore the nurse will program the IV pump for 83 mL/h, and the 1000 mL of LR will be infused over 12 hours.

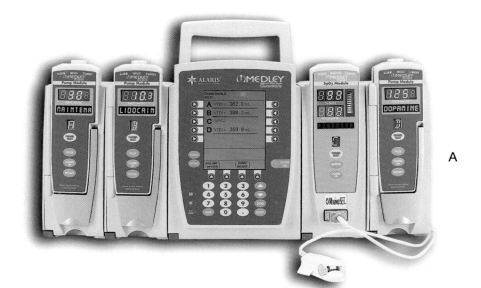

A

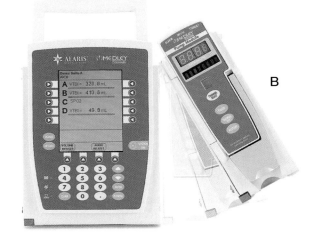

FIGURE 16-6 A, Medley™ Medication Safety System. **B,** Example of the Medley™ pump module attached to the Medley programming module. (From ALARIS Medical Systems, Inc., San Diego, CA.)

B

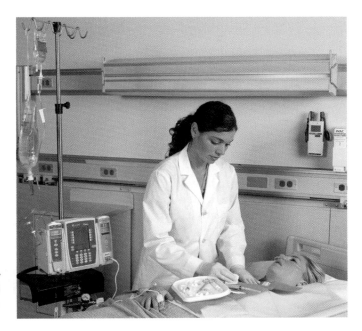

FIGURE 16-7 Medley™ Medication Safety System being used on a patient in a critical care setting. (From ALARIS Medical Systems, Inc., San Diego, CA.)

Intravenous Flow Rates **CHAPTER 16**   351

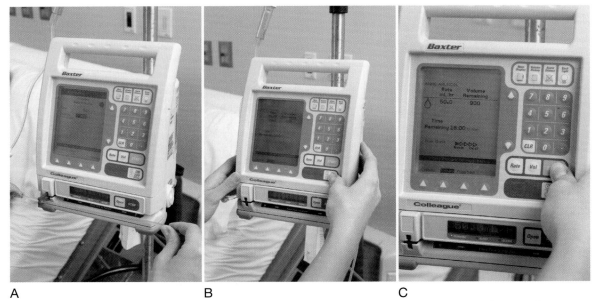

A   B   C

FIGURE 16-8 Baxter infusion pump. **A,** Insert IV tubing into chamber of control mechanism. **B,** Select rate and volume to be infused. **C,** Press start button. (From Elkin MK, Perry PA, Potter AG: *Nursing interventions and clinical skills,* ed 3, St Louis, 2004, Mosby.)

Infusion of IV Medications with an IV Pump

In some situations the health care professional will be required to infuse medications using an IV pump. Whether the medication is an electrolyte replacement, an antiinfective agent, or another type of medication to be infused by IVPB, the health care professional needs to calculate the rate, in milliliters per hour, for which the IV pump should be programmed.

Example 1:   Dilute potassium 40 mEq in 250 mL of D_5W and administer IV now. The facility's policy states to infuse potassium at a rate of 10 mEq/h. How many milliliters per hour should the IV pump be programmed for to infuse the potassium at a rate of 10 mEq/h?

Using the ratio-proportion method:

Calculate mL/h.

(Formula setup) $40 \text{ mEq} : 250 \text{ mL} :: 10 \text{ mEq} : x \text{ mL}$

(Calculate) $40x = 2500$

$$x = \frac{2500}{40}$$

$$x = 62.5 \text{ or } 63 \text{ mL}$$

Therefore the nurse will program the IV pump for 63 mL/h, and the potassium will be infused at 10 mEq/h as stated in the facility's policy. (NOTE: Follow your facility's policy when you calculate the rate for any electrolyte replacement.)

Using the $\dfrac{D}{A} \times Q = x$ mL/h method:

Calculate mL/h.

(Formula setup) $\dfrac{10 \text{ mEq}}{40 \text{ mEq}} \times 250 \text{ mL} = x \text{ mL}$

(Cancel) $\dfrac{\overset{1}{\cancel{10 \text{ mEq}}}}{\underset{4}{\cancel{40 \text{ mEq}}}} \times 250 \text{ mL} = x \text{ mL}$

(Calculate) $\dfrac{1}{4} \times 250 \text{ mL} = \dfrac{250}{4} = 62.5 \text{ or } 63 \text{ mL/h}$

Example 2: Administer 1 g of vancomycin over 60 minutes. The vancomycin is dissolved in 100 mL of D_5W. How many milliliters per hour should the IV pump be programmed for?

The formula: $\dfrac{\text{Total volume in milliliters}}{\text{Total time in hours}} = x \text{ mL/h}$

a. Convert minutes to hours.

60 min : 1 h

b. Calculate mL/h.

(Formula setup) $\dfrac{100 \text{ mL}}{1 \text{ h}} = 100 \text{ mL/h}$

The nurse will program the IV pump for 100 mL/h, and the 100 mL of vancomycin will be infused over 1 hour (60 minutes).

Example 3: The physician orders Kefzol 1 g dissolved in 50 mL of D_5W to be infused over 30 minutes. The IVPB may be given using an IV pump. How many milliliters per hour should the IV pump be programmed for to infuse the Kefzol over 30 minutes?

a. Convert minutes to hours.

1 h : 60 min :: x h : 30 min

$60x = 30$

$x = \dfrac{30}{60} = 0.5 \text{ h}$

b. Calculate mL/h.

(Formula setup) $\dfrac{50 \text{ mL}}{0.5 \text{ h}} = 100 \text{ mL/h}$

Saline and Heparin Locks

Saline and heparin locks are commonly used in a variety of health care settings. A saline lock is an IV catheter that is inserted into a peripheral vein. It may be used for medications or fluids, usually on an intermittent basis. The use of a saline lock prevents the patient from having to endure numerous venipunctures. Also, when fluid is not being infused, the patient enjoys greater mobility and freedom of movement. Each institution will have its own policy concerning the use and care of saline locks. The locks may be flushed with 2 to 3 mL of normal saline solution (Figures 16-9 and 16-10). Central line ports that are not being used for fluid or medication

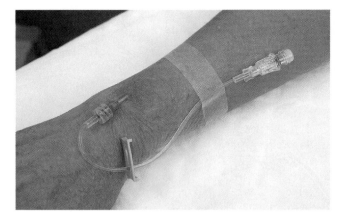

FIGURE 16-9   Example of a saline lock. (From Potter PA, Perry AG: *Fundamentals of nursing*, ed 6, St Louis, 2005, Mosby.)

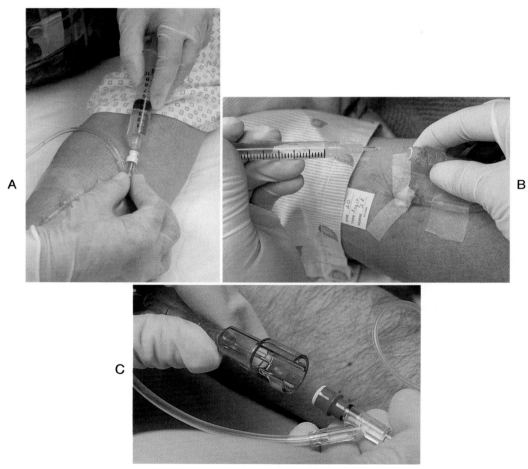

FIGURE 16-10   **A to C,** Examples of needleless systems used within intravenous lines. (From Elkin MK, Perry PA, Potter AG: *Nursing interventions and clinical skills*, ed 3, St Louis, 2004, Mosby.)

administration are heparin locks. The locks will be flushed with a heparin flush solution of 10 units of heparin per 1 mL. This practice is called *heparinization*, and it prevents clotting of the heparin lock.

Central Venous Catheters

Occasionally, a patient will need a central venous catheter. Central venous catheters are indwelling, semipermanent central lines that are inserted into the right atrium of the heart via the cephalic, subclavian, or jugular vein (Figure 16-11).

This type of catheter may be required for clients who need frequent venipuncture, long-term IV infusions, hyperalimentation, chemotherapy, intermittent blood transfusions, or antibiotics. These catheters may be referred to as *triple lumen catheters* or *Hickman lines*.

Central venous catheter management involves flushing the catheter with 2.5 mL of heparin (10 units/mL) when the catheter access is routinely capped or clamped after blood draws. Please consult your institution's procedure or policy guidelines about central venous line flushes. If continuous fluids are ordered, these fluids **must** be regulated via an infusion pump. All central venous catheter management must be done under the supervision of a registered nurse.

The central venous catheter site must be assessed regularly. The catheter site should always remain sterile under an occlusive dressing that is changed according to the institution's procedure regarding central venous catheters.

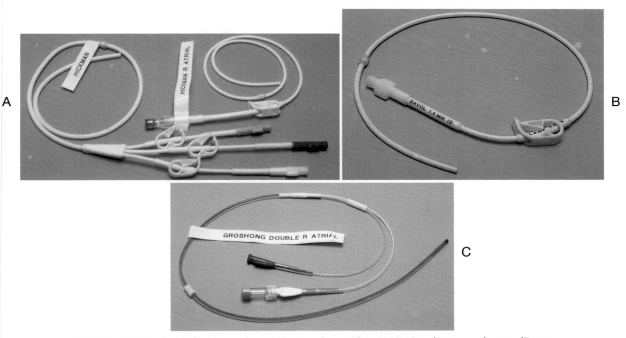

FIGURE 16-11   A, Hickman catheter. **B,** Broviac catheter. **C,** Groshong catheter. (From Clayton BD, Stock YN: *Basic pharmacology for nurses,* ed 13, St Louis, 2004, Mosby. Courtesy Chuck Dresner.)

Patient-Controlled Analgesia

Patient-controlled analgesia (PCA) or a PCA pump involves patients giving themselves an IV narcotic by pressing a button. This IV narcotic is given at intervals via an infusion pump (Figure 16-12). Only a registered nurse can be accountable for dispensing analgesia to be given in this manner. In addition, only a registered nurse can administer a PCA loading dose. For safety, most institutions now require that two registered nurses verify the PCA drug, dosage, and rate programmed into the machine.

Several considerations are crucial in the administration of PCA. IV narcotics may cause depressed respirations, hypotension, sedation, dizziness, and nausea or vomiting in the patient. The patient must not be allergic to the narcotic, must be able to understand and comply with instructions, and must have a desire to use the PCA, since *only* the patient can press the button to dispense the dose. The materials needed for infusion include a PCA pump, PCA tubing, a PCA pump key, a narcotic injector vial, and maintenance IV fluids through which the IV narcotic will be infused.

Example 1:   The physician orders morphine sulfate 1 mg every 10 minutes to a maximum of 30 mg in 4 hours. Morphine concentration is 1 mg/mL per 30-mL injector vial. What is the pump setting?

1 mg/10 min, 4-hour limit, is 30 mg

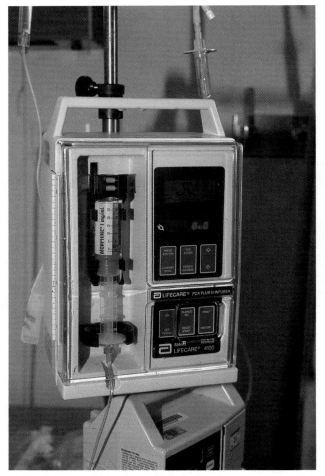

FIGURE 16-12   Patient-controlled analgesia infusion pump. (From Elkin MK, Perry PA, Potter AG: *Nursing interventions and clinical skills,* ed 3, St Louis, 2004, Mosby.)

Example 2: The physician orders hydromorphone 0.2 mg every 15 minutes to a maximum of 2 mg in 4 hours. Hydromorphone concentration is 1 mg/mL per 30-mL injector vial. What is the pump setting?

0.2 mg/15 min, 4-hour limit, is 2 mg

Complete the following work sheet, which provides for practice in the calculation of IV solutions and IVPB by either the IV pump or gravity. Check your answers. If you have difficulties, go back and review the necessary material. When you feel ready to evaluate your learning, take the first posttest. Check your answers. An acceptable score as indicated on the posttest signifies that you have successfully completed the chapter. An unacceptable score signifies a need for further study before taking the second posttest.

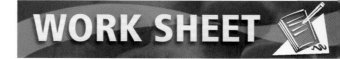

Directions: The IV fluid or medication order is listed in each problem. Calculate the IV flow rates using the appropriate formula. Show your work. Follow your instructor's rules on rounding final answers.

1. The physician orders 500 mL of dextran to be infused over 24 hours. How many milliliters per hour should the IV pump be programmed for? _____

2. A patient with genital herpes has an order for acyclovir 400 mg IVPB q8 h. The acyclovir is dissolved in 100 mL 0.9% NS and is to be infused over 1 hour. How many milliliters per hour should the IV pump be programmed for? _____

3. Amikacin 80 mg is ordered IVPB q12 h. The amikacin is dissolved in 100 mL D_5W and is to be infused over 30 minutes. With a tubing drop factor of 15 gtt/mL, how many drops per minute should be given? _____

4. 3000 mL of total parenteral nutrition (TPN) is ordered to be infused from 1900 to 0700. How many milliliters per hour should the IV pump be programmed for? _____

5. Mr. McCane, who has peptic ulcer disease, has Pepcid 20 mg in 100 mL D_5W ordered q12 h. The Pepcid is to be infused over 30 minutes. With a tubing drop factor of 10 gtt/mL, how many drops per minute should be given? _____

6. A malnourished patient has an order for 500 mL of Intralipid 10% to be infused over 6 hours. How many milliliters per hour should the IV pump be programmed for? _____

7. An order is received to infuse penicillin G 4,000,000 units in 100 mL of D_5W q12 h. The tubing drop factor is 10 gtt/mL. The penicillin should be infused over 60 minutes. How many drops per minute should be given? _____

8. Mrs. Ruiz has hypokalemia. The physician orders potassium 60 mEq in 250 mL of D_5W. The facility's policy states to infuse the potassium at 20 mEq/h. How many milliliters per hour should the IV pump be programmed for? _____

9. A postoperative patient has Kefzol 1 g ordered q8 h. The Kefzol is dissolved in 50 mL of D_5W and is to be infused over 30 minutes. The tubing drop factor is 60 gtt/mL. How many drops per minute should be given? _____

10. A postoperative patient has an order for 1000 mL of D_5LR over 10 hours. How many milliliters per hour should the IV pump be programmed for? _____

11. Mrs. England has sepsis and has an order for Kefzol 1 g in 50 mL of D$_5$W IVPB over 15 minutes. The drop factor is 60 gtt/mL. How many drops per minute should be given? _____

12. A patient with a methicillin-resistant *Staphylococcus aureus* infection has Cipro 400 mg in 200 mL D$_5$W ordered. The pharmacy recommends that the Cipro be infused at a rate of 200 mg/h with an IV pump. How many milliliters per hour should the IV pump be programmed for? _____

13. A patient with anuria has an order for 1000 mL of 0.9% NS to be infused over 1 hour. The tubing drop factor is 10 gtt/mL. How many drops per minute should be given? _____

14. After his operation Mr. Chambers has an order for 1000 mL of D$_5$W 0.45 NS with 20 mEq of potassium to be infused over 8 hours. How many milliliters per hour should the IV pump be programmed for? _____

15. After a total hip replacement, a patient has an order for Toradol 60 mg IVPB q6 h over 15 minutes. The Toradol is diluted in 25 mL of D$_5$W. The tubing drop factor is 15 gtt/mL. How many drops per minute should be given? _____

16. A terminal patient has an order for Dilaudid at 0.5 mg/h by continuous drip. Given a bag with a concentration of 20 mg Dilaudid in 100 mL of D_5W, how many milliliters per hour should the IV pump be programmed for? _____

17. A patient with peptic ulcer disease has an order for Pepcid 20 mg IVPB q12 h over 15 minutes. The Pepcid is diluted in 25 mL of D_5W. The tubing drop factor is 20 gtt/mL. How many drops per minute should be given? _____

18. Mr. Russell, who has alcoholism, has an order for magnesium sulfate 2 g in 100 mL of D_5W. The pharmacy recommends that the magnesium be infused at a rate of 1 g/h with an IV pump. How many milliliters per hour should the IV pump be programmed for? _____

19. A patient with aplastic anemia has an order for 1 unit of packed red blood cells (250 mL) to be infused. The facility's policy states to infuse the blood over 4 hours. The tubing drop factor is 20 gtt/mL. How many drops per minute should be given? _____

20. Ms. Tung has an order for 500 mL of 0.9% NS IV over 4 hours for oliguria. The drop factor is 10 gtt/mL. How many drops per minute should be given? _____

21. A patient with hypokalemia has an order for 40 mEq of potassium to be infused IV now. The potassium is diluted in 200 mL of D_5W. The facility's policy states to infuse IV potassium at a rate of 10 mEq/h. How many milliliters per hour should the IV pump be programmed for? _____

22. A patient with Crohn's disease has an order for TPN from 2200 to 0800. The total volume of the TPN bag is 1350 mL. How many milliliters per hour should the IV pump be programmed for? _____

23. Mr. Goldberg, who has hypomagnesemia, receives an order for magnesium sulfate 2 g in 50 mL D_5W IV. The pharmacist recommends that the magnesium be infused at 1 g/h. How many milliliters per hour should the IV pump be programmed for? _____

24. An immunosuppressed patient with herpes simplex virus 1 has acyclovir 700 mg in 200 mL of D_5W ordered to infuse over 1 hour. How many milliliters per hour should the IV pump be programmed for? _____

25. A patient with anasarca has albumin 25% 50 mL ordered over 30 minutes. The tubing drop factor is 20 gtt/mL. How many drops per minute should be given? _____

26. After the patient in question 25 receives her albumin, the physician orders Lasix 100 mg in 50 mL of D$_5$W to be given over 30 minutes. How many milliliters per hour should the IV pump be set for? _____

27. A patient with multiple antibiotic allergies has a urinary tract infection. Amikacin 250 mg IVPB q8 h is ordered over 1 hour. The amikacin is dissolved in 200 mL of D$_5$W. The drop factor is 20 gtt/mL. How many drops per minute should be given? _____

28. After an operation Mrs. Avery is hemorrhaging and has Amicar 8 g over 8 hours ordered. The Amicar is diluted in 500 mL of 0.9% NS. How many milliliters per hour should the IV pump be set for? _____

29. A patient with rapid atrial flutter has an order for Cardizem at 5 mg/hr. The Cardizem concentration is 200 mg in 250 mL of 0.9% NS. How many milliliters per hour should the IV pump be set for? _____

30. A malnourished patient has folic acid 1 mg in 50 mL of 0.9% NS ordered to infuse over 30 minutes. An IV pump is not available. The nurse chooses a tubing with a 60 gtt/mL drop factor. How many drops per minute should be given? _____

31. Vancomycin 1250 mg in 250 mL of D$_5$W is ordered to infuse over 2 hours. How many milliliters per hour should the IV pump be set for? _____

32. A patient has a blood urea nitrogen of 52 with oliguria and a blood pressure of 90/50 mm Hg. The physician orders 1000 mL of 0.9% NS to be infused over 10 hours. How many milliliters per hour should the IV pump infuse? _____

33. Using the Parkland formula, the fluid requirements for a severe burn patient reveal that 9600 mL should be infused over 8 hours. How many milliliters per hour should the IV pump be set for? _____

34. Mr. Cortez has IV immunoglobulin G (IgG) 100 mL ordered over 3 hours. How many milliliters per hour should the IV pump be set for? _____

35. A patient with rapid atrial fibrillation has an order for diltiazem at 20 mg/hr. The diltiazem concentration is 100 mg in 100 mL of 0.9% NS. How many milliliters per hour should the IV pump be set for? _____

36. A stat dose of Zosyn 3.375 mg in 100 mL of 0.9% NS is ordered to be given over 15 minutes. How many milliliters per hour should the nurse program the IV pump for? _____

Answers on pp. 554–556.

Name _____

Date _____

ACCEPTABLE SCORE ___14___

YOUR SCORE _____

POSTTEST 1

Directions: The IV fluid order is listed in the problem. Calculate the appropriate infusion rate for each problem. Follow your instructor's rules on rounding final answers.

1. A patient with hypotension has an order for 500 mL of Plasmanate to be infused over 2 hours. How many milliliters per hour should the IV pump be programmed for? _____

2. An order is received to infuse amphotericin B 240 mg in 500 mL D_5W over 4 hours. How many milliliters per hour should the IV pump be programmed for? _____

3. An NPO patient has an order for 0.9% NS at 120 mL/h. The drop factor is 12 gtt/mL. How many drops per minute should be given? _____

4. A postpartum patient is to receive 1500 mL of LR over the next 8 hours. How many milliliters per hour should the IV pump be programmed for? _____

5. After a burn injury Mr. Warren is to receive 500 mL of blood plasma over 4 hours. The tubing drop factor is 15 gtt/mL. How many drops per minute should be given? _____

6. A patient is admitted with pernicious anemia. The physician orders a unit of packed red blood cells (250 mL) to be infused over 3 hours. The tubing drop factor is 12 gtt/mL. How many drops per minute should be given? _____

7. Ms. Chandar has an order for 500 mL of LR over 6 hours. The tubing drop factor is 15 gtt/mL. How many drops per minute should be given? _____

8. A patient with hypomagnesemia has an order for infusion of magnesium sulfate 4 g diluted in 250 mL D_5W. Policy states that the magnesium be infused at a rate of 2 g/h. How many milliliters per hour should the IV pump be programmed for? _____

9. Mr. Simpson has an order for NS to be infused at 150 mL/h after a transesophageal echocardiogram. The tubing drop factor is 60 gtt/mL. How many drops per minute should be given? _____

10. A patient has an order for 2500 mL of TPN to be infused over 24 hours. How many milliliters per hour should the IV pump be programmed for? _____

11. A patient with hypokalemia and hypophosphatemia has an order for potassium phosphate 30 milliosmole in 200 mL of 0.9% NS IV. The facility's policy states to infuse the potassium phosphate at 10 mMos/h. How many milliliters per hour should the IV pump be programmed for? _____

12. A postoperative patient has an order for ceftazidime 1 g in 25 mL of D$_5$W over 15 minutes. The tubing drop factor is 60 gtt/mL. How many drops per minute should be given? _____

13. Mr. Anderson has metastatic cancer. The physician orders morphine sulfate 15 mg/h IV. Given a bag with a concentration of 100 mg of morphine sulfate in 200 mL of D$_5$W, how many milliliters per hour should the IV pump be programmed for? _____

14. A patient with a methicillin-resistant *S. aureus* infection has an order for vancomycin 1.5 g in 200 mL of D$_5$W IVPB q12 h. The physician orders the vancomycin to be infused over 4 hours. How many milliliters per hour should the IV pump be programmed for? _____

15. Mrs. Marx, who has sepsis, has an order for Timentin 3.1 g in 100 mL of D$_5$W IVPB over 1 hour. The drop factor is 60 gtt/mL. How many drops per minute should be given?

Answers on pp. 557–558.

Name _____

Date _____

ACCEPTABLE SCORE __14__

YOUR SCORE _____

POSTTEST 2

Directions: The IV fluid order is listed in each problem. Calculate the appropriate infusion rate for each problem. Follow your instructor's rules on rounding final answers.

1. A patient with poor wound healing has ascorbic acid 300 mg in 200 mL of 0.9% NS ordered to be infused over 6 hours. How many milliliters per hour should the IV pump be programmed for? _____

2. Cefoxitin 2 g q8 h IVPB is ordered for Mrs. Graham, who has osteomyelitis. The cefoxitin is dissolved in 50 mL of D_5W and is to be infused over 30 minutes. The tubing drop factor is 10 gtt/mL. How many drops per minute should be given? _____

3. A patient with iron-deficiency anemia has an order for iron dextran 100 mg in 200 mL of 0.9% NS over 6 hours. How many milliliters per hour should the IV pump be programmed for? _____

4. Mr. Sanchez has hypotension and receives an order for 500 mL of 0.9% NS over 3 hours. The tubing drop factor is 10 gtt/mL. How many drops per minute should be given? _____

5. Your patient with a gastrointestinal bleed has an order for 1 unit of whole blood (500 mL) to be given over 3 hours. The tubing drop factor is 15 gtt/mL. How many drops per minute should be given? _____

6. An order for a patient with hypocalcemia states to infuse 1 g of calcium chloride 10% over 30 minutes. The calcium chloride is diluted in 50 mL of 0.9% NS. How many milliliters per hour should the IV pump be programmed for? _____

7. A terminal patient has morphine sulfate ordered at 8 mg/h. The medication concentration is morphine 100 mg diluted in 100 mL of D_5W. How many milliliters per hour should the IV pump be programmed for? _____

8. Mrs. Watkins, who has undergone hip replacement, has an order for Toradol 30 mg q6 h. The Toradol is diluted in 50 mL of 0.9% NS and is to be infused over 15 minutes. The tubing drop factor is 60 gtt/mL. How many drops per minute should be given? _____

9. A patient with severe nausea and vomiting has a one-time order for Zofran 8 mg IVPB over 15 minutes. The Zofran is diluted in 50 mL of D_5W. The tubing drop factor is 15 gtt/mL. How many drops per minute should be given? _____

10. A postoperative patient has an order for 1000 mL of LR over 6 hours. How many milliliters per hour should the IV pump be programmed for? _____

11. Mr. Nakamura experiences bradypnea after intrathecal administration of anesthesia. An order for Narcan 0.4 mg/h is written. Given a bag with a concentration of 8 mg in 100 mL of 0.9% NS, how many milliliters per hour should the IV pump be programmed for? _____

12. A patient with a total gastrectomy has TPN ordered to be infused from 2200 to 0600. The total volume of the TPN bag is 1200 mL. How many milliliters per hour should the IV pump be programmed for? _____

13. A postoperative patient has an order for Kefzol 1 g in 25 mL of D₅W over 15 minutes. The medication will be infused with an IV pump. How many milliliters per hour should the IV pump be programmed for? _____

14. Ms. Pailey has oliguria and receives an order for 1000 mL of 0.9% NS over 3 hours. The tubing drop factor is 10 gtt/mL. How many drops per minute should be given? _____

15. An NPO patient has an order for 1000 mL of D₅W 0.45% NS with 30 mEq of potassium over 12 hours. How many milliliters per hour should the IV pump be programmed for?

Answers on pp. 558–559.

Refer to Advanced Calculations: Intravenous Calculations and Patient-Controlled Analgesia on the enclosed CD for additional help and practice problems.

Critical Care Intravenous Flow Rates

Linda K. Fluharty, MSN, RN

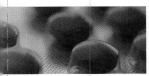

LEARNING OBJECTIVES

On completion of the materials provided in this chapter, you will be able to perform computations accurately by mastering the following mathematical concepts:

1 Calculating the IV flow rate of medications in units per kilogram per hour or international units per hour

2 Calculating the IV flow rate of medications in units per kilogram per hour (weight-based heparin)

3 Calculating the IV flow rate of medications in milligrams per minute

4 Calculating the IV flow rate of medications in micrograms per minute

5 Calculating the IV flow rate of medications in micrograms per kilogram per minute

6 Calculating the milligrams per minute of medications from the IV flow rate

7 Calculating the micrograms per minute of medications from the IV flow rate

8 Calculating the micrograms per kilogram per minute of medications from the IV flow rate

Critically ill patients in a hospital often receive special medications that are very potent and therefore need to be monitored closely. Some of these medications, such as regular insulin or heparin, may be ordered as a set amount of the drug measured in units to be infused over a given period. Other drugs used in the critical care setting may be ordered to be infused by amount of drug per kilogram of body weight per minute. These are called **titrations.** They are based on the manufacturer's provided recommended dosage and the patient's body weight measured in kilograms. In most health care institutions, these situations will occur in the emergency department, an intensive care unit, or a step-down unit. It is extremely important to accurately monitor the flow of these medications; therefore an intravenous (IV) machine is required. Because of the nature of these drugs, route of administration, and state of the patient, the importance of accuracy in calculating the drug dosage and IV flow rates cannot be overemphasized. It is truly a matter of life and death.

The following sections focus on medications that are ordered by units per hour, international units per hour, micrograms per kilogram per minute (mcg/kg/min), micrograms per minute (mcg/min), and milligrams per minute (mg/min). All the following medications *must* be delivered with an IV controller or pump for safe administration. Since infusion pumps are set by milliliters per hour (mL/h), the health care provider needs to be familiar with the steps to convert the ordered drug dosage to milliliters per hour.

Facilities that administer medications with a hemodynamic effect usually have IV controllers that allow the health care professional to program medication rates with a decimal. Therefore answers should be **rounded to the nearest tenth decimal place.**

IV Administration of Medications by Units/Hour or International Units/Hour

Example 1:   200 units of regular insulin have been added to 500 mL of 0.9% normal saline (NS). The order states to infuse the regular insulin IV at 10 units/h. The nurse needs to calculate how many milliliters per hour the IV pump should be programmed for.

Using the Ratio-Proportion Method

(Formula setup)   200 units : 500 mL :: 10 units : x mL

$$200x = 5000$$

$$x = \frac{5000}{200}$$

$$x = \frac{25}{1}$$

$$x = 25 \text{ mL}$$

Therefore the nurse will program the IV pump for 25 mL/h to infuse the insulin at 10 units/h.

Using the $\frac{D}{A} \times Q$ Method

(Formula setup) $\dfrac{10 \text{ units}}{200 \text{ units}} \times 500 \text{ mL} = x \text{ mL}$

(Cancel) $\dfrac{10 \text{ units}}{\underset{2}{200 \text{ units}}} \times \overset{5}{500} \text{ mL} = x \text{ mL}$

(Calculate) $\dfrac{50}{2} = 25 \text{ mL}$

CHAPTER 17 Critical Care Intravenous Flow Rates

Example 2: 25,000 units of heparin have been added to 250 mL of dextrose 5% in water (D_5W). The order is to infuse the heparin drip at 2000 units/h. The health care provider needs to calculate how many milliliters per hour to program the IV pump for.

Using the Ratio-Proportion Method

(Formula setup)   25,000 units : 250 mL :: 2000 units : x mL

$$25,000x = 500,000$$

$$\frac{\cancel{25,000}x}{\cancel{25,000}} = \frac{500,\cancel{000}}{25,\cancel{000}}$$

$$x = \frac{500}{25}$$

$$x = 20 \text{ mL}$$

Therefore the nurse will program the IV pump for 20 mL/h to deliver the heparin at 2000 units/h.

Using the $\dfrac{D}{A} \times Q$ Method

(Formula setup) $\dfrac{2000 \text{ units}}{25,000 \text{ units}} \times 250 \text{ mL} = x \text{ mL}$

(Cancel) $\dfrac{2000 \text{ }\cancel{units}}{\underset{100}{\cancel{25,000} \text{ }\cancel{units}}} \times \overset{1}{\cancel{250}} \text{ mL} = x \text{ mL}$

(Calculate) $\dfrac{2000 \text{ mL}}{100} = 20 \text{ mL}$

IV ADMINISTRATION OF WEIGHT-BASED HEPARIN

Many facilities order heparin for a patient based on the patient's weight. The rationale behind this is that a patient who weighs 50 kg requires a different dose of heparin than the patient who weighs 100 kg to achieve a therapeutic dose. Weight-based heparin orders require two calculations: (1) the calculation for the heparin IV bolus and (2) the calculation for the heparin drip in milliliters per hour.

Weight-Based Heparin Protocol (Example)

1. Bolus dose of 70 units/kg, rounded to the nearest 100 units (e.g., 6850 units would be rounded to 6900 units).
2. Begin infusion of heparin at 17 units/kg/h (25,000 units/250 mL = 100 units/mL).
3. Obtain partial thromboplastin time (PTT) every 6 hours and adjust the infusion using the following scale:

PTT Result	Heparin Dosing
<35	Bolus 70 units/kg and increase drip by 4 units/kg/h
35-54	Bolus 35 units/kg and increase drip by 3 units/kg/h
55-85	Therapeutic—no change
86-100	Decrease drip by 2 units/kg/h
>100	Hold infusion 1 hour; decrease drip by 3 units/kg/h, then restart drip

Example: The order is to start a heparin infusion using the heparin protocol. The patient's weight is 143 lb. The nurse needs to do two calculations: the heparin bolus and the rate, in milliliters per hour, at which to program the IV pump.

Bolus. The protocol calls for 70 units/kg, rounded to the nearest hundredth.

    a. Convert pounds to kilograms.

      (Formula setup)   2.2 lb : 1 kg :: 143 lb : x kg

$$2.2x = 143$$

$$\frac{2.2x}{2.2} = \frac{143}{2.2}$$

$$x = 65 \text{ kg}$$

    b. Calculate the units required for the IV bolus.

      (Formula setup)   1 kg : 70 units :: 65 kg : x units

$$x = 70 \times 65$$

$$x = 4550 \text{ or } 4600 \text{ units IV bolus}$$

IV Infusion. The protocol states 17 units/kg/h, rounded to the nearest tenth.

    a. Calculate how many units are needed for a patient weighing 65 kg.

      (Formula setup)   1 kg : 17 units/h :: 65 kg : x units/h

$$x = 17 \times 65$$

$$x = 1105 \text{ units/h are required for a 65-kg patient}$$

    b. Calculate mL/hr for the IV pump

Using the Ratio-Proportion Method

    (Formula setup)   100 units : 1 mL :: 1105 units : x mL

$$100x = 1105$$

$$\frac{100x}{100} = \frac{1105}{100}$$

$$x = 11.05 \text{ or } 11.1 \text{ mL/h (rounded to the nearest tenth)}$$

Therefore the nurse will set the IV pump for 11.1 mL/h to infuse the heparin at 17 units/kg/h.

Using $\frac{D}{A} \times Q$ Method

    (Formula setup) $\dfrac{1105 \text{ units}}{100 \text{ units}} \times 1 \text{ mL} = x \text{ mL}$

    (Cancel) $\dfrac{1105 \ \cancel{\text{units}}}{100 \ \cancel{\text{units}}} \times 1 \text{ mL} = x \text{ mL}$

    (Calculate) $\dfrac{1105}{100} = 11.05 \text{ or } 11.1 \text{ mL/h (rounded to the nearest tenth)}$

IV Administration of Medications by Milligram/Minute

Example: Lidocaine 1 g has been added to 500 mL of D_5W. The order states to infuse the lidocaine at 2 mg/min. The nurse needs to calculate the rate, in milliliters per hour, at which to set the IV pump.

$$\text{The formula:} \quad \frac{\text{Desired mg/min} \times 60 \text{ min/h}^*}{\text{Medication concentration (mg/mL)}}$$

*60 min/h is a constant fraction in the formula and represents the equivalency of 60 min = 1 h.

When this formula is used, the answer will always be expressed in milliliters per hour because the pair of values in milligrams will cancel each other, as will the pair of values in minutes.

    a. Convert total g in the IV bag to mg.

$$1 \text{ g} = 1000 \text{ mg}$$

    b. Calculate mL/h.

(Formula setup) $\quad \dfrac{2 \text{ mg/min} \times 60 \text{ min/h}}{2 \text{ mg/mL}} = x \text{ mL/h}$

(Cancel) $\quad \dfrac{\overset{1}{\cancel{2}} \text{ mg/min} \times 60 \text{ min/h}}{\underset{1}{\cancel{2}} \text{ mg/mL}} = x \text{ mL/h}$

(Calculate) $\quad \dfrac{1 \times 60}{1} = 60 \text{ mL/h}$

IV Administration of Medications by Microgram/Minute

Example: 50 mg of nitroglycerin has been added to 500 mL of 0.9% NS. The order is to infuse the nitroglycerin at 5 mcg/min. The nurse needs to calculate the rate, in milliliters per hour, at which to set the IV pump.

$$\text{The formula:} \quad \frac{\text{Ordered mcg/min} \times 60 \text{ min/h}}{\text{Medication concentration (mcg/mL)}}$$

When this formula is used, the answer will always be expressed in milliliters per hour because the pair of values in milligrams will cancel each other, as will the pair of values in minutes.

    a. Convert total mg in the IV bag to mcg.

$$1 \text{ mg} : 1000 \text{ mcg} :: 50 \text{ mg} : x \text{ mcg}$$

$$x = 50,000 \text{ mcg}$$

    b. Calculate the concentration (mcg/mL) by dividing the total mcg by the total amount of fluid in the IV bag.

$$\frac{50,000 \text{ mcg}}{500 \text{ mL}} = 100 \text{ mcg/mL}$$

c. Calculate the mL/h.

(Formula setup) $\dfrac{5\ \text{mcg/min} \times 60\ \text{min/h}}{100\ \text{mcg/mL}} = x\ \text{mL/h}$

(Cancel) $\dfrac{\overset{1}{\cancel{5\ \text{mcg/min}}} \times 60\ \cancel{\text{min/h}}}{\underset{20}{\cancel{100\ \text{mcg/mL}}}} = x\ \text{mL/h}$

(Calculate) $\dfrac{1 \times 60}{20} = \dfrac{60}{20} = 3\ \text{mL/h}$

IV Administration of Medications by Microgram/Kilogram/Minute

Example: 800 mg of dopamine is added to 250 mL of 0.9% NS. The order is to begin the infusion at 3 mcg/kg/min. The patient's weight is 70 kg. The nurse needs to calculate the rate, in milliliters per hour, at which to set the IV pump.

The formula for calculating the mL/h is:

$$\dfrac{\text{Ordered mcg/kg/min} \times \text{Patient's weight in kg} \times 60\ \text{min/h}}{\text{Medication concentration (mcg/mL)}}$$

When this formula is used, the result will always be expressed in milliliters per hour because the pair of values in micrograms cancel each other, as do the pair of values in kilograms and the pair of values in minutes.

a. Before the medication concentration can be determined, the total mg in the IV bag must be converted to mcg.

$$1\ \text{mg} : 1000\ \text{mcg} :: 800\ \text{mg} : x\ \text{mcg}$$

$$x = 800{,}000\ \text{mcg}$$

b. Determine the concentration (mcg/mL) by dividing the total mcg in the IV bag by the total amount of fluid in the IV bag.

$$\dfrac{800{,}000\ \text{mcg}}{250\ \text{mL}} = \dfrac{3200\ \text{mcg}}{1\ \text{mL}} = 3200\ \text{mcg/mL}$$

c. Calculate mL/h.

(Formula setup) $\dfrac{3\ \text{mcg/kg/min} \times 70\ \text{kg} \times 60\ \text{min/h}}{3200\ \text{mcg/mL}} = x\ \text{mL/h}$

(Cancel) $\dfrac{3\ \cancel{\text{mcg/kg/min}} \times 70\ \cancel{\text{kg}} \times 60\ \cancel{\text{min/h}}}{3200\ \cancel{\text{mcg/mL}}} = x\ \text{mL/h}$

(Calculate) $\dfrac{3 \times 70 \times 60}{3200} = \dfrac{12{,}600}{3200} = 3.93\ \text{or}\ 3.9\ \text{mL/h}$

Converting Milliliter/Hour to the Dose the Patient Is Receiving

Calculations for critical care medications do not stop with taking and order and calculating milliliters per hour. A nurse may receive in report, "Mr. Douglas is receiving dopamine at 15 mL/h, which is around 10 mcg/kg/min." Since the nurse administering the medication during the upcoming shift is the final link in safety, this nurse needs to be able to take the milliliters per hour and calculate the exact dose of dopamine the patient is receiving. This situation can also be applied to medications that are ordered in milligrams per minute and micrograms per minute.

Calculating Milligram/Minute from Milliliter/Hour

Example: A patient is receiving lidocaine at 60 mL/h. The concentration of lidocaine is 1 g in 500 mL of D$_5$W. The nurse needs to calculate the milligrams per minute the patient is receiving.

$$\text{The formula: } \frac{\text{Concentration (mg/mL)} \times \text{Rate (mL/h)}}{60 \text{ min/h}}$$

When this formula is used, the answer will always be expressed in milligrams per minute because the pair of values in milliliters cancel each other, as do the pair of values in hours.

    a. Convert total g in the IV bag to mg.

        1 g = 1000 mg

    b. Calculate the concentration (mg/mL).

$$\frac{1000 \text{ mg}}{500 \text{ mL}} = 2 \text{ mg/mL}$$

    c. Calculate the mg/min.

(Formula setup) $\dfrac{2 \text{ mg/mL} \times 60 \text{ mL/h}}{60 \text{ min/h}}$

(Cancel) $\dfrac{\overset{1}{2 \text{ mg/\cancel{mL}} \times 60 \text{ \cancel{mL/h}}}}{\underset{1}{60 \text{ min/\cancel{h}}}}$

(Calculate)   2 mg/min

Calculating Microgram/Minute from Milliliter/Hour

Example: A patient is receiving nitroglycerin at 3 mL/h. The concentration of nitroglycerin is 50 mg in 500 mL of 0.9% NS. The nurse needs to calculate the micrograms per minute the patient is receiving.

$$\text{The formula: } \frac{\text{Concentration (mcg/mL)} \times \text{Rate (mL/h)}}{60 \text{ min/h}}$$

When this formula is used, the answer will always be expressed in micrograms per minute because the pair of values in milliliters cancel each other, as do the pair of values in hours.

    a. Convert total mg in the IV bag to mcg.

(Formula setup)   1 mg : 1000 mcg :: 50 mg : x mcg

                 $x = 1000 \times 50$

                 $x = 50,000$ mcg

    b. Calculate the concentration (mcg/mL).

$$\frac{50,000 \text{ mcg}}{500 \text{ mL}} = 100 \text{ mcg/mL}$$

c. Calculate the mcg/min.

(Formula setup) $$\frac{100 \text{ mcg/mL} \times 3 \text{ mL/h}}{60 \text{ min/h}}$$

(Cancel) $$\frac{\overset{1}{\cancel{100 \text{ mcg/\cancel{mL}} \times 3 \text{ \cancel{mL}/\cancel{h}}}}}{\underset{20}{\cancel{60} \text{ min/\cancel{h}}}}$$

(Calculate) $$\frac{100}{20} = 5 \text{ mcg/min}$$

Calculating Microgram/Kilogram/Minute from Milliliter/Hour

Example: A patient is receiving dopamine at 12 mL/h. The concentration of dopamine is 200 mg in 250 mL of 0.9% NS. The nurse needs to calculate the micrograms per kilogram per minute the patient is receiving. The patient's weight is 70 kg.

The formula: $$\frac{\text{Concentration (mcg/mL)} \times \text{Rate (mL/h)}}{60 \text{ min/h} \times \text{Weight (kg)}}$$

When this formula is used, the answer will always be expressed in micrograms per kilogram per minute because the pair of values in milliliters cancel each other, as do the pair of values in hours.

a. Convert total mg in the IV bag to mcg.

(Formula setup)   1 mg : 1000 mcg :: 200 mg : x mcg

$x = 1000 \times 200$

$x = 200,000$ mcg

b. Calculate the concentration (mcg/mL).

$$\frac{200,000 \text{ mcg}}{250 \text{ mL}} = 800 \text{ mcg/mL}$$

c. Calculate the mcg/kg/min.

(Formula setup) $$\frac{800 \text{ mcg/mL} \times 12 \text{ mL/h}}{60 \text{ min/h} \times 70 \text{ kg}}$$

(Cancel) $$\frac{\overset{1}{\cancel{800 \text{ mcg/\cancel{mL}} \times 12 \text{ \cancel{mL}/\cancel{h}}}}}{\underset{5}{\cancel{60} \text{ min/\cancel{h}} \times 70 \text{ kg}}}$$

(Calculate) $$\frac{800}{5 \times 70} = \frac{800}{350} = 2.28 \text{ or } 2.3 \text{ mcg/kg/min}$$

Complete the following work sheet, which provides for practice in the calculation of critical care IV flow rates. Check your answers. If you have difficulties, go back and review the necessary material. An acceptable score as indicated on the posttest signifies that you have successfully completed the chapter. An unacceptable score signifies a need for further study before taking the second posttest.

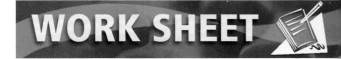

Directions: The IV fluid order is listed in each problem. Calculate the IV flow rates using the appropriate formula required for the problem.

1. Mr. Sinks has undergone aortic valve repair and has orders for heparin at 1000 units/h. The concentration is heparin 25,000 units in 250 mL of 0.9% NS. How many milliliters per hour should the IV pump be programmed for? _____

2. You have an order for your patient with diabetes to receive regular insulin IV at 12 units/h. The concentration is insulin 100 units in 250 mL of 0.9% NS. How many milliliters per hour should the IV pump be programmed for? _____

3. The insulin order for the patient in problem 2 is reduced to 8 units/h. How many milliliters per hour should the IV pump be programmed for? _____

4. A patient who has undergone mitral valve repair has heparin ordered at 1000 units/h. The concentration is heparin 10,000 units in 500 mL of D_5W. How many milliliters per hour should the IV pump be programmed for? _____

5. The physician orders dobutamine at 12 mcg/kg/min for Mrs. White, who weighs 75 kg. The concentration is dobutamine 1 g in 250 mL of D_5W. How many milliliters per hour should the IV pump be programmed for? _____

6. Mr. Baxter is having chest pain and has an order for nitroglycerin at 10 mcg/min. The concentration is nitroglycerin 100 mg in 500 mL of D_5W. How many milliliters per hour should the IV pump be programmed for? _____

7. The physician orders dopamine at 5 mcg/kg/min. The concentration is dopamine 2 g in 250 mL of 0.9% NS. The patient's weight is 80 kg. How many milliliters per hour should the IV pump be programmed for? _____

8. Ms. Moreno has a brachial thrombus and has streptokinase ordered at 100,000 international units/h. The concentration is 250,000 international units of streptokinase in 45 mL of 0.9% NS. How many milliliters per hour should the IV pump be programmed for? _____

9. The physician has ordered amiodarone at 0.5 mg/min. The concentration is amiodarone 900 mg in 500 mL of D₅W. How many milliliters per hour should the IV pump be programmed for? _____

10. Your patient with malignant hypertension is ordered to have nitroprusside at 3 mcg/kg/min. The concentration is nitroprusside 50 mg in 250 mL of D₅W. The patient's weight is 70 kg. How many milliliters per hour should the IV pump be programmed for? _____

11. A patient with heart failure has dobutamine ordered at 10 mcg/kg/min. The patient weighs 100 kg. The concentration is dobutamine 2 g in 500 mL of D₅W. How many milliliters per hour should the IV pump be programmed for? _____

12. Mr. Nast has propofol ordered at 30 mcg/kg/min. The propofol concentration is 15 mg/mL. The patient's weight is 75 kg. How many milliliters per hour should the IV pump be programmed for? _____

13. A patient with a ventricular dysrhythmia has procainamide ordered at 4 mg/min. The concentration is procainamide 2 g in 250 mL of D_5W. How many milliliters per hour should the IV pump be programmed for? _____

14. Mrs. Waters, who has been resuscitated, has Levophed ordered at 10 mcg/min. The concentration is Levophed 2 mg in 250 mL of 0.9% NS. How many milliliters per hour should the IV pump be programmed for? _____

15. A patient with a dysrhythmia has an order for amiodarone 0.75 mg/min. The concentration is amiodarone 900 mg in 500 mL D_5W. How many milliliters per hour should the IV pump be programmed for? _____

16. A patient with hypotension has a vasopressor ordered at 15 mcg/min. The concentration is vasopressor 4 mg in 250 mL of D_5W. How many milliliters per hour should the IV pump be programmed for? _____

17. Mrs. Roberts has lidocaine ordered at 2 mg/min. The concentration is lidocaine 2 g in 250 mL of D₅W. How many milliliters per hour should the IV pump be programmed for? _____

18. A patient with deep vein thrombosis has an order for a heparin infusion at 750 units/h. The heparin bag has a concentration of 25,000 units in 500 mL of D₅W. How many milliliters per hour should the IV pump be programmed for? _____

19. A patient with diabetic ketoacidosis has an order for insulin at 10 units/h. The insulin comes in a concentration of 100 units in 100 mL of 0.9% NS. How many milliliters per hour should the IV pump be programmed for? _____

20. The physician orders dopamine at 10 mcg/kg/min. The concentration is dopamine 2 g in 250 mL of 0.9% NS. The patient's weight is 90 kg. How many milliliters per hour should the IV pump be programmed for? _____

21. Mr. Diaz is admitted to your ICU with dopamine infusing at 13.5 mL/h. His weight is 75 kg. The dopamine concentration is 1 g in 250 mL of D_5W. At what rate, in micrograms per kilogram per minute, is the dopamine infusing? _____

22. A patient with heart failure has nitroglycerin infusing at 3 mL/h. The nitroglycerin concentration is 100 mg in 500 mL of D_5W. At what rate, in micrograms per minute, is the nitroglycerin infusing? _____

23. A patient with supraventricular tachycardia has amiodarone infusing at 17 mL/h. The amiodarone concentration is 900 mg in 500 mL of D_5W. At what rate, in milligrams per minute, is the amiodarone infusing? _____

24. Ms. Hart requires mechanical ventilation and is agitated. Propofol is infusing at 9 mL/h. The patient's weight is 75 kg. The propofol concentration is 15 mg/mL. At what rate, in micrograms per kilogram per minute, is the propofol infusing? _____

25. Mr. Simon is admitted with angina. Nitroglycerin is infusing at 5 mL/h. The nitroglycerin concentration is 50 mg in 250 mL of D_5W. How many micrograms per minute is the patient receiving? _____

26. A patient with uncontrolled atrial fibrillation is receiving amiodarone at 20 mL/h. The amiodarone concentration is 900 mg in 500 mL of D$_5$W. How many milligrams per minute is the patient receiving? _____

27. Mr. McCormick is receiving dopamine at 15 mL/h by IV pump. The patient weighs 80 kg. The dopamine concentration is 2 g in 500 mL of D$_5$W. Calculate the micrograms per kilogram per minute. _____

28. A patient is receiving nitroglycerin at 10 mL/h by IV pump. The nitroglycerin concentration is 100 mg in 250 mL of D$_5$W. Calculate the micrograms per minute. _____

29. A patient is receiving amiodarone at 15 mL/h by IV pump. The amiodarone concentration is 900 mg in 250 mL of D$_5$W. Calculate the milligrams per minute. _____

30. Ms. Nesbitt is receiving lidocaine at 15 mL/h by IV pump. The lidocaine concentration is 1 g in 500 mL of 0.9% NS. Calculate the milligrams per minute. _____

31. The physician orders heparin per protocol (use protocol on p. 377). The patient's weight is 60 kg.

    Bolus:

    Infusion:

32. Six hours after the heparin protocol is begun (question 31), the aPTT returns at 98 seconds. Using the protocol on p. 377, does the heparin need to be changed? _____

    Bolus:

    Infusion:

33. The physician orders heparin per protocol (use protocol on p. 377). The patient's weight is 80 kg. Calculate the heparin bolus and infusion.

    Bolus:

    Infusion:

34. Six hours after the heparin protocol is begun (question 33), the aPTT returns at 48 seconds. Using the protocol on p. 377, does the heparin need to be changed? _____

    Bolus:

    Infusion:

35. Mr. Vargas has supraventricular tachycardia and has a maintenance infusion of Brevibloc 100 mcg/kg/min ordered. The Brevibloc concentration is 10 mg/mL. The patient's weight is 80 kg. At what rate, in milliliters per hour, should the IV pump be set?

Answers on pp. 559–562.

Name _____

Date _____

ACCEPTABLE SCORE ___14___

YOUR SCORE _____

POSTTEST 1

Directions: The IV fluid order is listed in each problem. Calculate the appropriate rate for each problem.

1. Your patient with diabetes has an order for regular insulin IV at 9 units/h. The concentration is insulin 500 units in 500 mL of 0.9% NS. How many milliliters per hour should the IV pump be programmed for? _____

2. Mrs. Allen has deep vein thrombosis and has an order for heparin at 800 units/h. The concentration is heparin 50,000 units in 500 mL of D_5W. How many milliliters per hour should the IV pump be programmed for? _____

3. Your patient with hypertension has orders for Nipride at 5 mcg/kg/min. The concentration is Nipride 100 mg in 250 mL of D_5W. The patient weighs 62 kg. How many milliliters per hour should the IV pump be programmed for? _____

4. Mr. Marshall, who is admitted with pulmonary edema, has dobutamine ordered at 5 mcg/kg/min. The concentration is dobutamine 1 g in 250 mL of 0.9% NS. The patient's weight is 50 kg. How many milliliters per hour should the IV pump be programmed for? _____

5. A patient with an acute myocardial infarction has IV nitroglycerin ordered at 20 mcg/min. The concentration is nitroglycerin 50 mg in 250 mL of D$_5$W. How many milliliters per hour should the IV pump be programmed for? _____

6. A patient with a ventricular dysrhythmia has lidocaine ordered at 3 mg/min. The concentration is lidocaine 2 g in 500 mL of D$_5$W. How many milliliters per hour should the IV pump be programmed for? _____

7. Mrs. Morales has been resuscitated and now has Levophed ordered at 5 mcg/min. The concentration is Levophed 1 mg in 250 mL of 0.9% NS. How many milliliters per hour should the IV pump be programmed for? _____

8. An intubated patient has propofol ordered at 25 mcg/kg/min. The concentration of propofol is 10 mg/mL. The patient's weight is 50 kg. How many milliliters per hour should the IV pump be programmed for? _____

9. A patient with a thrombosis is to receive heparin at 1050 units/h. The concentration is heparin 25,000 units in 250 mL of D$_5$W. How many milliliters per hour should the IV pump be programmed for? _____

10. Mrs. Green, who has atrial fibrillation, has amiodarone ordered at 0.5 mg/min. The concentration is amiodarone 900 mg in 250 mL of D$_5$W. How many milliliters per hour should the IV pump be programmed for?

11. A patient with a blood pressure of 240/120 mm Hg is receiving nitroprusside at 63 mL/h. The patient's weight is 70 kg. The nitroprusside concentration is 50 mg in 250 mL of D$_5$W. How many micrograms per kilogram per minute of nitroprusside is infusing? _____

12. A patient is receiving lidocaine at 45 mL/h after being defibrillated for ventricular fibrillation. The lidocaine concentration is 2 g in 500 mL of 0.9% NS. How many milligrams per minute of lidocaine is the patient receiving? _____

13. Mr. Messer is receiving vasopressin at 15 mL/h. The vasopressin concentration is 4 mg in 250 mL. How many micrograms per minute of vasopressin is the patient receiving? _____

14. A patient has hypotension after cardiac arrest. Dopamine is infusing at 15 mL/h. The patient's weight is 80 kg. The dopamine concentration is 2 g in 500 mL of D$_5$W. How many micrograms per kilogram per minute is the patient receiving? _____

15. Begin heparin per protocol (use protocol example on p. 377). Patient's weight is 105 kg.

Bolus:

Infusion:

Answers on pp. 563–564.

Name _____

Date _____

ACCEPTABLE SCORE __14__

YOUR SCORE _____

POSTTEST 2

Directions: The IV fluid order is listed in each problem. Calculate the rate needed in each problem to deliver the correct dose.

1. A patient with hypotension has dopamine ordered at 3 mcg/kg/min. The patient weighs 85 kg. The concentration is dopamine 2 g in 500 mL of D_5W. How many milliliters per hour should the IV pump be programmed for? _____

2. A patient with a pulmonary embolus has an order for streptokinase to be infused at 100,000 international units/h. The concentration is streptokinase 750,000 international units in 200 mL of 0.9% NS. How many milliliters per hour should the IV pump be programmed for? _____

3. Ms. Farmer, who has tachycardia, has an order for Brevibloc to be started at 50 mcg/kg/min. The concentration is Brevibloc 5 g in 500 mL of D_5W. The patient weighs 80 kg. How many milliliters per hour should the IV pump be programmed for? _____

4. A patient with a ventricular dysrhythmia has an order for amiodarone at 0.5 mg/min. The concentration is amiodarone 900 mg in 250 mL of D_5W. How many milliliters per hour should the IV pump be programmed for? _____

5. Mr. Wu has an order for a vasopressor at 10 mcg/min. The concentration is vasopressor 4 mg in 500 mL of D$_5$W. How many milliliters per hour should the IV pump be programmed for? _____

6. A patient has an order for procainamide at 4 mg/min. The concentration is procainamide 2 g in 500 mL of D$_5$W. How many milliliters per hour should the IV pump be programmed for? _____

7. Mrs. Davis has an order for dobutamine at 7 mcg/kg/min. The concentration is dobutamine 1 g in 200 mL of 0.9% NS. The patient's weight is 55 kg. How many milliliters per hour should the IV pump be programmed for? _____

8. A patient in shock has an order for Isuprel to be infused at 2 mcg/min. The concentration is Isuprel 1 mg in 500 mL of D$_5$W. How many milliliters per hour should the IV pump be programmed for? _____

9. Your patient has a blood clot in his arm, and the physician has ordered heparin to be infused at 1500 units/h. The concentration is heparin 20,000 units in 200 mL of D_5W. How many milliliters per hour should the IV pump be programmed for? _____

10. Mr. Powers has diabetic ketoacidosis and receives an order for regular insulin to be infused at 8 units/h. The concentration is insulin 50 units in 100 mL of 0.9% NS. How many milliliters per hour should the IV pump be programmed for? _____

11. Begin heparin per protocol (use protocol example on p. 377). The patient's weight is 75 kg.

Bolus:

Infusion:

12. Ms. Shepard's blood pressure is 60/30 mm Hg. Levophed is infusing at 75 mL/h. The Levophed concentration is 2 mg in 250 mL of 0.9% NS. How many micrograms per minute of Levophed is infusing? _____

13. A patient with ventricular tachycardia is receiving procainamide at 30 mL/h. The procainamide concentration is 2 g in 250 mL of D$_5$W. How many milligrams per minute of procainamide is infusing? _____

14. A hypotensive patient is receiving dopamine at 3 mL/h. The patient's weight is 80 kg. The dopamine concentration is 2 g in 250 mL of 0.9% NS. How many micrograms per kilogram per minute of dopamine is infusing? _____

15. Mr. Flores is receiving nitroprusside at 50 mL/h by IV pump. The patient's weight is 60 kg. The nitroprusside concentration is 50 mg in 250 mL of D$_5$W. Calculate the micrograms per kilogram per minute.

Answers on pp. 564–565.

 Refer to Advanced Calculations on the enclosed CD for additional help and practice problems.

Pediatric Dosages

Mary Ann Reklau, MSN, RN, CPNP

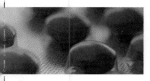

LEARNING OBJECTIVES

On completion of the materials provided in this chapter, you will be able to perform computations accurately by mastering the following mathematical concepts:

1 Converting the weight of a child from pounds to kilograms

2 Converting the neonate and infant weight from grams to kilograms

3 Performing pediatric dosage calculations

4 Calculating the single or individual dose of medications

5 Determining whether the prescribed dose is safe and therapeutic

6 Calculating a safe and therapeutic 24-hour dosage range

7 Calculating the single dose range from a 24-hour dosage range

8 Determining whether the actual dosage (in milligrams per kilograms per 24 hours) is safe to administer

9 Calculating pediatric IV solutions

10 Administering IV medications to pediatric patients

11 Calculating the daily fluid requirements for infants and young children

12 Calculating the body surface area (BSA) for medication administration

Children are more sensitive than adults to medications because of their weight, height, physical condition, immature systems, and metabolism. Nurses who administer medications to infants and children must be vigilant in determining whether the patient is receiving the correct medication. The correct dose is one of the six rights of drug administration: right patient, medication, route, time, dose, and documentation.

The physician or provider will prescribe the medication to be delivered. However, the nurse is responsible for detecting any errors in calculation of dosage, as well as for preparing the medication and administering the drug. The nurse needs to be aware that pediatric dosages are often less than 1 mL; therefore a tuberculin syringe is used for accurate dosing.

Pediatric medications are calculated using the infant or child's kilogram weight. The dosages have been established by the drug companies. Safe and therapeutic (S&T) dosages are readily available from a reliable source such as *The Harriet Lane Handbook*.

The child who weighs more than 45 kg **may** receive adult dosages. If the calculated dose is greater than the recommended adult dose, DO NOT administer the medication. A child should not receive higher doses than those recommended for the adult, ever. Many drugs have a "do not exceed" or "max. dose" in 24 hours listed; this must always be considered.

Additionally, the physician or pharmacist may use the child's body surface area (BSA) to calculate a dosage of medication to administer. The BSA calculation may be used when an established dosage has not been determined by the drug company, as with some anticancer or specialized drugs.

In general, pediatric dosages are rounded to the nearest tenth. A few exceptions are presented later in the chapter.

KILOGRAM CONVERSIONS

Converting Pounds to Kilograms

The formula: 2.2 lb = 1 kg

Infant's and young children's weight in pounds must be converted to kilograms to accurately calculate medication doses and daily fluid requirements. S&T drug dosages have been established using kilogram weights.

Always round the kilogram weight to the nearest tenth, NOT a whole number.

Example 1: An infant weighs 24 lb. Convert the infant's weight to kilograms.

Proportion

2.2 lb : 1 kg :: 24 lb : x kg

2.2 : 1 :: 24 : x

$2.2x = 24$

$x = \dfrac{24}{2.2}$

$x = 10.9$ kg

Formula Setup

$$\dfrac{2.2 \text{ lb}}{1 \text{ kg}} = \dfrac{24 \text{ lb}}{x \text{ kg}}$$

$2.2x = 24$

$x = 10.9$ kg

Example 2: A child weighs 47 lb. Convert the child's weight to kilograms.

2.2 lb : 1 kg :: 47 lb : x kg

2.2 : 1 :: 47 : x

2.2x = 47

$x = \dfrac{47}{2.2}$

x = 21.36 kg or 21.4 kg (rounded to the nearest tenth)

$\dfrac{2.2 \text{ lb}}{1 \text{ kg}} = \dfrac{47 \text{ lb}}{x \text{ kg}}$

2.2x = 47

x = 21.4 kg

Converting Grams to Kilograms

The formula: 1000 g = 1 kg

Newborn (neonate) and some infant weights are measured in grams. Converting grams to kilograms is done as shown below or by simply dividing the number of grams by 1000.

Example 1: A neonate weighs 2300 g. Convert to kilograms.

1000 g : 1 kg :: 2300 g : x kg

1000 : 1 :: 2300 : x

1000x = 2300

x = 2.3 kg

Example 2: A newborn weighs 4630 g at birth. Convert to kilograms.

1000 g : 1 kg :: 4630 g : x kg

1000 : 1 :: 4630 : x

1000x = 4630

x = 4.63 kg, or 4.6 (rounded to the nearest tenth)

Practice Problems. Convert pounds and grams to kilograms.

1. 27 lb ÷ 2.2   _12.3_ kg
2. 38 lb   _17.3_ kg
3. 52 lb   _23.6_ kg
4. 5220 g   _5.2_ kg
5. 3202 g   _3.2_ kg
6. 72 lb   _32.7_ kg
7. 16 lb   _7.3_ kg
8. 92 lb   _41.8_ kg

Answers

1. 12.3 kg	4. 5.2 kg	7. 7.3 kg
2. 17.3 kg	5. 3.2 kg	8. 41.8 kg
3. 23.6 kg	6. 32.7 kg	

PEDIATRIC DOSAGE CALCULATIONS

In pediatric dosage calculations, you can use a formula or proportion method.

Proportion   or   **Formula**

mg : mL :: mg : x mL $\dfrac{mg}{mL} \times \dfrac{mg}{mL}$

Example 1:   The physician orders Benadryl 12.5 mg po q4-6 h prn for itching. The nurse has available Benadryl 25 mg/5 mL. How many milliliters would be needed to administer 12.5 mg? Show math.

25 mg : 5 mL :: 12.5 mg : x mL $\dfrac{25 \text{ mg}}{5 \text{ mL}} \times \dfrac{12.5 \text{ mg}}{x \text{ mL}}$ $\dfrac{12.5}{25} \times 5 = 2.5$

$x = 2.5$ mL

$x = 2.5$ mL

Example 2:   The physician orders morphine 15 mg by intravenous (IV) piggyback (IVPB) now. You have available morphine 10 mg/mL. How much would you give? Show math.

10 mg : 1 mL :: 15 mg : x mL $\dfrac{10 \text{ mg}}{1 \text{ mL}} \times \dfrac{15 \text{ mg}}{x \text{ mL}}$ $\dfrac{15}{10} \times 1 = 1.5 \, m\ell$

$x = 1.5$ mL

$x = 1.5$ mL

CALCULATING THE SINGLE OR INDIVIDUAL DOSE (MILLIGRAMS/DOSE)

Medications such as acetaminophen and ibuprofen are administered as a single dose. This means that each time the infant or child receives the medication, it is calculated in a single or individual dose based on the kilogram weight.

Most of the medications prescribed in this manner are prn medications, which are given as needed for relief of symptoms such as pain, nausea, and fever. Again, the manufacturer of the drug has established an S&T dosage or range. The nurse is responsible for administering the single dose that is S&T. Therefore it is helpful for the nurse to know how the ordered dose is derived.

To **determine the correct single dose** for the child, you must **calculate the correct dose.** A systematic approach is helpful in determining the S&T dose range:
- Change the child's weight in pounds to kilograms.
- Find the recommended dosage in a reliable source.
- Multiply the kilogram weight by the recommended dose(s).
- The answer is the individual or single dose *(mg/dose)* of medication to be given each time the child receives the medication.

Example 1:   A child weighs 22 lb. The child needs acetaminophen for pain and fever.

    a. **Weight**   22 lb = 10 kg
    b. **Recommended**   10 to 15 mg/kg/dose q4-6 h
    c. **Calculation**

      10 mg : 1 kg :: x mg : 10 kg   15 mg : 1 kg :: x mg : 10 kg

      10 : 1 :: x : 10   15 : 1 :: x : 10

      $x = 100$ mg/dose $x = 150$ mg/dose

The child may receive 100 to 150 mg each time he or she is given acetaminophen. This is the single or individual dose. The dose is both S&T for this child.

- A dose smaller than 100 mg is considered **safe but may not be therapeutic for the child's weight.**
- Doses larger than 150 mg are considered too much for the child's weight and may **exceed the therapeutic range.**

Example 2: Calculate an S&T dose range of ibuprofen for a child who weighs 36 lb. Ibuprofen is available as 100 mg/5 mL. How many milliliters would you need to administer for the ordered dose to be S&T?

$$\frac{36}{2.2} = 16.4 \times 5$$
$$\times 10$$
$$81.8 \text{ mg or } 164 \text{ mg}$$

   a. **Weight**   36 lb = 16.4 kg
   b. **Recommended** 5 to 10 mg/kg/dose q6-8 h
   c. **Calculations**

5 mg : 1 kg :: x mg : 16.4 kg   10 mg : 1 kg :: x mg : 16.4

5 : 1 :: x : 16.4   10 : 1 :: x : 16.4

x = 82 mg/dose x = 164 mg/dose

The S&T single dose range for this child is 82 to 164 mg/dose.

   d. Now perform dosage calculations for the single dose range using the 100 mg/5 mL strength:

100 mg : 5 mL :: 82 mg : x mL   100 mg : 5 mL :: 164 mg : x mL

x = 4.1 mL $\frac{82}{100} \times 5$ x = 8.2 mL

DETERMINE WHETHER THE PRESCRIBED DOSE IS SAFE AND THERAPEUTIC (MILLIGRAMS/KILOGRAM/DOSE)

This method will **determine whether the child is receiving an S&T dosage** of the drug that is prescribed by the physician. The nurse must determine whether the ordered dose is within the recommended range.

Even though the physician has prescribed the medication to be given, it is the nurse's responsibility to determine whether the dose is S&T to administer to the child. This is done by **dividing the ordered dosage by the child's weight in kilograms (mg/kg/dose).** A systematic approach is needed.

- Obtain the child's weight in kilograms.
- Obtain the ordered dosage.
- Divide the ordered dose by the child's weight.
- The answer is the mg/kg/dose (for each dose administered).
- Check your drug book to determine whether the ordered dose is S&T (in the recommended dosage range).

Example: The doctor has ordered 210 mg of acetaminophen q4-6 h for pain and fever for a postoperative child. The child weighs 39 lb. The recommended dose range for acetaminophen is 10 to 15 mg/kg/dose q4-6 h. Acetaminophen is supplied as 160 mg/5 mL.

Is the ordered dose S&T to administer? If the dose ordered is S&T to administer, how many milliliters will be needed?

   a. **Weight**   39 lb = 17.7 kg
   b. **Ordered**   210 mg q4-6 h

   c. **Calculation** $\dfrac{210 \text{ mg/dose}}{17.7 \text{ kg}} = 11.86$ or 11.9 mg/kg/dose

   d. **Recommended** 10 to 15 mg/kg/dose

The patient will receive 11.9 mg/kg/dose. Yes, it is safe to administer the acetaminophen because it is within the S&T dosage range of 10 to 15 mg/kg/dose.

    e. Perform dosage calculation using 160 mg/5 mL concentration:

$$160 \text{ mg} : 5 \text{ mL} :: 210 \text{ mg} : x \text{ mL}$$

$$160x = 1050$$

$$x = 6.6 \text{ mL rounded to the nearest tenth}$$

Remember to round all doses to the nearest tenth.

Exceptions: Round all narcotics, antiepileptics, and cardiac medications to *nearest hundredth*. Medications that may be rounded to the nearest hundredth include phenobarbital, morphine, dilantin, digoxin, and anticancer drugs.

CALCULATE THE 24-HOUR DOSAGE (RANGES)

Many drugs are calculated based on the recommended 24-hour dose, then divided into single doses to be given every 12, 8, 6, or 4 hours or as recommended by the drug manufacturers. These divided time schedules vary, and the physician, nurse practitioner, or physician's assistant will order the medication based on the recommended schedules.

Antibiotics especially are given this way. Additionally, an antibiotic may be given in dosages or ranges that have been found to be effective for the child's diagnosis. The physician chooses how often the medication is to be delivered. An example of an antibiotic with many dosing choices is ampicillin.

Recommended dosages for ampicillin may be any of the following:

<2 kg	50 to 100 mg/kg/24 h/q8 h
>2 kg	100 to 200 mg/kg/24 h/q8 h
Mild to moderate infection	100 to 200 mg/kg/24 h/q6 h
Severe infection	200 to 400 mg/kg/24 h/q4-6 h

The physician must determine the dosage to be given to the infant or child. If an infant or child is diagnosed with otitis media (OM), then the physician may choose the dosage of antibiotic in the mild to moderate range. However, if an infant is admitted with a diagnosis of fever of undetermined origin, sepsis, or meningitis, then the physician may decide to prescribe a larger dosage of the antibiotic, as in the severe infection range.

Knowing the diagnosis is helpful in determining whether the infant or child will be receiving S&T dosages of antibiotics. Nurses who administer antibiotics or antiinfectives can learn how to determine the doses needed for the patient. **However, only the physician, advanced practice nurse, or physician assistant can prescribe and order the infant's or child's medications.**

Example 1: An infant is admitted to the hospital to rule out sepsis. The infant weighs 8 lb. Ampicillin is prescribed. Calculate an S&T 24-hour dosage range for this infant with a possible severe infection.

    a. **Weight**   8 lb = 3.6 kg

    b. **Recommended**   200 to 400 mg/kg/24 h q4-6 h

    c. **Calculation**   3.6 kg × 200 mg/kg/24 h = 720 mg/24 h

                                 3.6 kg × 400 mg/kg/24 h = 1440 mg/24 h

    d. **24-hour dosage range**   720 to 1440 mg/24 h

This means the infant can receive 720 to 1440 mg of ampicillin in a 24-hour period.

Example 2: The child weighs 35 lb and is diagnosed with OM. The physician prescribes amoxicillin. Calculate an S&T 24-hour dosage range for this patient.

a.	**Weight**	35 lb = 15.9 kg
b.	**Recommended**	25 to 50 mg/kg/24 h two or three times a day
		Adult dosage 250 to 500 mg/dose two times a day
c.	**Calculation**	15.9 kg × 25 mg/kg/24 h = 397.5 mg/24 h
		15.9 kg × 50 mg/kg/24 h = 795 mg/24 h
d.	**24-hour dosage range**	397.5 to 795 mg/24 h

The child may receive 397.5 to 795 mg/24 h of amoxicillin. **Remember not to exceed the adult dose or "max" dose.** The physician will now decide how often the child will receive the medication. This is called the individual or single dose, based on 24 hours.

CALCULATE THE INDIVIDUAL DOSE OR SINGLE DOSE (MILLIGRAMS/KILOGRAM/24 HOURS DIVIDED)

The physician will now determine how often the antibiotic will be administered as a single or individual dose. First determine the 24-hour dosage range. Then divide the 24-hour dosage into single doses (the number of times per day the medications is to be given).

- This is the individual dose each time the patient receives the medication.
- These times are established by the drug companies (e.g., q4 h, q6 h, q8 h, q12 h, or every day).
- **As long as the dose does not exceed the maximum dose established in 24 hours and the dose does not exceed the adult dose, then it can be given safely.**
- The physician will decide how often the medication is to be given.

Example 1: A child weighs 22 lb. The physician prescribes ampicillin 100 to 200 mg/kg/24 h divided q6 h. Calculate the individual dose for ampicillin.

a.	**Weight**	22 lb = 10 kg	
b.	**Recommended**	100 to 200 mg/kg/24 h divided q6 h	
c.	**Calculation**	10 kg × 100 mg/kg/24 h = 1000 mg/24 h	
		10 kg × 200 mg/kg/24 h = 2000 mg/24 h	
d.	**Divided q6 h (4 doses in 24 h)**	$\dfrac{1000\ mg/24\ h}{4\ doses/24\ h}$	$\dfrac{2000\ mg/24\ h}{4\ doses/24\ h}$
e.	**Single dose range**	250 to 500 mg/dose	

Example 2: A child weighs 60 lb. The physician orders cefuroxime. The recommended dosage is 75 to 100 mg/kg/24 h q8 h. What is the S&T dosage or range for this child?

a.	**Weight**	60 lb = 27.3 kg	
b.	**Recommended**	75 to 100 mg/kg/24 h q8 h	
c.	**Calculation**	27.3 kg × 75 mg/kg/24 h = 2047.5 mg/24 h	
		27.3 kg × 100 mg/kg/24 h = 2730 mg/24 h	
d.	**Divided q8 h (3 doses in 24 h)**	$\dfrac{2047.5\ mg/24\ h}{3\ doses/24\ h}$	$\dfrac{2730\ mg/24\ h}{3\ doses/24\ h}$
e.	**Single dose range**	682.5 to 910 mg/dose	

DETERMINE THE ACTUAL MILLIGRAMS/KILOGRAM/24 HOURS OR DOSE/KILOGRAM/24 HOURS

The nurse must understand how to *prove* that the patient is actually receiving an S&T dosage or range. When a physician prescribes a medication, he or she has a range from which to choose. As a nurse, you need to check to see whether the medication falls within the recommended dosage or range. This is important because medication doses are patient-weight specific.

Determining the actual milligrams per kilogram per 24 hours that the patient is receiving is done simply by dividing the actual milligrams to be given in 24 hours by the patient's weight. Remember that the physician has already prescribed the medication based on the recommended dose in milligrams per kilogram per 24 hours. **For nurses, knowing how to prove S&T dosing is critical.**

To determine (prove) whether the patient is receiving an S&T dosage, the nurse will need to:
- Obtain the infant's or child's kilogram weight.
- Obtain the medication order.
- Determine the amount of medication the child will receive in the 24-hour period (the 24-hour dosage).
- **Divide the prescribed 24-hour dosage by the patient's weight.**
- Compare the ordered dosage with the recommended dosage.

There is no need to calculate a dosage range, since the physician has already done this.

Example 1: A 4-year-old child is receiving vancomycin 220 mg q6 h IV via syringe pump. She weighs 48 lb. Recommended dosage is 40 to 60 mg/kg/24 h q6 h.

How many milligrams per kilogram per 24 hours is this child receiving? Is the ordered dosage S&T?

    a. **Weight**   48 lb = 21.8 kg
    b. **Ordered**   Vancomycin 220 mg q6 h
    c. **24-hour dosage**   220 mg × 4 doses = 880 mg/24 h

    d. **mg/kg/24 h** $\dfrac{\text{24-h dose}}{\text{Weight (kg)}} = \dfrac{880 \text{ mg/24 h}}{21.8 \text{ kg}} = 40.36$ or 40.4 mg/kg/24 h

    e. **Recommended**   40 to 60 mg/kg/24 h q6-8 h

The patient is receiving 40.4 mg/kg/24 h, which is within the S&T range.

Example 2: A 75-lb patient is receiving 900 mg of ampicillin IVPB q6 h. How many milligrams per kilogram per 24 hours is the patient receiving? Is the dosage S&T?

    a. **Weight**   75 lb = 34.1 kg
    b. **Ordered**   Ampicillin 900 mg IVPB q6 h
    c. **24-hour dosage**   900 mg × 4 doses = 3600 mg/24 h

    d. **mg/kg/24 h** $\dfrac{3600 \text{ mg/24 h}}{34.1 \text{ kg}} = 105.6$ mg/kg/24 h

    e. **Recommended**   100 to 200 mg/kg/24 h q6-8 h

The patient is receiving an S&T dose at 105.6 mg/kg/24 h. Between 100 and 200 mg/kg/24 h is safe.

CALCULATING PEDIATRIC IV SOLUTIONS

Pediatric patients require smaller volumes of IV fluids and medications than adults. An IV pump, a buretrol (soluset), or both may be used for the pediatric patient. Each facility has guidelines for preparing and administering IV solutions and medications to the pediatric patient. Also, for a pediatric patient, IV tubing with a drop factor of 60 gtt/mL is usually recommended.

The concentration of the IV medication is also an important factor in medication administration. Administering a medication with a higher concentration than recommended is avoided because of the vein irritation that can result.

Example 1: Infuse 100 mL of 0.9% NS over 5 hours to a 6-month-old child. How many milliliters per hour should the IV pump be programmed for?

The formula: $\dfrac{\text{Total volume to be infused}}{\text{Total time in hours}} = x \text{ mL/h}$

(Formula setup) $\dfrac{100 \text{ mL}}{5 \text{ h}} = 20 \text{ mL/h}$

Example 2: Infuse 150 mL of D$_5$LR over 3 hours to a 3-year-old child. How many milliliters per hour should the IV pump be programmed for?

(Formula setup) $\dfrac{150 \text{ mL}}{3 \text{ h}} = 50 \text{ mL/h}$

If an IV pump is not used, IV fluids may be given by gravity. In this case, the formula is

$\dfrac{\text{Total volume to be given}}{\text{Total time in minutes}} \times \text{Tubing drop factor} = x \text{ gtt/min}$

Example 3: Infuse 200 mL lactated Ringer's solution (LR) over 4 hours to an 8-year-old child. The tubing drop factor is 60 gtt/mL. How many drops per minute of LR should be infused?

(Formula setup) $\dfrac{200 \text{ mL}}{\underset{4}{240 \text{ min}}} \times \overset{1}{60} \text{ gtt/mL} = x \text{ gtt/min}$

$\dfrac{200}{4 \text{ min}} \times 1 \text{ gtt} = 50 \text{ gtt/min}$

Example 4: Infuse 500 mL of D$_5$W over 8 hours to a 14-year-old child. The tubing drop factor is 60 gtt/mL. How many drops per minute of D$_5$W should be infused?

a. Convert hours to minutes.
 1 h : 60 min :: 8 h : x min

 $x = 480$ min

b. Calculate gtt/min.

(Formula setup) $\dfrac{500 \text{ mL}}{\underset{8}{480 \text{ min}}} \times \overset{1}{60} \text{ gtt/mL} = x \text{ gtt/min}$

$\dfrac{500}{8 \text{ min}} \times 1 \text{ gtt} = 62.5 \text{ or } 63 \text{ gtt/min}$

ADMINISTRATION OF IV MEDICATIONS TO PEDIATRIC PATIENTS

The formulas to calculate the administration rate of IV medications to pediatric patients are not different from those used for adults. The difference in administration of medications to a pediatric patient lies in the volume of solution used. Pediatric patients require a smaller volume of IV solutions; therefore care must be taken to give the medication at the recommended infusion concentration. Using a concentration that is higher than recommended may result in vein irritation and phlebitis. Unit policies and IV drug books provide the guidelines needed for appropriate concentration of IV medications for the pediatric patient.

If the medication is to be infused with an IV pump, the formula would be

$$\frac{\text{Total volume to be infused}}{\text{Total time for infusion in hours}} = x \text{ mL/h}$$

If the medication is to be infused with a buretrol (soluset) by gravity (Figure 18-1), then the formula would be

$$\frac{\text{Total volume to be infused}}{\text{Total time for infusion in minutes}} \times \text{Drop factor} = x \text{ gtt/min}$$

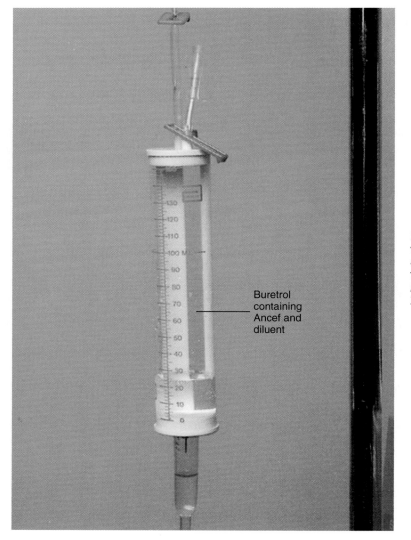

Buretrol containing Ancef and diluent

FIGURE 18-1 Dilution of Ancef in volume-control device, also known as a buretrol or soluset. (Modified from Potter PA, Perry AG: *Fundamentals of nursing,* ed 6, St Louis, 2005, Mosby.)

Example 1: An 18-month-old child has Ancef 450 mg q4 h IVPB over 15 minutes ordered. The child weighs 19 kg. The maximum recommended infusion concentration is 50 mg/mL. The vial of medication has a concentration of Ancef 250 mg/mL. How many milliliters of medication will provide 450 mg? _____ How many milliliters of IV solution need to be added to the medication to equal the recommended final concentration? _____ How many milliliters per hour should the IV pump be programmed for? _____

    a. Calculate volume of medication to withdraw from the vial.

       (Formula setup) $250 \text{ mg} : 1 \text{ mL} :: 450 \text{ mg} : x \text{ mL}$

$$250x = 450$$

$$x = \frac{450}{250}$$

$$x = 1.8 \text{ mL}$$

Therefore the nurse would withdraw 1.8 mL from the vial to administer 450 mg of Ancef.

    b. Calculate the volume of IV solution to provide the recommended final concentration.

       The formula: $\text{Ordered dose} \times \dfrac{1 \text{ mL}}{\text{Recommended concentration}} = x \text{ mL}$

       (Formula setup) $450 \text{ mg} \times \dfrac{1 \text{ mL}}{50 \text{ mg}} = 9 \text{ mL}$

Therefore to the 1.8 mL of Ancef, the nurse must add enough IV solution to give a TOTAL of 9 mL.

$$9 \text{ mL} - 1.8 \text{ mL} = 7.2 \text{ mL}$$

    1. Add 1.8 mL of Ancef to an empty buretrol.
    2. Add 7.2 mL of compatible IV fluid diluent to make a total volume of 9 mL.

$$
\begin{array}{r}
1.8 \text{ mL} \\
+ \quad 7.2 \text{ mL} \\
\hline
9.0 \text{ mL}
\end{array}
$$

    Final concentration: 50 mg/mL

    c. Calculate the milliliters per hour to program the IV pump.

       (Formula setup) $\dfrac{9 \text{ mL}}{0.25 \text{ h}} = 36 \text{ mL/h}$

Therefore the nurse would program the IV pump for 36 mL/h to infuse the Ancef over 15 minutes.

Example 2: A child weighing 30 kg has an order for nafcillin 850 mg IVPB q6 h over 10 minutes. The nafcillin vial gives a concentration of 250 mg/mL. The recommended infusion concentration of nafcillin is 100 mg/mL. How many milliliters of medication will provide 850 mg of nafcillin? _____ How many milliliters of IV solution need to be added to the medication to equal the recommended final concentration? _____ How many drops per minute should the IVPB be programmed for? _____

a. Calculate the volume of medication to withdraw from the vial.

(Formula setup)   250 mg : 1 mL :: 850 mg : x mL

$$250x = 850$$

$$x = \frac{850}{250}$$

$$x = 3.4 \text{ mL}$$

Therefore the nurse will withdraw 3.4 mL from the vial to administer 850 mg of nafcillin.

b. Calculate the volume of IV solution to provide the recommended final concentration

(Formula setup) $850 \text{ mg} \times \dfrac{1 \text{ mL}}{100 \text{ mg}} = 8.5 \text{ mL}$

Therefore to the 3.4 mL of nafcillin, the nurse must add IV solution to give a **TOTAL** of 8.5 mL.

$$8.5 \text{ mL} - 3.4 \text{ mL} = 5.1 \text{ mL}$$

Therefore the nurse will add an additional 5.1 mL of IV solution to the 3.4 mL of nafcillin to give a total of 8.5 mL.

c. Calculate gtt/min (a buretrol or soluset has a drop factor of 60 gtt/mL).

(Formula setup) $\dfrac{8.5 \text{ mL}}{10 \text{ min}} \times 60 \text{ gtt/mL} = x \text{ gtt/min}$

$$\frac{510}{10} = x \text{ gtt/min}$$

$$x = 51 \text{ gtt/min}$$

CALCULATION OF DAILY FLUID REQUIREMENTS FOR THE PEDIATRIC PATIENT

Maintenance fluids are those fluids needed daily for bodily function. Overhydration or dehydration (underhydration) can pose a great danger to the infant or young child. Therefore understanding daily fluid requirements is essential for the pediatric nurse. Use the formula below to calculate daily requirements.

PEDIATRIC FLUID REQUIREMENTS	
Patient weight	Maintenance fluid requirements in 24 hours
0–10 kg	100 mL/kg/24 h
10–20 kg	1000 mL + 50 mL/kg (for every kg >10 kg)
>20 kg	1500 mL + 20 mL/kg (for every kg >20 kg)

Modified from Hockenberry MJ, Wilson D, Winkelstein ML: *Wong's essentials of pediatric nursing*, ed 7, St Louis, 2005, Mosby, p 841.

To calculate the milliliters per hour, as when the patient receives IV fluids, simply divide the calculated amount of fluids required in 24 hours by 24 to obtain the amount of fluids needed per hour (see formula below).

Example 1: An infant weighs 20 pounds. Calculate the hourly IV fluid rate for this infant.

      a. **Weight**   20 lb = 9.1 kg

      b. **Calculation**   9.1 kg × 100 mL/kg/24 h = 910 mL/24 h

      c. **Daily fluid requirement**   910 mL/24 h

      d. **IV fluid formula:**

$$\frac{\text{Total volume to be infused}}{\text{Total time for infusion in hours}} = x \text{ mL/h}$$

      e. **Calculation** $\dfrac{910 \text{ mL}}{24 \text{ h}} = 37.9 \text{ mL/h}$

      f. **Fluids per hour**   37.9 mL/h

Example 2: A child weighs 19.3 kg. Calculate the hourly IV fluid rate for this child.

      a. **Weight**   19.3 kg

      b. **Calculation**

                                 First 10 kg = 1000 mL
                                 Remaining 9.3 kg × 50 mL/kg = 465 mL
                                 1000 mL + 465 mL = 1465 mL/24h

      c. **Daily fluid requirement**   1465 mL/24 h

      d. **IV fluid formula** $\dfrac{1465 \text{ mL}}{24 \text{ h}} = 61$

      e. **Fluid per hour**   61 mL/hr

NOTE: These rules apply to infants and young children.

Fluid requirements are 2000 to 3000 mL/24 h for the adult and for the child who approaches adult weight. Never exceed adult fluid requirements in a 24-hour period.

BODY SURFACE AREA CALCULATIONS

Body surface area (BSA) is determined by using a child's height and weight along with the West nomogram. If the child has a normal height and weight for his or her age, the BSA may be ascertained by the weight alone. For example, in Figure 18-2 showing the West nomogram, you can see that a child who weighs 70 lb has a BSA of 1.10 m².

When using the West nomogram, take a few minutes to assess the markings of each column. Note that the markings are not at the same intervals throughout each column.

If the child is not of normal height and weight for his or her age, an extended use of the nomogram is required. The far right column is for weight measured in pounds and kilograms. The far left column is for height measured in centimeters and inches. Place a ruler on the nomogram and draw a line connecting the height and weight points. Where the line crosses the surface area (SA) column, the SA in square meters (m²) will be indicated.

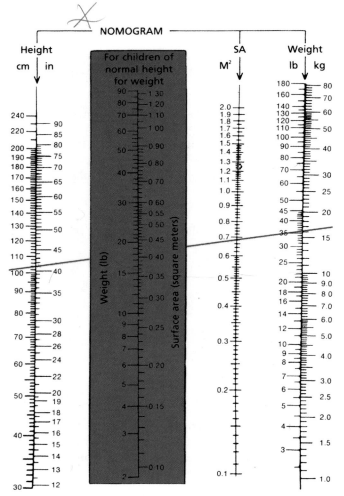

FIGURE 18-2 West nomogram for estimation of body surface areas in children. A straight line is drawn between height and weight. The point where the line crosses the surface area *(SA)* column is the estimated body surface. (From Behrman RE, Kleigman RM, Jenson HB, editors: *Nelson textbook of pediatrics,* ed 17, Philadelphia, 2004, Saunders.)

Practice Problems. Using the West nomogram, state the BSA in square meters for each child of normal height and weight listed below:

1. Child weighs 22 lb.   BSA = _____

2. Child weighs 4 lb.   BSA = _____

3. Child weighs 75 lb.   BSA = _____

4. Child weighs 10 lb.   BSA = _____

5. Child weighs 32 lb.   BSA = _____

Answers
1. 0.46 m²
2. 0.15 m²
3. 1.15 m²
4. 0.27 m²
5. 0.62 m²

Calculation of Dosage Based on Body Surface Area

The calculation of dosage may be based on BSA. The BSA method provides a means of converting an adult dosage to a safe pediatric dosage. There are three steps to the calculation with this method.

1. Determine the child's weight in kilograms.
2. Calculate the BSA in square meters. The formula for this calculation is as follows:

$$\frac{4 \text{ W (Child's weight in kilograms)} + 7}{\text{W (Child's weight in kilograms)} + 90} = \text{BSA in square meters}$$

3. Calculate the pediatric dosage using the following formula. The formula is based on the premise that an adult who weighs 140 lb has a BSA of 1.7 m².

$$\frac{\text{BSA in square meters}}{1.7} \times \text{Adult dose} = \text{Child's dose}$$

Example: Child weighs 24 lb and the adult dose is 100 mg.

    a. First, convert the child's weight to kilograms.

$$2.2 \text{ lb} : 1 \text{ kg} :: 24 \text{ lb} : x \text{ kg}$$

$$2.2 : 1 :: 24 : x$$

$$2.2x = 24$$

$$x = 10.9 \text{ kg}$$

The child weighs approximately 10.9 kg.

    b. Next, calculate the child's BSA in m².

$$\frac{4(10.9) + 7}{10.9 + 90} = \frac{43.6 + 7}{10.9 + 90} = \frac{50.6}{100.9} = 0.5$$

Child's BSA = 0.5 m²

    c. Finally, calculate the appropriate dosage for this child.

$$\frac{0.5}{1.7} \times 100 = 29.4 \text{ mg}$$

Practice Problems. Calculate the following children's dosages.

1. Child weighs 40 lb, adult dose = 300 mg.   Child's dose = _____
2. Child weighs 65 lb, adult dose = 30 mL.   Child's dose = _____
3. Child weighs 20 lb, adult dose = 50 mg.   Child's dose = _____
4. Child weighs 90 lb, adult dose = 10 mL.   Child's dose = _____
5. Child weighs 14 lb, adult dose = 2 g.   Child's dose = _____

Answers
1. 132 mg
2. 18.5 mL
3. 13 mg
4. 7.65 mL
5. 0.4 g

Practice Problems. Using the West nomogram, calculate the BSA for each child with the following heights and weights:

1. Child weighs 6 kg, height is 110 cm.   BSA = _____
2. Child weighs 5 lb, height is 19 in.   BSA = _____
3. Child weighs 25 kg, height is 70 cm.   BSA = _____
4. Child weighs 30 lb, height is 90 cm.   BSA = _____
5. Child weighs 160 lb, height is 200 cm.   BSA = _____

Answers
1. 0.41 m²
2. 0.18 m²
3. 0.74 m²
4. 0.58 m²
5. 2.0 m²

Complete the following work sheet, which provides for extensive practice in the calculation of pediatric dosages. Check your answers. If you have difficulties, go back and review the necessary material. When you feel ready to evaluate your learning, take the first posttest. Check your answers. An acceptable score as indicated on the posttest signifies that you have successfully completed this chapter. An unacceptable score signifies a need for further study before taking the second posttest.

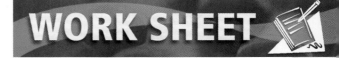

Directions: The medication order is listed at the beginning of each problem. Calculate the child's weight in kilograms, determine the safe recommended dosage or range, determine the safety of the order, and calculate the drug dose. Show your work.

1. The physician orders Keflex 250 mg po four times a day for a child weighing 50 lb. You have Keflex 250-mg capsules. The recommended daily po dosage for a child is 25 to 50 mg/kg/day in divided doses q6 h. a. Child's weight is _____ kg. b. What is the safe recommended dosage or range for this child? _____ c. Is the order safe? _____ d. If yes, how many capsules will you administer? _____

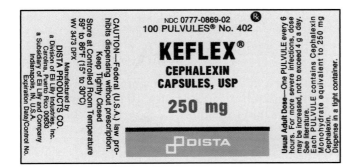

2. The physician orders Lanoxin 12.5 mg po daily for an infant weighing 6 lb 8 oz. You have Lanoxin 0.05 mg/mL. The recommended daily dosage for an infant is 0.035 to 0.06 mg/kg/day in divided doses two times a day. a. Child's weight is _____ kg. b. What is the safe recommended dosage or range for this child? _____ c. Is the order safe? _____ d. If yes, how many milliliters will you administer? _____

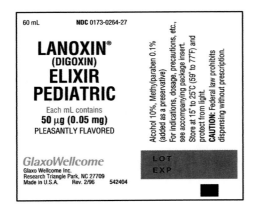

3. The physician orders Benadryl 25 mg IV q6 h for a child weighing 50 lb. You have available Benadryl 12.5 mg/mL. The recommended daily dosage for a child weighing more than 12 kg is 5 mg/kg/24 h in four divided doses. a. Child's weight is _____ kg. b. What is the safe recommended single dosage for this child? _____ c. Is the order safe? _____ d. If yes, how many milliliters will you prepare? _____

4. Calculate the 24-hour maintenance fluids for a child who weighs 28 lb.
a. _____ b. How many milliliters per hour are needed to program the pump to deliver the maintenance fluids? _____

5. The physician orders Omnicef 70 mg po twice a day for a child weighing 22 lb. The recommended dosage for Omnicef is 14 mg/kg/24 h twice a day for 10 days for skin infections. It is available as 125 mg/5 mL. a. Child's weight is _____ kg. b. Is the order safe? Prove your answer. _____ c. If the dose is S&T, how many milliliters are needed to deliver the ordered dose? _____

6. The physician orders Cipro 300 mg q12 h po for a child weighing 30.3 kg. You have Cipro 250 mg/5 mL. The recommended oral dosage is 20 to 30 mg/kg/24 h q12 h. a. Child's weight is _____ kg. b. What is the S&T 24-hour dosage range for this child? _____ c. What is the single dose range for this child? _____ d. How many milliliters are needed to deliver the ordered dose? _____

7. The physician orders Orapred 45 mg twice a day po for an asthmatic child weighing 94 lb. You have Orapred 15 mg/5 mL. The recommended oral dosage is 0.5 to 2 mg/kg/24 h divided twice a day. Maximum dosage is not to exceed 80 mg/24 h. a. Child's weight is _____ kg. b. What is a safe dosage range for this child? _____ c. Is the order safe? _____ d. Would you administer this medication as dosed? If not, why not?
_____

8. The physician orders Dilantin 60 mg po q12 h for a child weighing 40 lb. You have Dilantin 30-mg chewable tablets available. The recommended oral dosage for a child is 5 to 7 mg/kg/24 h in divided doses q12 h. a. Child's weight is _____ kg. b. What is the safe 24-hour dosage range for this child? _____ c. Is the order safe? _____ d. If yes, how many chewtabs will you administer? _____

9. A child is to receive vancomycin 750 mg IVPB q6 h. The child weighs 68 lb. The recommended dosage of vancomycin is 40 to 60 mg/kg/24 h. a. Child's weight is _____ kg. b. What dose per kilogram per 24 hours is the child receiving? _____ c. Is the order safe? _____

10. The physician orders Amoxil 300 mg po q12 h for a child weighing 42 lb. You have Amoxil 125 mg/5 mL. The recommended oral dosage is 25 to 50 mg/kg/24 h q12 h. a. Child's weight is _____ kg. b. What is the safe single dose range for this child? _____ c. How many milliliters are needed to deliver the ordered dose? _____

11. The physician orders 100 mL D₅W bolus IV to run over 30 minutes to a 3-year-old child. The drop factor of the tubing is 60 gtt/mL (microdrip). How many drops per minute are needed to deliver the bolus of D₅W? _____

12. The physician orders Tegretol 150 mg po three times a day for a child weighing 58 lb. You have Tegretol 100 mg/5 mL. The recommended oral dosage for a child is 10 to 20 mg/kg/24 h divided in doses three times a day. a. Child's weight is _____ kg. b. What is the safe single dose range for this child? _____ c. Is the order safe? _____ d. If yes, how many milliliters are needed? _____

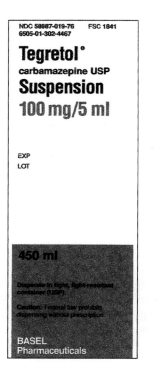

NDC 58887-019-76   FSC 1841
6505-01-302-4467

Tegretol°
carbamazepine USP
Suspension
100 mg/5 ml

EXP
LOT

450 ml

Dispense in tight, light-resistant
container (USP).

Caution: Federal law prohibits
dispensing without prescription

BASEL
Pharmaceuticals

13. Calculate the 24-hour maintenance fluid requirements for a child who weighs 72 lb.
a. Child's weight is _____ kg. b. The maintenance fluid requirements are _____.
c. How many milliliters per hour are needed to deliver the maintenance fluids? _____

14. The physician orders ibuprofen 100 mg for a child who weighs 52 lb. Recommended dose for ibuprofen is 5 to 10 mg/kg/dose q6 h. It is available as 100 mg/5 mL. a. Child's weight is _____ kg. b. What is a safe individual dose range for this child? _____ c. How many milliliters are needed to deliver the ordered dose? _____

15. The physician orders Kefzol 350 mg po q6 h for a child weighing 81 lb. You have Kefzol 500 mg/5 mL. The recommended daily oral dosage is 25 to 50 mg/kg/24 h divided q6 h. a. Child's weight is _____ kg. b. What is the safe recommended single dose range for this child? _____ c. Is the order safe? _____ d. If yes, how many milliliters will you prepare? _____

16. The physician orders Tagamet 60 mg po q8 h for an infant weighing 16 lb. Tagamet 300 mg/5 mL is available. The recommended daily oral dosage is 15 to 20 mg/kg/24 h divided q8 h. a. Child's weight is _____ kg. b. What is the safe recommended dosage or range for this child? _____ c. Is the order safe? _____ d. How many milligrams per kilogram per 24 hours is the child receiving? _____ e. If the ordered dosage is safe, how many milliliters will you administer? _____

17. The physician orders prednisone 8 mg po q12 h for a child weighing 19 lb. You have prednisone syrup 5 mg/5 mL. The recommended oral dosage is 0.5 to 2 mg/kg/24 h given once daily or divided and given in two doses per day. a. Child's weight is _____ kg. b. What is a safe single dose range for this child? _____ c. Is the order safe? _____ d. If yes, how many milliliters will you draw up? _____

18. The physician orders Ancef 400 mg IV q8 h for a child weighing 32 lb. You have Ancef 330 mg/mL. The recommended daily IV dosage for a child is 100 mg/kg/24 h in divided doses q6-8 h. a. Child's weight is _____ kg. b. What is the safe recommended dosage or range for this child? _____ c. Is the order safe? _____ d. If yes, how many milliliters will you prepare? _____

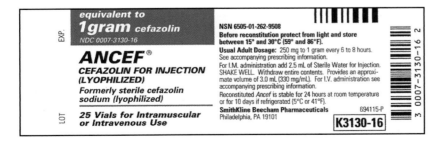

19. The order is to infuse 250 mL of D_5W over 3 hours to an 11-year-old child. How many milliliters per hour should the IV pump be programmed for? _____

20. A 25-kg child has an order for gentamicin 40 mg IVPB twice a day over 20 minutes. The concentration of the vial states 10 mg/mL. The recommended infusion concentration is 2 mg/mL. a. How many milliliters of medication will provide 40 mg of gentamicin? _____ b. How many milliliters of IV solution need to be added to the medication to equal the recommended final concentration? _____ c. How many drops per minute of gentamicin should be infused? _____

Answers on pp. 565–572.

Name _____

Date _____

ACCEPTABLE SCORE __49__

YOUR SCORE _____

POSTTEST 2

Directions: The medication order is listed at the beginning of each problem. Calculate the child's weight in kilograms, determine the S&T dosage or range, determine the safety of the order, and calculate the drug dosage. Show your work.

1. A child is to receive vancomycin 450 mg IVPB q6 h. The patient weighs 70 lb on admission. The recommended dosage is 40 to 60 mg/kg/24 h q6 h. a. Child's weight is _____ kg. b. How many milligrams per kilogram per 24 hours is the patient receiving? _____ c. Is the order S&T? Prove. _____

2. The physician orders Dilantin 100 mg po q12 h for a child weighing 62 lb. You have Dilantin 125/5 mL on hand. The recommended daily oral dosage for a child is 7 to 8 mg/kg/24 h in divided doses two or three times per day. a. Child's weight is _____ kg. b. What is a safe 24-hour dosage range for this child? _____ c. What is the single dose range for this child? _____ d. Is the prescribed dose safe to administer? _____ e. If yes, how many milliliters will you administer? _____

N 0071-2214-20   *Shake Well*

Dilantin-125®
(Phenytoin Oral Suspension, USP)

125 mg per 5 mL potency

Important—Another strength available; verify unspecified prescriptions.

Caution—Federal law prohibits dispensing without prescription.

8 fl oz (237 mL)

PARKE-DAVIS
Div of Warner-Lambert Co/ Morris Plains, NJ 07950 USA   2214G013

Shake well before using.

Each 5 mL contains phenytoin, 125 mg with a maximum alcohol content not greater than 0.6 percent.

Usual Dose—Adults, 1 teaspoonful three times daily; Children, see package insert.

See package insert for complete prescribing information.

Store below 30° C (86° F). Protect from freezing.

Keep this and all drugs out of the reach of children.

Exp date and lot

6505-00-890-1110

3. The physician orders Amoxil 400 mg po q12 h for a child weighing 58 lb. You have Amoxil suspension 250 mg/5 mL. The recommended daily oral dosage for a child is 25 to 50 mg/kg/24 h in divided doses q12 h. a. Child's weight is _____ kg. b. What is the safe 24-hour dosage range for this child? _____ c. What is the single dose range for this child? _____ d. How many milligrams per kilogram per 24 hours is the patient receiving with this order? _____ e. How many milliliters are needed to deliver the ordered dose? _____

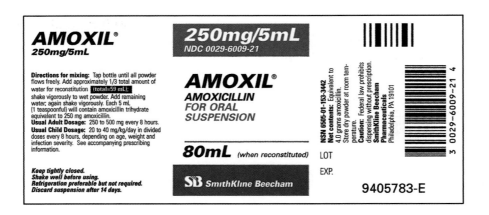

4. The physician orders Keflex 500 mg po q6 h for a 99-lb school-age child. Available is Keflex 250-mg capsules. The recommended daily oral dosage is 50 to 100 mg/kg/24 h divided q6 h. Maximum dosage is not to exceed 2 g/24 h. a. Child's weight is _____ kg. b. How many milligrams per kilogram per 24 hours is this child receiving? _____ c. Is the order safe? _____ d. If yes, how many capsules will you administer? _____

5. The physician orders Omnicef 200 mg po q12 h for a child weighing 66 lb. Omnicef is available as 125 mg/5 mL. Recommended dosage is 14 mg/kg/24 h divided q12 h. a. Child's weight is _____ kg. b. How many milligrams per kilogram per 24 hours is the child receiving? _____ c. Is the order safe? _____ d. If yes, how many milliliters are needed? _____

6. A neonate weighs 2012 g. He is to receive ampicillin 100 to 200 mg/kg/24 h divided q6 h IV per syringe for otitis media. a. Child's weight is _____ kg. b. What 24-hour dosage range is needed? _____ c. What single dose range is needed? _____

7. The physician orders Amoxil 180 mg po q8 h for a 35-lb child. Available is Amoxil 125 mg/5 mL. Recommended dosage is 25 to 50 mg/kg/24 h divided q6-8 h. a. Child's weight is _____ kg. b. How many milligrams per kilogram per 24 hours is the child receiving? _____ c. Is the order safe? _____ d. If yes, how many milliliters are needed? _____

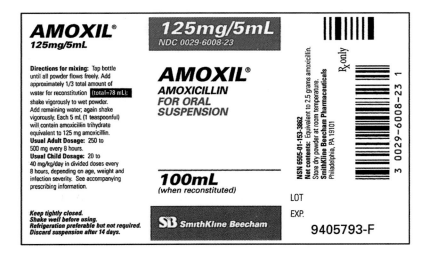

8. An infant is to receive 150 mL of whole blood over 3 hours. Using a microdrip (60 gtt/mL), how many drops per minute are needed? _____

9. The physician orders vancomycin 330 mg po q6 h for a 74-lb child. You have vancomycin 250 mg/5 mL. The recommended daily oral dosage is 40 mg/kg/24 h divided q6 h. a. Child's weight is _____ kg. b. How many milligrams per kilogram per 24 hours is the child receiving? _____ c. Is the order safe? _____ d. If yes, how many milliliters are needed? _____

10. The physician orders morphine sulfate 0.9 mg IV q4 h for pain. Available is morphine sulfate 0.5 mg/mL. The child weighs 20 lb. The recommended single dose is 0.1 to 0.2 mg/kg q4 h. a. Child's weight is _____ kg. b. What is the safe dose range for this child? _____ c. Is the order safe? _____ d. If yes, how many milliliters will you draw up? _____

11. The physician orders an infusion of 200 mL of D₅LR over 3 hours to a 6-year-old child. How many milliliters per hour should the IV pump be programmed for? _____

12. A 60-kg child has an order for vancomycin 500 mg IVPB to be delivered over a 1- to 2-hour period. The vial concentration is 50 mg/mL. The recommended infusion concentration is 5 mg/mL. a. How many milliliters of medication will provide 500 mg of vancomycin? _____ b. How many milliliters of IV solution need to be added to the medication to equal the recommended concentration? _____ c. How many drops per minute of vancomycin should be infused? _____

13. The physician orders Lanoxin 0.013 mg po twice a day for an infant weighing 3036 g. The recommended oral dosage for Lanoxin is 6 to 10 mcg/kg/24 h divided q12 h. Available is Lanoxin elixir 50 mcg/mL. a. Child's weight is _____ kg. b. What is an S&T 24-hour dosage range for this infant? _____ c. What is a safe single dose range for this infant? _____ d. Is the order safe? _____ e. If yes, how many milliliters will you give? _____

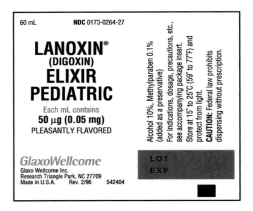

14. Calculate the single dose range of acetaminophen for an infant who weighs 9 lb. Acetaminophen is available as 80 mg/0.8 mL, and the safe dose range is 10 to 15 mg/kg/dose q6 h. a. Infant's weight is _____ kg. b. What is the single dose range? _____ c. How many milliliters are needed to deliver the calculated dose range? _____

15. Phenobarbital elixir 72 mg po daily is ordered for a child who weighs 37 lbs. Phenobarbital is supplied as 20 mg/5 mL. Recommended dosage is 4 to 6 mg/kg/24 h one or two times per day. a. Child's weight is _____ kg. b. What is the 24-hour dosage range needed for this child? _____ c. Is the order safe? _____ d. If yes, how many milliliters will you administer? _____

Answers on pp. 576–580.

 Refer to Introducing Pediatric Calculations on the enclosed CD for additional help and practice problems.

Drug Administration Considerations

CHAPTERS

Automated Medication Dispensing Systems

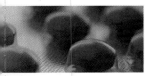

LEARNING OBJECTIVES

On completion of the materials provided in this chapter, you will be able to:

1 Recognize an automated medication dispensing system

2 Identify the advantages of using an automated medication dispensing system

Health care delivery systems continue to strive to improve the accuracy and efficiency of the delivery of medications to patients. In recent years, more and more hospitals and other care center areas have moved to the use of automated medication dispensing systems.

Each patient care unit is provided with a special cabinet that houses the medications that will be dispensed from that unit. The medications in the machine are usually listed by both their trade and generic names. This feature helps expedite location of the medications by the nurse. These cabinets are connected to the central pharmacy for order verifications and accuracy, as well as for automation of usage reports that are provided for many facets of the medication process. Depending on the vendor chosen by the institution, a variety of medications may be housed in the cabinet, ranging from only controlled substances to inclusion of first doses, as-needed (prn) doses, and regularly scheduled medications.

Having a wide range of medications within the patient care area allows a quick response to changes in a patient's condition. For example, a new medication order does not require a special trip to the central pharmacy to obtain the needed medication, allowing the new drug regimen to be initiated quickly. With a computerized system, the patient has the added benefit of more time being available to the nurse for all aspects of patient care, and the pharmacist has more time to confer with physicians and resource nurses and to analyze drug studies and usage.

An automatic drug dispensing system also leads to a reduction in medication errors. This is especially true as vendors market new options that allow only the designated drawer housing the medication that is being given at that time to open. The automated medication dispensing system also enhances patient satisfaction. This is especially evident in postsurgical patients or patients with cancer who require the administration of pain medications in a timely manner. Pain medications are usually controlled substances that require the nurse to first locate and obtain the narcotic keys from a peer, then open the narcotic supply, find and remove the right medication, relock the supply area, sign out the controlled substance, and then take the medication to the patient for administration. With an automated system, the nurse is able to access the medication from the cabinet and confirm the accuracy of the controlled substance count immediately. The medication may then be given quickly to the patient with the least amount of time and effort expended (Figure 19-1). All these systems are password secured. Each nurse has a password or

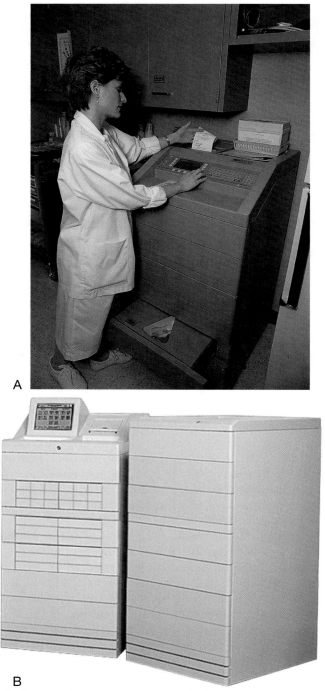

A

B

FIGURE 19–1 A, Nurse using computer-controlled dispensing system. **B,** Medstation automated drug dispensing system. (**A,** From Potter P, Perry A: *Fundamentals of nursing,* ed 6, St Louis, 2005, Mosby. **B,** From Pyxis Corporation, San Diego, Calif.)

CHAPTER 19 Automated Medication Dispensing Systems

ID number. Continuous documentation occurs while the cabinet is in use. The nurse can review records, but at the same time the cabinet records how long the nurse has been "logged in." This is important for quality control and evaluation of nursing actions in relation to patient care.

Another advantage of an automated medication dispensing system is reduction in the time required for end-of-shift narcotic counts. This count is performed by two nurses, usually one from the ending shift and one from the starting shift. It is also standard practice that until the narcotic count is completed and correct, all staff who are ending their shift may not leave. This results in staff dissatisfaction and unnecessary overtime costs that can be better spent on actual patient care. This scenario is prevented because automated systems require the confirmation of the count of controlled substance medications after each withdrawal.

These medication dispensing systems are also beneficial for patients who are transferred from one unit to another. The medications are already housed in the cabinet if it is one that has been expanded to include most patient medications (Figure 19-2). This allows the patient's continued progress by eliminating delays in obtaining medications.

Some of the systems currently on the market interface with the health care system's program for charting medications. With some dispensing systems, charting is done at the cabinet in the unit, whereas other manufacturers are designing programs to document the administration of medication at the bedside. With the automatic documentation of the administration of the patient's medications, the nurse is not required to return to the paper medication administration record and manually chart that the medicine has been given.

There are some disadvantages to the automated dispensing systems. Because some of the drawers have open compartments, it is possible for the wrong medication to be placed in the drawer. This makes the three medicine checks the nurse performs when he or she prepares a

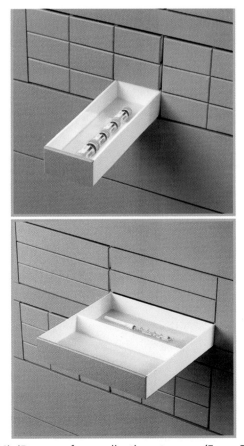

FIGURE 19–2 Pyxis MiniDrawers for medication storage. (From Pyxis Corporation, San Diego, Calif.)

patient's medicines absolutely paramount. Technology is *not* perfect, and mistakes can and do occur in the delivery of medication. The pharmacy, as the cabinet is being restocked, or another nurse may have mishandled the medications while searching the drawers for the medication that is currently needed. If the machine houses all of the patient medications, lines may form when several nurses need to obtain patient medications at the same time. The nurse needs to be well organized and plan ahead for access to the cabinet.

As health care facilities continue to monitor costs and at the same time strive to improve patient and staff satisfaction, the use of automated medication dispensing systems will become more widespread. This is a new area in which nursing students will need to become knowledgeable and competent because the accurate and efficient delivery of medications is one of the most important tasks of patient care that the nurse is required to perform.

 Refer to Safety in Medication Administration: Pyxis and Bar Code on the CD for additional help.

Special Considerations for the Administration of Medications to the Elderly

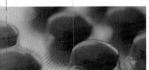

LEARNING OBJECTIVES

On completion of the materials provided in this chapter, you will be able to:

1 Understand the implications of the physiological changes of aging and their effect on medication administration to the elderly

2 Understand the special problems and issues related to medication administration to the elderly

People are now living longer than at any period in history, and we are continuing to increase our knowledge of how to protect our health and prevent illness. By practicing good health habits, such as proper diet, an exercise program, and a positive attitude, people are enjoying better health. As research continues, cures and maintenance regimens for major health problems are being found. Life expectancy continues to increase. "Old-old" persons over the age of 85 are the most rapidly increasing portion of the population in the United States. This group is also using more of the nation's health care resources.

Aging is a normal process, beginning at infancy and continuing throughout the life cycle. Aging is not the cause of specific diseases, but certain chronic illnesses are more prevalent in the elderly and may lead to additional health problems. Chronic illnesses usually require an increase in drug use to control the symptoms or progression of the condition.

Changes Experienced by the Elderly

Biological and physiological changes that affect all body systems occur and conflict with the action of some medications. Medication problems are more likely to occur in the older age-group. These problems can be drug interactions, adverse reactions, drug and food interactions, or medication errors. Reflexes slow, and the body is unable to adapt quickly to changes in temperature. A decrease in the sense of touch may be a safety issue. There is a decrease in saliva, which may slow the absorption of buccal medications. Some elderly persons may have difficulty swallowing, especially large tablets. An advantage of aging is a diminished sense of taste: elderly people may have no difficulty with some of the bitter-tasting medications.

Biological and physiological changes also affect the metabolism and excretion of drugs. Chronic conditions, such as hypertension, diabetes, heart conditions, and arthritis, interfere with homeostasis and may cause medications to be less effective. Absorption is affected by age-related changes in the motility of the gastrointestinal tract. A decrease in motility may cause an increase in drug actions. Many elderly persons resort to the regular use of laxatives. Laxatives increase the motility of the gastrointestinal tract and therefore allow less time for the prescribed medication to be absorbed.

Changes in cardiac output may also decrease the flow of blood to the liver and kidneys. Another major change with aging is the decrease in renal function. This may lead to medications being removed from the body more slowly and perhaps less completely.

A decrease in body weight of many elderly persons is reason to reassess the dosages of medications ordered. The patient's actual weight should be used to validate the correct dosage of each drug. Many drug reference manuals now list the appropriate dosages for geriatric, pediatric, and adult patients. At times it may be difficult to select a proper site for an injection. This is because of a decrease in muscle mass. However, an advantage to aging may be a decrease in the perception of pain from injections because of a decrease in some sensory perceptions.

These changes, in concert with a person's genetic programming, add to the severity of health problems in the elderly. It is difficult for a person who has had an active life to deal with these changes. The nurse must be understanding to help an elderly person adapt to a limited lifestyle.

Physical illness often affects a person's mental state, adding to anxiety and further deterioration. Occasionally, an elderly person feels unable to make the most basic decisions. The nurse, in collaboration with other members of the health care team, can help the patient, the family, and the persons responsible for giving care to understand the process of change or aging. For example, Alzheimer's disease negatively affects a person's ability to safely assume responsibility for taking his or her own medications, especially as the stages advance. It is important for family members and caregivers to be aware of this.

Problems of the Elderly

Some older persons are in the habit of visiting an internist for an annual physical examination. Because the elderly have more aches and pains than those in other age-groups, they may also visit a physician in family practice to deal with minor problems. If these aches and pains do not resolve, they may visit a third physician. If each physician writes prescriptions, the patient may be prescribed several medications that duplicate actions or cause drug interaction or overdosage.

The patient should be encouraged to visit only one physician unless referred to a specialist. If the patient visits another physician, he or she should prepare a list of all medications taken routinely or as needed and give it to the new physician. The physician can then prescribe medication and instruct the patient to stop taking duplicate medications or those that cause drug interactions.

Older patients should be encouraged to have all their prescriptions filled at the same pharmacy. This allows the pharmacist to have a complete listing of the medications that have been prescribed. The pharmacist is then able to monitor for adverse interactions of the patient's medicines. When an older patient uses many different pharmacies, this safety check does not occur.

Inadequate income is a major problem for many older people. To lower medical costs, they may take less than the prescribed amount of a prescription drug so that it will last longer. They may also stop taking the medication if they perceive it to be ineffective. They may go to the drug store and buy nonprescription drugs. Such drugs will save a physician's fee and are less expensive than prescription drugs, but they may be ineffective. However, the patient may perceive them to be a cure. Another method used to lower costs of drugs is to take medication prescribed for a family member or friend. Misuse of drugs is widespread among the elderly and may cause various problems, such as fluid imbalance, nutritional disturbances, and psychological or neurological problems. The elderly may also experience a deterioration in their eyesight. There are many magnifying tools that can help them continue to administer the correct dose of their medication.

As older persons become forgetful, they may not take their medications or may not take them at the prescribed time. Often family members find medication bottles on the floor, and they do not know whether the medication was taken.

When it becomes unsafe for an elderly person to stay at home alone, a day-care center can relieve the pressure on family members. People enjoy being with others of their age to discuss memories and similar experiences. They can join in crafts and activities as they wish. There are opportunities to discuss thoughts and concerns with personnel at the center. Then the medication regimen can be continued during the day, and meals can be served and activities planned. Activities at the center stimulate the elderly and give them something interesting to discuss at home in the evening.

More elderly persons elect to live in their own homes rather than in a retirement home or a nursing home. Sometimes they share their home with someone near their age. If an elderly person or couple cannot care for themselves, they may choose to share their home with an individual or a couple who will not only be homemakers but also give care as needed. Apart from providing a home for the ones giving care, the elderly person may provide monetary compensation.

Medical Alert System

A medical alert system is a valuable tool for a homebound person living alone or for times when the caregiver must be away. It is also used in retirement homes. In an emergency a button is pushed on the monitoring system or on a device on a chain worn by the patient. The system alerts medical personnel to the emergency situation. Such a system gives a feeling of security to homebound persons and their families.

Medications for the Elderly in the Home

When purchasing medications from a pharmacy, elderly persons should request that childproof containers *not* be used. Containers that are available to prepare medications for a day or a week at a time should be purchased and used (Figure 20-1). Such containers have a special compartment for each hour the medications are to be given. The time can be written on the lid of the individual compartment and easily removed if the time changes. These containers are especially helpful if someone outside the home assists the patient in preparing medications.

An appointment book with the day and date, a spiral notebook, or a writing tablet with the day and date added can be used as an efficient and safe way to plan medications taken in the home. The medications and the times they are to be taken each day are listed. The entry is crossed off after the medication has been taken (Box 20-1). The used medication sheet is discarded and a new one is completed each day.

The Visiting Nurse

At times when the patient, the family, or the person giving care believes that an assessment of the patient's health status is needed, a request can be made to the physician for assistance from a visiting nurse. The visiting nurse provides skilled care and consultation in the home under the supervision of the patient's physician.

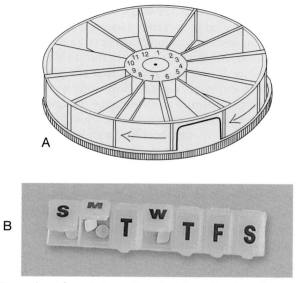

FIGURE 20-1 Examples of containers that hold medications for a day **(A)** or a week **(B)** at a time. **(B,** From Elkin MK, Perry AG, Potter PA: *Nursing interventions and clinical skills,* ed 3, St Louis, 2004, Mosby.)

BOX 20-1 ■ MEDICATION SHEET EXAMPLE

Thursday, March 25
Motrin 300 mg after each meal
  ~~8:00~~ AM 1:00 PM 6:00 PM
Naprosyn 250 mg two times a day
  ~~8:00~~ AM 4:00 PM
Persantin 25 mg two times a day
  10:00 AM 6:00 PM
Lanoxin 40 mg daily
  10:00 AM
Mylanta 2 tablespoons after meals

The nurse assesses the patient's condition, gives nursing care as needed, and helps the family and the person giving care to better understand the patient. The nurse should review the patient's medication regimen with the person giving care. If some time has elapsed since the medication was ordered, the nurse should review the medication orders with the physician. The service provided by the visiting nurse will help the patient and family feel secure that the patient is receiving optimum health care in the home.

Medication Errors with the Elderly

The elderly at home are more prone to medication errors than those in health care facilities. The most common error is that of omission. This may be because of the cost of medication or the person's forgetfulness. Other medication errors involve an incorrect dosage, wrong time, or misunderstanding of directions.

The decrease in gross and fine motor skills may affect how well the packaging of medications can be handled. For example, arthritis may make it difficult for a patient with insulin-dependent diabetes to draw up and self-administer the correct dose of insulin. If the patient is unable to self-administer, then a family member, friend, or caretaker will need to be taught.

It is important for the nurse to make certain that elderly patients understand the directions for taking their medications safely. Many elderly persons are hearing impaired to some degree. The nurse should ask the patient to verbally repeat the instructions. Older people, beginning with middle age, often are also visually impaired. It is necessary to make certain they can read the labels of their drugs, and any written directions should be printed in a large, easy-to-read format. Written directions for later reference should always be provided, since the patient may forget.

Medication errors with the elderly can be reduced if time is taken to explain the reason for the medication, its importance, and how it works. This is especially important if timing is critical in maintaining a therapeutic blood level of the medication. Some elderly patients fear becoming addicted to their medication because they do not understand its purpose.

A careful and complete drug history, including illicit drugs, should be obtained from all patients, but especially older ones. This history should include over-the-counter drugs, alternative medicines, supplements, and large doses of vitamins. Many people think that all of these products are completely safe. However, they may be unaware of the negative interactions that may occur if these products are taken with other medicines that have been prescribed by their physician.

Alcohol is one of the most abused drugs in the elderly population. The combination of alcohol and certain medicines may be a problem for the chronic drinker and the occasional drinker. The nurse's assessment should include the patient's use of alcohol. This information should be validated with other family members.

Medications for the Elderly in the Hospital

Professional nurses will plan nursing care for older patients in the hospital. As our older population continues to increase, nurses will be employed not only in hospitals and nursing homes but also in day-care centers and retirement communities. Nurses will work with the patient and the family and other health care practitioners, including the physician, dietitian, pharmacist, occupational therapist, social worker, and clinical nurse specialist or nurse practitioner.

Although the physician orders the medications and the pharmacist prepares them, the nurse is responsible for administering the medication to the patient. It is important that the right amount of the right medicine be given to the right patient at the right time in the right way. The patient must also be observed for reactions. The physician must be notified if drug reactions occur. The nurse must record the date, time, medication, dosage, and route of administration. It is important to follow the six rights of medication administration with the elderly, as with all other patients (Box 20-2).

Before administering the medication to the patient, the nurse should tell the patient the name of the drug and why it was prescribed. The nurse must also be certain that the medication was taken. Sometimes an older patient may hold the medication in the mouth and then remove it after the nurse leaves the bedside. The patient may save the medication in case he or she needs it later. This could cause an overdose.

BOX 20-2 ■ SIX RIGHTS OF MEDICATION ADMINISTRATION

1. Drug
2. Dose
3. Patient
4. Route
5. Time
6. Documentation

The nurse should observe the patient after administering the medication for any unusual symptoms and record these observations on the patient's chart. The patient's physician must be notified if serious symptoms occur.

Administration of medications is one of the nurse's most important responsibilities. However, without good skin care, oral hygiene, body alignment, exercise, and a well-balanced diet, the patient will not maintain the potential for health and a satisfying life. Care of the whole person is essential for health and well-being.

Remember, the elderly should be viewed as experienced and mature adults, no matter what the functional state of the body. Older adults are using the Internet more and more for health education information. Older adults are capable of learning, but their learning is most successful when there is no time constraint. Allow plenty of time for their learning to take place, and relate the new material to something familiar, if possible. For these reasons discharge planning needs to be done *before the day of discharge*. When teaching the elderly, use visual material, simple language, and large print and involve their support persons. The elderly should be encouraged to administer their own medications in the hospital if possible. This allows the nurse to answer questions and assess the level of learning that has occurred.

Home Care Considerations in the Administration of Medications

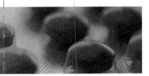

LEARNING OBJECTIVES

On completion of the materials provided in this chapter, you will be able to:

1 Understand the unique issues of nursing practice in a home care setting

2 Understand the administration of IV therapy in a home care setting

HOME HEALTH NURSING

Home health nursing is one of the fastest growing sectors in the health care industry. High-quality nursing care is being delivered to patients in their homes to promote cost-effective health care. These services may be provided on a scheduled or intermittent basis. Home health care is often more conducive to restoring or maintaining a patient's quality of life than care in a hospital or other facility. Patient satisfaction may also be increased by being at home rather than separated from family in an acute care setting.

Nurses working in the field of home care enjoy increased autonomy of practice. They must have a medical-surgical background (usually 1 year of clinical experience) and be able to demonstrate expert critical thinking skills. These skills include assessment, communication, judgment, and problem solving. Home care nurses need to be self-directed. Their patients are more likely to need specialized care because of the shortened length of stays in hospitals, resulting in an increased use of technology in the home. These nurses need to be independent and innovative in their practice. The technical skills required of them are often the same as for nurses working in intensive care units. Many states require home care agencies to have nurses available 24 hours a day.

Home care nursing may involve dressing changes, tracheostomy and ventilator care, patient and family teaching, bathing, rehabilitation services, and hospice care. However, the home infusion market is the area of greatest growth in home care. This involves the administration and management of medications in the home. Administration of intravenous (IV) medications at home costs substantially less than it would in a hospital. The design of portable infusion pumps has improved the safety, accuracy, and ease of home infusion therapy (Figures 21-1 and 21-2).

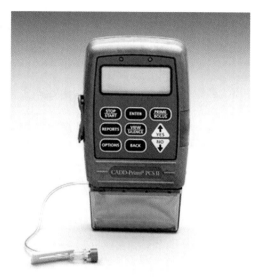

FIGURE 21-1 Patient-controlled analgesia pump with cassette. (From Deltec, Inc., St. Paul, Minn.)

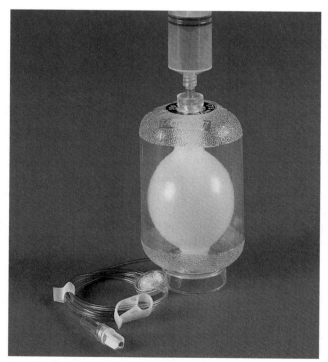

FIGURE 21-2 MedFlo Postoperative Pain Management System ambulatory infusion device. (From Smith & Nephew Endoscopy, Andover, Md.)

The principles of medication administration are the same in the home setting as in a hospital. The physician writes the order for the medication. Medication calculations are done in exactly the same way as discussed earlier in this book. The guiding principles include the six rights of medication administration (Box 21-1). The nurse must follow the rights as discussed in Chapter 10, Interpretation of the Physician's Orders.

BOX 21-1 ■ SIX RIGHTS OF MEDICATION ADMINISTRATION

1. Drug
2. Dose
3. Patient
4. Route
5. Time
6. Documentation

The sixth right of *documentation* is also required in home administration of medications. This is not only for a legal record; it also plays a significant role in cost reimbursement and payments. The nurse needs to be very knowledgeable about home health care policies. This information is then used to provide the clinical documentation that results in the greatest amount of reimbursement for the patient.

IV THERAPY IN THE HOME

Central Venous Catheter

A central venous catheter (CVC) is often used in home care. The CVC may be used for antibiotic therapy, fluid replacement, chemotherapy, hyperalimentation, narcotic pain control, and delivery of blood components. These devices prevent repeated venipunctures in the treatment of patients with cancer, malnutrition, and long-term antibiotic needs. Central lines may also be used for drawing blood from a patient without another needlestick.

Different brand names for CVCs include the *Hickman, Broviac,* and *Groshong*. The line is placed by a physician using sterile technique, after local or general anesthesia has been induced. The line is threaded into a subclavian or jugular vein or superior vena cava. The catheter is sutured on the outside of the body to secure placement. Before the line is used for administration of fluids or medications, a radiograph is obtained to confirm appropriate placement. A subclavian catheter is for short-term use of less than 60 days. Tunneled catheters, such as a Hickman, are for long-term use of 1 to 2 years (Figure 21-3).

Peripherally Inserted Central Catheter

A current trend in home care is to favor the use of a peripherally inserted central catheter (PICC). The line is inserted peripherally by a physician or specially certified nurse at the bedside, using strict aseptic technique. This catheter is used for 1 to 8 weeks of therapy. Placement should be confirmed by radiography.

Implantable Venous Access Devices, or Ports

An implantable or subcutaneous port is placed in the subcutaneous layer beneath the skin. The port is seen as a raised area 0.2 inch beneath the skin (Figures 21-4 and 21-5). The dome of the port is made of a self-sealing silicone septum. This access device may be used for long-term therapy of 1 to 2 years.

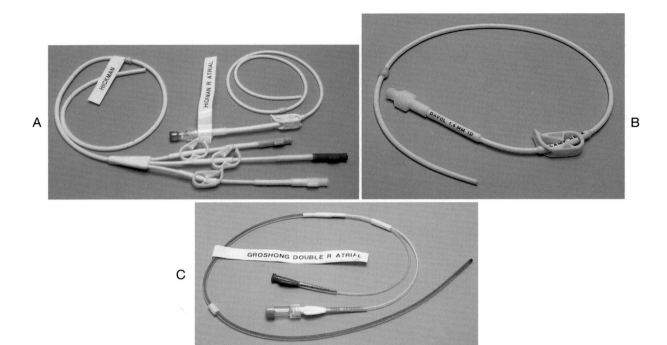

FIGURE 21-3 **A,** Hickman catheter. **B,** Broviac catheter. **C,** Groshong catheter. (From Clayton BD, Stock YN: *Basic pharmacology for nurses,* ed 13, St Louis, 2004, Mosby. Courtesy Chuck Dresner.)

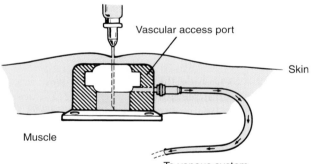

FIGURE 21-4 Example of an implantable vascular access device. (From Potter PA, Perry AG: *Fundamentals of nursing,* ed 6, St Louis, 2005, Mosby.)

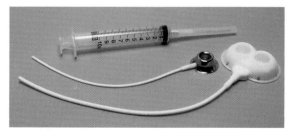

FIGURE 21-5 Silicone venous catheters with infusion ports. (From Clayton BD, Stock YN: *Basic pharmacology for nurses,* ed 13, St Louis, 2004, Mosby. Courtesy Chuck Dresner.)

Landmark Midline Venous Access Device

The midline catheter follows the same principle as other PICCs with one exception. This catheter is inserted into the antecubital area and is advanced into the upper veins of the arm. It does not advance into the chest area. Therefore placement does not require a confirmation by radiography.

The Landmark catheter is constructed of a material called *Aquavan*. This catheter is introduced by an over-the-needle method. After catheter placement, the Aquavan material absorbs fluid from the blood and softens. At the same time, the gauge expands and provides an increased flow rate. This catheter should also be placed using strict aseptic technique.

Implications for Home Care Nursing

With home IV therapy, it is important that the nurse treating the patient be aware of the care and precautions required for an IV line. Routine dressing changes and assessment of the insertion site and area are mandatory. Assessment for infiltration and signs and symptoms of infection are necessary also. Education of the patient and the family is vital for the successful use of home IV therapies. Routine line care must be performed accurately to prevent clotting and infection. The patient also needs to be assessed for systemic complications such as circulatory overload and an air embolus. The routine care will be delineated by the physician and by agency policies.

For home infusion therapy to be successful, the patient and family need to be informed and educated. The areas to include are medication information, how to administer and manage the IV fluids, what complications may occur and how to handle them, principles of infection control, operation of equipment, and clear guidelines as to when to notify the physician. With physicians, nurses, patients, and families working together, true continuity of care may be attained in the home.

ACCEPTABLE SCORE ___86___

YOUR SCORE _____

Directions: This test contains 40 questions with a total of 90 points (pts) possible. Each of the seven separate case sections includes a variety of patient diagnoses. Test items focus on medication dosages, medication calculations, and medication transcription. Use the forms provided, and mark syringes where indicated.

CASE 1 *(20 PTS)*

Mr. Jones is transferred to your floor from the ICU. You receive Mr. Jones and look over his orders. It is 1700 on 2/3/11. Refer to the physician's order sheet and medication profile sheet on p. 450 for the following questions. Show your work where applicable.

1. Mr. Jones complains of pain to his incision. Percocet tablets are ordered on the physician's order sheet. Percocet is supplied in single tablets issued from the pharmacy. Give _____

(1 pt)

2. What regularly scheduled medications would Mr. Jones receive at 0900 each day? Include the amount of medication. a. _____ b. _____ c. _____ d. _____

(4 pts)

3. How much IV fluid will Mr. Jones receive every 8 hours? _____ mL

(1 pt)

PHYSICIAN'S ORDERS

Mr. Jones

1. ADDRESSOGRAPH BEFORE PLACING IN PATIENT'S CHART ▶
2. INITIAL AND DETACH COPY EACH TIME PHYSICIAN WRITES ORDERS
3. TRANSMIT COPY TO PHARMACY
4. ORDERS MUST BE DATED AND TIMED

☐ Inpatient   ☐ Outpatient

DATE	TIME	ORDERS	TRANS BY
		Diagnosis: S/P Coronary Art. Bypass Graff Weight: 184.5 lb Height: 5'11"	
		Sensitivities/Drug Allergies: NKDA	
2/3/11	2250	1. Transfer to step-down unit from ICU	
		2. VS q.4. h. $\times$ 24 hours then q. 8 hours	
		3. Up in chair 3$\times$day, asst. to walk in hall 2$\times$day	
		4. Intake and output q. 8 hours	
		5. Daily WT.	
		6. TED Hose	
		7. Incentive spirometer q.1 h. while awake	
		8. Diet: 3 g Na^+, low cholesterol	
		9. Percocet $\overset{..}{ii}$ tabs p.o. q.4 h. p.r.n. pain	
		10. Tylenol gr x p.o. q.4 h. p.r.n. pain or Temp. >38°C	
		11. MOM 30 mL p.o. q.day p.r.n. constipation	
		12. Mylanta 30 mL p.o. q.4 h. p.r.n. indigestion	
		13. Restoril 15 mg p.o. at bedtime p.r.n. insomnia	
		14. O_2 3 L per nasal cannula	
		15. IVF: D_5 $\frac{1}{2}$ NS @ 50^{mL}/$_{hr}$, maximum 1200 mL IVF/day	
		16. Digoxin 0.25 mg p.o. daily	
		17. E.C. ASA gr. v p.o. daily	
		18. Cimetidine 300 mg p.o. three times a day	
		19. Lasix 20 mg I.V. q.8 h.	
		20. Slow-K 10 meq p.o. twice a day	
		21. Labs A_7, CBC, CXR q. a.m.	
		M. Doctor, M.D.	

Do Not Write Orders If No Copies Remain; Begin New Form   Copies Remaining

MEDICAL RECORDS COPY			**PHYSICIAN'S ORDERS**						T-5
B-CLIN. NOTES	E-LAB	G-X-RAY	K-DIAGNOSTIC	M-SURGERY	Q-THERAPY	T-ORDERS	W-NURSING	Y-MISC.	

4. Transcribe each as-needed (prn) medication from the physician's orders. Include date, medication, dose, route, interval, and time schedule.

(5 pts)

		dose	route	interval											
		dose	route	interval											
		dose	route	interval											
		dose	route	interval											
		dose	route	interval											

5. Transcribe each regularly scheduled medication from the physician's order sheet. Include date, medication, dose, route, interval, and time schedule.

(5 pts)

		dose	route	interval											
		dose	route	interval											
		dose	route	interval											
		dose	route	interval											
		dose	route	interval											

6. Mr. Jones complains of insomnia at 2300. What prn medication is available for him? _____

(1 pt)

7. It is time to give Mr. Jones his Lasix. You have a premixed intravenous piggyback (IVPB) of Lasix 20 mg in 50 mL of normal saline solution (NS). Infusion time is 30 minutes. Drop factor is 60 gtt/mL. How many drops per minute will you administer? _____

(1 pt)

8. Mr. Jones complains of constipation. What medication will you give? _____ How much will you administer? _____

(1 pt)

9. What regularly scheduled medication would Mr. Jones receive at 0800 each day? Include the amount of medication. Give _____

(1 pt)

Mrs. Smith is received by you from the recovery room. You review her orders. It is 1700 on 2/3/11. Refer to the physician's order sheet on p. 454 for the following questions. Show your work where applicable.

1. What regularly scheduled medications would Mrs. Smith receive at 0900 each day? Include the amount of each medication. a. _____ b. _____

(2 pts)

2. Mrs. Smith complains of nausea. You have Phenergan 25 mg/2 mL available. How many milliliters will you administer? _____

(1 pt)

3. How much intravenous (IV) fluid will Mrs. Smith receive per shift? _____ Per day? _____

(2 pts)

PHYSICIAN'S ORDERS

Mrs. Smith

1. ADDRESSOGRAPH BEFORE PLACING IN PATIENT'S CHART ▶
2. INITIAL AND DETACH COPY EACH TIME PHYSICIAN WRITES ORDERS
3. TRANSMIT COPY TO PHARMACY
4. ORDERS MUST BE DATED AND TIMED

☐ Inpatient ☐ Outpatient

DATE	TIME	ORDERS	TRANS BY
2/3/11	1650	Diagnosis: S/P Thyroidectomy Weight: 146.0 lb Height: 5'10"	
		Sensitivities/Drug Allergies: PCN	
		STATUS: ASSIGN TO OBSERVATION ☐ ; ADMIT AS INPATIENT ☐	
		1. Transfer to ward from recovery room.	
		2. VS q.1 hour ×2 hours, then q.4 hours	
		3. HOB ↑45 degrees	
		4. Up in chair 3× day, support head and neck	
		5. Intake and output q. 8 hours	
		6. Incentive spirometer q.1 hour while awake	
		7. Diet: Full liquid	
		8. Demerol 25 mg I.M. q.4 hours p.r.n. pain	
		9. Phenergan 12.5 mg. q.4 hours p.r.n. nausea	
		10. Tylenol gr x p.o. q.4 hours p.r.n. pain or Temp >38°C	
		11. Restoril 15 mg p.o. at bedtime p.r.n. insomnia	
		12. O_2 4 L per nasal cannula	
		13. IVF: NS 75$^{mL}/_h$	
		14. Synthroid 0.15 mg. p.o. daily	
		15. Tagamet 300 mg. p.o. daily	
		16. Labs: Ca^+ q. 8 hours × 3 days	
		A$_7$, CBC q. a.m.	
		17. JP drains × 2 to bulb suction, record output q. 8 hours	
		M. Doctor, M.D.	

Do Not Write Orders If No Copies Remain; Begin New Form   Copies Remaining

MEDICAL RECORDS COPY		**PHYSICIAN'S ORDERS**							T-5
B-CLIN. NOTES	E-LAB	G-X-RAY	K-DIAGNOSTIC	M-SURGERY	Q-THERAPY	T-ORDERS	W-NURSING	Y-MISC.	
						███			

4. Mrs. Smith complains of insomnia at 2200. Restoril is supplied in 30-mg tablets. Give _____ tablet(s).

(1 pt)

5. What prn medications are available for complaints of pain? a. _____ b. _____

(2 pts)

6. Your patient complains of pain shortly after she is received on the ward from the recovery room. Demerol is available 100 mg/2 mL for injection. How many milliliters will you administer? _____

(1 pt)

7. Your patient has a fever of 38.6° C. You have Tylenol 325-mg tablets available. How many tablets will you administer? _____

(1 pt)

8. Transcribe all regularly scheduled medications from the physician's orders. Include date, medication, dose, route, interval, and time schedule.

(2 pts)

	dose	route	interval									
	dose	route	interval									

Mrs. Hutsen is received by you after vaginal delivery childbirth without complications. Refer to the physician's order sheet for the following questions. Show your work where applicable.

	PHYSICIAN'S ORDERS	Mrs. Hutsen
	1. ADDRESSOGRAPH BEFORE PLACING IN PATIENT'S CHART ▶	
	2. INITIAL AND DETACH COPY EACH TIME PHYSICIAN WRITES ORDERS	
	3. TRANSMIT COPY TO PHARMACY	
	4. ORDERS MUST BE DATED AND TIMED	☐ Inpatient ☐ Outpatient

DATE	TIME	ORDERS	TRANS BY
4/27/11	0815	Diagnosis: S/P Childbirth Weight: 146.0 lb Height: 5'8"	
		Sensitivities/Drug Allergies: PCN	
		STATUS: ASSIGN TO OBSERVATION ☐ ; ADMIT AS INPATIENT ☐	
		1. Diet: Regular	
		2. Activity: Up ad lib $\bar{c}$ assistance as needed	
		3. Vital signs: Routine	
		4. Breast care: per protocol manual breast pump if desired.	
		5. Incentive spirometer ×10 breaths q.1 h. while awake	
		6. May shower as desired	
		7. If pt. unable to void within 8 h. or fundus boggy, bladder distended, or uterus displaced, may in and out cath.	
		8. Notify M.D. if unable to void 6 h. after catheterization.	
		9. Call physician for temp >38.5°C, urinary output <240 mL/shift.	
		10. DSLR 50mL/h, may D/C I.V. when tolerating p.o. well.	
		11. FeSO$_4$ 0.3 g p.o. twice daily	
		12. Percocet p.o. q.6 h. p.r.n. pain	
		13. Tucks to peri-area p.r.n. at bedside.	
		14. Senokot $\frac{\cdot}{\top}$ p.o. daily p.r.n.	
		15. Tylenol 650 mg p.o. q.4 h. p.r.n. mild pain or fever	
		M. Doctor, M.D.	

Do Not Write Orders If No Copies Remain; Begin New Form   Copies
Remaining

MEDICAL RECORDS COPY			**PHYSICIAN'S ORDERS**					**T-5**
B-CLIN. NOTES	E-LAB	G-X-RAY	K-DIAGNOSTIC	M-SURGERY	Q-THERAPY	T-ORDERS	W-NURSING	Y-MISC.

1. What regularly scheduled medication would your patient receive each day? Include the amount. _____

   (2 pts)

2. Your patient is tolerating oral intake well. Her IV fluid was stopped 2 hours before the evening shift (1500-2330) ended. How many milliliters did the patient receive on the evening shift? _____ mL.

   (1 pt)

3. Your patient complains of pain and has ibuprofen ordered. Ibuprofen is supplied as 1200-mg tablets. How many tablets will you administer? _____

   (1 pt)

4. Transcribe all prn medications from the physician's orders. Include date, medication, dose, route, interval, and time schedule.

   (5 pts)

	dose	route	interval									
	dose	route	interval									
	dose	route	interval									
	dose	route	interval									
	dose	route	interval									

J. Todd is received on your floor with a diagnosis of acute lymphocytic leukemia. Refer to the physician's order sheet for the following questions. Show your work where applicable.

	PHYSICIAN'S ORDERS		
			Jason Todd
1. ADDRESSOGRAPH BEFORE PLACING IN PATIENT'S CHART ▶			
2. INITIAL AND DETACH COPY EACH TIME PHYSICIAN WRITES ORDERS			
3. TRANSMIT COPY TO PHARMACY			
4. ORDERS MUST BE DATED AND TIMED			☐ Inpatient ☐ Outpatient

DATE	TIME	ORDERS	TRANS BY
10/13/11	0800	Diagnosis: Acute Lymphocytic Leukemia Weight: 12.73 kg Height: 3'0"	
		Sensitivities/Drug Allergies: Codeine	
		STATUS: ASSIGN TO OBSERVATION [＿＿＿＿]； ADMIT AS INPATIENT [＿＿＿＿]	
		1. Diet: Regular	
		2. Activity: ↑chair three times a day, Ø rigorous play activity	
		3. O_2–Biox to keep sats >93%	
		4. Vital signs: q.4 h.	
		5. I+O q. 8 hours	
		6. Daily WT.	
		7. IVF: $D_5 \frac{1}{2}$ NS 25^{ml}/$_h$	
		8. Allopurinol 50 mg. p.o. three times a day	
		9. Theophylline 16 mg p.o. q.6 h.	
		10. Prednisone 2 mg/kg/day	
		11. Vincristine 5 mg/m² in 50 ml of NaCl × $\frac{\div}{1}$ now	
		12. MVI $\frac{\div}{1}$ q.day p.o.	
		13. Compazine 0.07 mg/kg I.M. q.day p.r.n. nausea	
		14. Tylenol 120 mg p.o. three times a day p.r.n. pain	
		15. Call physician SBP >140<90, DBP >90<40, Temp. >38.5 °C, SOB,	
		urinary output <200 ^{ml}/shift, any problems	
		16. Labs: CBC c̄ diff., A₇, plts., CXR q.day	
		M. Doctor, M.D.	

Do Not Write Orders If No Copies Remain; Begin New Form   Copies Remaining

MEDICAL RECORDS COPY	**PHYSICIAN'S ORDERS**							T-5
B-CLIN. NOTES	E-LAB	G-X-RAY	K-DIAGNOSTIC	M-SURGERY	Q-THERAPY	T-ORDERS	W-NURSING	Y-MISC.

COMPREHENSIVE POSTTEST

1. Transcribe all regularly scheduled medications. Include date, medication, dose, route, interval, and time schedule.

(4 pts)

		dose	route	interval								
		dose	route	interval								
		dose	route	interval								
		dose	route	interval								
		dose	route	interval								

2. Transcribe all prn medications. Include date, medication, dose, route, interval, and time schedule.

(2 pts)

		dose	route	interval								
		dose	route	interval								

3. Your patient requires theophylline 16 mg po q6 h. You have theophylline elixir 11.25 mg/mL available. Give _____ mL.

(1 pt)

4. Your patient requires the allopurinol dose now. You have allopurinol elixir 100 mg/mL available. Give _____ mL.

(1 pt)

5. Your patient receives prednisone 2 mg/kg/day. You have 10 mg/mL available. Calculate the patient's weight in kilograms and the correct dose. _____ kg. Give _____ mL.

(2 pts)

6. Your patient requires a vincristine dose now. The vincristine is supplied in 50 mL of NaCl to be infused over 60 minutes. Drop factor is 60 gtt/mL. Administer _____ gtt/min.

(1 pt)

7. Your patient complains of nausea. You have Compazine 1 mg/mL available. How many milliliters will you administer? _____ Mark the syringe at the appropriate amount.

(2 pts)

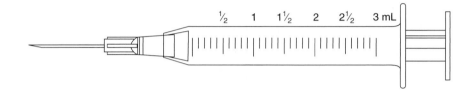

8. Your patient receives D$_5$ ½ NS at 25 mL/h. How much fluid will your patient receive during each 8-hour shift? _____ mL

(1 pt)

9. Your patient complains of pain. You have Tylenol elixir 360 mg/2 mL available. How many milliliters will you administer? _____

(1 pt)

CASE 5

Mr. Miller is received on your floor from the recovery room. Refer to the physician's order sheet for the following questions. Show your work where applicable.

PHYSICIAN'S ORDERS	Mr. Miller

1. ADDRESSOGRAPH BEFORE PLACING IN PATIENT'S CHART ▶
2. INITIAL AND DETACH COPY EACH TIME PHYSICIAN WRITES ORDERS
3. TRANSMIT COPY TO PHARMACY
4. ORDERS MUST BE DATED AND TIMED

☐ Inpatient ☐ Outpatient

DATE	TIME	ORDERS	TRANS BY
6/15/11	1600	Diagnosis: S/P Ⓡ total hip replacement Weight: 197 lb Height: 6'2"	
		Sensitivities/Drug Allergies: NKDA	
		STATUS: ASSIGN TO OBSERVATION ☐ ; ADMIT AS INPATIENT ☐	
		1. Diet: NPO til fully awake, then clear liquids	
		2. Activity: Bedrest, log roll side-back-side q.2 h.	
		3. Vital signs: q.4 h.	
		4. Overhead frame trapeze	
		5. Abductor pillow while in bed.	
		6. Incentive spirometer q.1 h. while awake.	
		7. Intake and output q.8 h.	
		8. Hemovacs to own reservoirs, record output q.1 h. × 6 h., then q.6 h.	
		9. I+O catheterization q.shift p.r.n. inability to void	
		10. Heparin 5000 units subcutaneous twice a day	
		11. Torecan 10 mg I.M. q.4 h. p.r.n. nausea	
		12. Mylanta 30 mL p.o. p.r.n. indigestion	
		13. Restoril 15 mg. p.o. at bedtime p.r.n. insomnia	
		14. Tylenol c̄ codeine p.o. 2 tabs q.4 h. p.r.n. pain	
		15. Morphine PCA 10 mg I.V. q.10 min to maximum 250 mg/4 h.	
		16. Dulcolax supp. $\frac{\cdot}{i}$ per rectum every shift prn constipation	
		17. Labs: CBC q.day × 3	
		18. Call orders: Hemovac output >500^{mL}/shift,	
		urinary output<250^{mL}/shift, Temp. >38.5° C, Hgb <10.0,	
		SBP >160<80, DBP >90<50	
		19. IVF: D$_5$ NS 50^{mL}/h	
		Cefuroxime 1g IVPB q.8 h.	
		M. Doctor, M.D.	

Do Not Write Orders If No Copies Remain; Begin New Form   Copies Remaining

MEDICAL RECORDS COPY	PHYSICIAN'S ORDERS							T-5
B-CLIN. NOTES	E-LAB	G-X-RAY	K-DIAGNOSTIC	M-SURGERY	Q-THERAPY	T-ORDERS	W-NURSING	Y-MISC.

1. Transcribe the regularly scheduled medication below. Include date, medication, dose, route, interval, and time schedule.

(2 pts)

╱											
	dose	route	interval								
╱											
	dose	route	interval								

2. Transcribe all prn medications ordered below. Include date, medication, dose, route, interval, and time schedule.

(7 pts)

╱											
	dose	route	interval								
╱											
	dose	route	interval								
╱											
	dose	route	interval								
╱											
	dose	route	interval								
╱											
	dose	route	interval								
╱											
	dose	route	interval								
╱											
	dose	route	interval								

3. Your patient requires 5000 units heparin subcutaneous. You have a vial containing 5000 units/mL. Give _____ mL. Mark the syringe at the appropriate amount.

(2 pts)

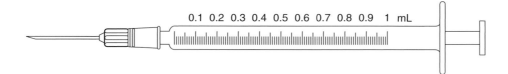

0.1 0.2 0.3 0.4 0.5 0.6 0.7 0.8 0.9 1 mL

4. Your patient requires a morphine sulfate patient-controlled analgesia (PCA) 10 mg every 10 minutes. You have a morphine sulfate syringe with 300 mg/30 mL available. How many milliliters will the patient receive every 10 minutes? _____ mL/10 min

(1 pt)

5. Your patient complains of nausea and requires Torecan as ordered. You have Torecan 20 mg/2 mL available per vial. Give _____ mL

(1 pt)

6. Your patient receives D$_5$ NS at 50 mL/h. How much IV fluid will your patient receive per 8-hour shift? _____ mL/shift Per day? _____ mL/day

(2 pts)

7. Your patient receives cefuroxime 1 g in 100 mL NS IVPB 30 minutes q8 h. Drop factor is 60 gtt/mL. _____ mL/h _____ mL/min _____ gtt/min

(3 pts)

Ms. Keys, admitted with a diagnosis of myocardial infarction, returns from the cardiac catheterization laboratory for a stent placement. Refer to the physician's order sheet and medication profile sheet for the following questions. Show your work where applicable.

PHYSICIAN'S ORDERS

Ms. Keys

1. ADDRESSOGRAPH BEFORE PLACING IN PATIENT'S CHART ▶
2. INITIAL AND DETACH COPY EACH TIME PHYSICIAN WRITES ORDERS
3. TRANSMIT COPY TO PHARMACY
4. ORDERS MUST BE DATED AND TIMED

☐ Inpatient ☐ Outpatient

DATE	TIME	ORDERS	TRANS BY
		Diagnosis: MI, s/p stent Weight: 168 lb Height: 5'5"	
		Sensitivities/Drug Allergies: PCN	
3/4/11	1100	1. Transfer to CCU	
		2. Diet: Healthy Heart	
		3. Activity: BR × 6 h, then dangle. If no bleeding from right groin	
		site, up ad lib	
		4. VS q15 min × 4, q30 min × 4, then every hour	
		5. Telemetry	
		6. EKG every morning × 2	
		7. Cardiac profile q8 h × 2 (1800 and 0200)	
		8. O$_2$ 2 L/min	
		9. Tylenol gr x po q4 h p.r.n. headache	
		10. ASA 325 mg po daily, start 3/5/11	
		11. Plavix 75 mg po daily, start 3/5/11	
		12. Nitroglycerin drip at 10 mcg/min	
		13. IV heparin per protocol	
		14. Metoprolol 12.5 mg p.o. twice a day Hold for SBP <80 mm Hg	
		15. Ambien 5 mg p.o. at bedtime p.r.n. sleep	
		16. Call for chest pain, any concerns	
		M. Doctor, M.D.	

Do Not Write Orders If No Copies Remain; Begin New Form   Copies Remaining

MEDICAL RECORDS COPY			**PHYSICIAN'S ORDERS**						T-5
B-CLIN. NOTES	E-LAB	G-X-RAY	K-DIAGNOSTIC	M-SURGERY	Q-THERAPY	T-ORDERS	W-NURSING	Y-MISC.	

---

1. Transcribe each regularly scheduled medication from the physician's order sheet. Include date, medication, dose, route, interval, and time schedule.

(3 pts)

		dose	route	interval									
		dose	route	interval									
		dose	route	interval									
		dose	route	interval									
		dose	route	interval									

2. Transcribe each prn medication from the physician's order sheet. Include date, medication, dose, route, interval, and time schedule.

(2 pts)

		dose	route	interval								
		dose	route	interval								

3. The nitroglycerin drip has a concentration of 50 mg/100 mL of 0.9% NS. How many milliliters per hour should the IV pump be programmed for? _____ mL/h

(1 pt)

4. Follow the heparin protocol in Chapter 17 for the following questions. The patient weighs 76.4 kg.

   a. How many units of heparin should be administered for the bolus? _____ units

(1 pt)

b. With the following vial of heparin, how many milliliters should the nurse administer? _____ mL

(1 pt)

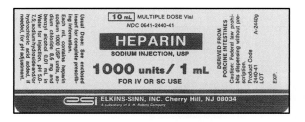

c. How many milliliters per hour should the IV pump be programmed for the heparin infusion? _____ mL/h

(1 pt)

5. The metoprolol comes in 25-mg tablets. How many tablets should be administered? _____

(1 pt)

6. Ms. Keys complains of a headache after the nitroglycerin is started. The Tylenol comes in 325-mg tablets. How many tablets should the nurse administer? _____

(1 pt)

A 5-day-old neonate is admitted to the pediatric unit. She is being breast-fed on demand and supplemented with Enfamil with iron Lipil.

		PHYSICIAN'S ORDERS		
		1. ADDRESSOGRAPH BEFORE PLACING IN PATIENT'S CHART ▶	Baby Jackson	
		2. INITIAL AND DETACH COPY EACH TIME PHYSICIAN WRITES ORDERS		
		3. TRANSMIT COPY TO PHARMACY		
		4. ORDERS MUST BE DATED AND TIMED	☐ Inpatient ☐ Outpatient	

DATE	TIME	ORDERS	TRANS BY
5/1/11	0200	Diagnosis: Fever, poor feeding, jaundice, possible sepsis Weight: 7 lb, 8 oz	
		Sensitivities/Drug Allergies: NKDA	
		STATUS: ASSIGN TO OBSERVATION [ ] ; ADMIT AS INPATIENT [ ]	
		1. Admit to pediatric unit	
		2. Cardiac apnea monitor with continuous Biox	
		3. Labs: CBC with diff, Chem 7, Blood cultures ×2, and	
		total bilirubin count @ 0600	
		4. I&O cath for colony count plus micro	
		5. Start IV fluids D_5 45% NS at 12 ^{mL}/h continuous until d/c.	
		6. Ampicillin 160 mg IV infuse over 20 minutes per syringe	
		pump q.8 h daily starting today	
		7. Gentamicin 12 mg IV infuse over 30 minutes per syringe pump once daily	
		8. Tylenol elixir 40 mg po q. 6 h. p.r.n. for fever >100.4° F axillary	
		9. Vital signs q.4 h	
		10. Weigh daily	
		11. Strict I&O	
		12. Diet: Breast milk, supplement with Enfamil with iron Lipil po ad lib	
		13. Activity: Up in Mom's arms ad lib	
		14. Call orders: Notify MD for: temp >100.6° or <95° F axillary,	
		pulse >180<100, resp >60<20, any problems or concerns	
		15. Notify MD for sats <92%	
		16. Humidity via isolette	
		M. Doctor, M.D.	

Do Not Write Orders If No Copies Remain; Begin New Form   Copies Remaining

MEDICAL RECORDS COPY	**PHYSICIAN'S ORDERS**							**T-5**
B-CLIN. NOTES	E-LAB	G-X-RAY	K-DIAGNOSTIC	M-SURGERY	Q-THERAPY	T-ORDERS	W-NURSING	Y-MISC.

1. Ampicillin is available as 500-mg powder to be reconstituted with 4.8 mL of sterile water for a final dilution of 250 mg/mL. Recommended dosage is 100 to 200 mg/kg/24 h q6-8 h.

   a. How many milligrams per kilogram per 24 hours of ampicillin is the neonate receiving? _____ mg/kg/24 h b. Is the order safe? _____ c. If yes, how many milliliters are needed to deliver the ordered dose? _____ mL

   (3 pts)

2. The neonate has a body temperature of 100.4° F axillary. Tylenol infant drops come as 80 mg/0.8 mL. How many milliliters are needed to deliver the ordered dose? _____ mL
   (1 pt)

3. This neonate is receiving IV fluids at 12 mL/h. How many milliliters are needed to deliver 6 hours of the ordered fluids? _____ mL
   (1 pt)

Answers on pp. 581-584.

Refer to the Comprehensive Posttest on the enclosed CD for further testing of your knowledge base for calculations of all the various types of dosage problems.

Glossary

Addends   the numbers to be added

Ampule   a sealed glass container; usually contains one dose of a drug

Buccal   between teeth and cheek

Canceling   dividing numerator and denominator by a common number

Capsule   a small soluble container for enclosing a single dose of medicine

Complex fraction   a fraction whose numerator, denominator, or both contain fractions

Decimal fraction   a fraction consisting of a numerator that is expressed in numerals, a decimal point that designates the value of the denominator, and the denominator, which is understood to be 10 or some power of 10

Decimal numbers   include an integer, a decimal point, and a decimal fraction

Denominator   the number of parts into which a whole has been divided

Difference   the result of subtracting

Dividend   the number being divided

Divisor   the number by which another number is divided

Dosage   the determination and regulation of the size, frequency, and number of doses

Dose   the exact amount of medicine to be administered at one time

Drug   a chemical substance used in therapy, diagnosis, and prevention of a disease or condition

Elixir   a clear, sweet, hydroalcoholic liquid in which a drug is suspended

Equivalent   equal

Extremes   the first and fourth terms of a proportion

Fraction   indicates the number of equal parts of a whole

Improper fraction   a fraction whose numerator is larger than or equal to the denominator

Infusion   the therapeutic introduction of a fluid into a vein by the flow of gravity

Injection   the therapeutic introduction of a fluid into a part of the body by force

Integer   a whole number

Intramuscular   within the muscle

Intravenous   within the vein

Invert   turn upside down

Lowest common denominator   the smallest whole number that can be divided evenly by all denominators within the problem

Means   the second and third terms of a proportion

Medicine   any drug

Milliequivalent   the number of grams of a solute contained in 1 mL of a normal solution

Minuend   the number from which another number is subtracted

Mixed number   a combination of a whole number and a proper fraction

Multiplicand   the number that is to be multiplied

Multiplier   the number that another number is to be multiplied by

Numerator   the number of parts of a divided whole

Oral dosage   a medication taken by mouth

Parenteral dosage   a dosage administered by routes that bypass the gastrointestinal tract; generally given by injection

Percent   indicates the number of hundredths

Product   the result of multiplying

Proper fraction   a fraction whose numerator is smaller than the denominator

Proportion   two ratios that are of equal value and are connected by a double colon, which symbolizes the word *as*

Quotient   the answer to a division problem

Ratio   the relationship between two numbers that are connected by a colon, which symbolizes the words *is to*

Reconstitution   the return of a medication to its previous state by the addition of water or other designated liquid

Subcutaneous   beneath the skin

Sublingual   under the tongue

Subtrahend   the number being subtracted

Sum   the result of adding

Suspension   a liquid in which a drug is distributed

Syrup   a sweet, thick, aqueous liquid in which a drug is suspended

Tablet   a drug compressed into a small disk

Topical   on top of the skin or mucous membrane

Unit   the amount of a drug needed to produce a given result

Vial   a glass container with a rubber stopper; usually contains a number of doses of a drug

Answer Key

PART I REVIEW OF MATHEMATICS

Review of Mathematics Pretest, pp. 3–6

1. $^{17}/_{24}$
2. $4^2/_{21}$
3. $4^9/_{40}$
4. 4.364
5. 34.659
6. $^{23}/_{30}$
7. $1^5/_6$
8. 1.053
9. 0.585
10. $1^5/_7$
11. 9
12. 1.827
13. 31.79484

14. $^{18}/_{25}$
15. $^2/_{15}$
16. $^{33}/_{80}$
17. 25.9924
18. 21.373
19. 6.4771
20. 0.003
21. 0.45
22. 0.0072
23. 0.058
24. 0.155
25. 0.8
26. 0.249

27. 2.99
28. 0.625
29. 0.68
30. $^3/_8$
31. $^1/_{20}$
32. 43.2%
33. $^{13}/_{20}$
34. 3 : 1000
35. 20%
36. 0.15
37. 292.5
38. 3 : 14

39. 9 : 16
40. 17 : 50
41. 400
42. 5
43. 24
44. $7^1/_5$ or 7.2
45. 20
46. 100
47. 500
48. 51
49. $2^1/_2$ or 2.5
50. 68

Chapter 1 Fractions—Pretest, pp. 7–8

1. $1^{10}/_{63}$
2. $10^2/_3$
3. $9^3/_4$
4. $5^9/_{16}$
5. $9^1/_{22}$
6. $7^8/_9$
7. $5^{23}/_{24}$
8. $^3/_{10}$

9. $^7/_8$
10. $2^5/_8$
11. $2^{17}/_{24}$
12. $1^5/_6$
13. $1^4/_5$
14. $1^5/_6$
15. $^1/_{15}$
16. 5

17. $7^{19}/_{63}$
18. $1^1/_{14}$
19. $^1/_{10,000}$
20. $4^5/_{18}$
21. $12^1/_{12}$
22. $2^{25}/_{28}$
23. $^5/_{16}$

24. $1^1/_3$
25. $33^1/_3$
26. $^7/_8$
27. $1^1/_3$
28. $^5/_9$
29. $1^7/_{10}$
30. 2

Chapter 1 Fractions—Work Sheet, pp. 21–24

Improper fractions to mixed numbers, p. 21

1. $1\frac{1}{3}$
2. 3
3. $3\frac{1}{5}$
4. $3\frac{1}{4}$
5. $1\frac{1}{2}$
6. $1\frac{1}{8}$
7. $1\frac{2}{3}$
8. $2\frac{1}{6}$
9. $3\frac{1}{2}$
10. $1\frac{3}{8}$
11. $3\frac{1}{2}$
12. $1\frac{3}{25}$

Mixed numbers to improper fractions, p. 21

1. $\frac{3}{2}$
2. $\frac{15}{4}$
3. $\frac{8}{3}$
4. $\frac{17}{6}$
5. $\frac{8}{5}$
6. $\frac{25}{7}$
7. $\frac{39}{8}$
8. $\frac{307}{100}$
9. $\frac{27}{10}$
10. $\frac{53}{8}$
11. $\frac{28}{25}$
12. $\frac{17}{4}$

Addition, p. 22

1. $1\frac{1}{2}$
2. $\frac{29}{35}$
3. $3\frac{19}{24}$
4. $3\frac{1}{4}$
5. $5\frac{13}{20}$
6. $3\frac{5}{39}$
7. $7\frac{5}{8}$
8. $6\frac{17}{22}$
9. $6\frac{4}{9}$
10. $6\frac{11}{30}$
11. 9
12. $8\frac{7}{30}$

Subtraction, pp. 22–23

1. $\frac{5}{21}$
2. $\frac{9}{16}$
3. $\frac{7}{48}$
4. $\frac{1}{2}$
5. $1\frac{1}{10}$
6. $1\frac{15}{16}$
7. $\frac{5}{8}$
8. $1\frac{1}{3}$
9. $2\frac{5}{8}$
10. $1\frac{5}{12}$
11. $1\frac{19}{24}$
12. $\frac{15}{16}$

Multiplication, p. 23

1. $\frac{4}{15}$
2. $\frac{7}{12}$
3. 4
4. $1\frac{1}{2}$
5. $8\frac{3}{4}$
6. $11\frac{7}{8}$
7. $12\frac{11}{16}$
8. $1\frac{25}{32}$
9. $\frac{1}{5}$
10. $\frac{3}{1000}$
11. $6\frac{5}{12}$
12. $3\frac{1}{9}$

Division, p. 24

1. $\frac{10}{21}$
2. $2\frac{1}{5}$
3. $1\frac{5}{9}$
4. $2\frac{1}{2}$
5. $1\frac{23}{26}$
6. $1\frac{7}{20}$
7. $1\frac{7}{11}$
8. $3\frac{47}{51}$
9. $3\frac{1}{2}$
10. $2\frac{5}{17}$
11. $2\frac{1}{16}$
12. $1\frac{1}{2}$

Chapter 1 Fractions—Posttest 1, pp. 25–26

1. $1\frac{1}{9}$
2. $\frac{17}{24}$
3. $5\frac{1}{12}$
4. $3\frac{2}{21}$
5. $\frac{39}{50}$
6. $8\frac{3}{20}$
7. $7\frac{7}{12}$
8. $\frac{9}{10}$
9. $\frac{5}{6}$
10. $\frac{3}{14}$
11. $1\frac{15}{16}$
12. $1\frac{31}{63}$
13. $5\frac{7}{10}$
14. $1\frac{1}{12}$
15. $\frac{9}{14}$
16. $2\frac{2}{5}$
17. 2
18. $3\frac{5}{24}$
19. $3\frac{1}{3}$
20. $14\frac{7}{10}$
21. $3\frac{18}{35}$
22. $\frac{7}{8}$
23. $1\frac{1}{15}$
24. 10
25. $\frac{2}{3}$
26. $1\frac{1}{4}$
27. $\frac{3}{5}$
28. $1\frac{7}{20}$
29. $4\frac{1}{2}$
30. $1\frac{3}{22}$

Chapter 1 Fractions—Posttest 2, pp. 27–28

1. $1\frac{1}{12}$
2. $4\frac{1}{10}$
3. $3\frac{2}{21}$
4. $5\frac{11}{40}$
5. $4\frac{19}{24}$
6. $11\frac{4}{5}$
7. $3\frac{1}{2}$
8. $\frac{1}{9}$
9. $1\frac{7}{8}$
10. $1\frac{5}{6}$
11. $2\frac{5}{16}$
12. $1\frac{1}{2}$
13. $3\frac{9}{10}$
14. $\frac{3}{5}$
15. $\frac{4}{21}$
16. $6\frac{1}{5}$
17. $1\frac{1}{3}$
18. $1\frac{17}{18}$
19. $\frac{1}{1000}$
20. 36
21. $3\frac{1}{2}$
22. $11\frac{1}{4}$
23. $\frac{27}{32}$
24. $\frac{21}{26}$
25. $6\frac{2}{9}$
26. $\frac{1}{49}$
27. $\frac{5}{8}$
28. $\frac{21}{32}$
29. $1\frac{11}{16}$
30. $1\frac{1}{8}$

Chapter 2 Decimals—Pretest, pp. 29–31

1. Four hundredths
2. One and six tenths
3. Sixteen and six thousand seven hundred thirty-four hundred thousandths
4. One and fifteen thousandths
5. Nine thousandths

6. 0.02	15. 84.565	24. 29.5336	33. $^{161}/_{500}$
7. 0.004	16. 1.078	25. 186.543	34. $^{1}/_{250}$
8. 1.6	17. 1.008	26. 0.2060	35. $^{17}/_{50}$
9. 2.082	18. 759.4	27. 17.95	36. 0.6
10. 0.003	19. 1.7	28. 0.01097	37. 0.67
11. 25.376	20. 10.946	29. 627	38. 0.006
12. 324.3	21. 0.0567	30. 0.0186	39. 0.35
13. 1012.867	22. 6.6472	31. $^{1}/_{125}$	40. 0.625
14. 150.6736	23. 1.9425	32. $^{1}/_{4}$	

Chapter 2 Decimals—Work Sheet, pp. 41–46

Writing numbers in words, p. 41

1. Two tenths
2. Nine and sixty-eight hundredths
3. Three ten thousandths
4. One thousand nine hundred sixty-eight and three hundred forty-two thousandths
5. Two hundredths

Decimal numbers with the greatest value, p. 41

1. 0.25	4. 0.68
2. 0.45	5. 1.8
3. 0.98	6. 7.44

Decimal numbers with the least value, p. 41

1. 0.6	4. 0.08
2. 0.0003	5. 0.007
3. 1.0022	6. 3.006

Addition, pp. 41–42

1. 41.755	4. 39.073	7. 26.62	9. 55.117
2. 372.675	5. 894.842	8. 37.9	10. 142.218
3. 40.9787	6. 67.137		

Subtraction, p. 42

1. 1257.87	4. 174.804	7. 0.461	9. 62.022
2. 1.849	5. 7.418	8. 0.988	10. 287.371
3. 0.71	6. 4.144		

Multiplication, p. 43

1. 16.25	5. 41.92	8. 409.0318
2. 609.6	6. 33.6	9. 0.15113
3. 52.052	7. 103.983	10. 23.5971
4. 56.1144		

Multiply by 10, p. 43

1. 0.9   **4.** 3
2. 2   **5.** 6.25
3. 1.8   **6.** 23.3

Multiply by 100, p. 43

1. 2.3   **4.** 12.5
2. 150   **5.** 865
3. 0.4   **6.** 7640

Multiply by 1000, p. 43

1. 200   **4.** 9650
2. 5   **5.** 460
3. 187   **6.** 489

Multiply by 0.1, p. 44

1. 3   **4.** 0.095
2. 0.069   **5.** 0.0138
3. 0.17   **6.** 0.567

Multiply by 0.01, p. 44

1. 0.0026   **4.** 0.112
2. 0.908   **5.** 0.00875
3. 0.055   **6.** 0.633

Multiply by 0.001, p. 44

1. 0.056   **4.** 0.0333
2. 0.01255   **5.** 0.009684
3. 0.1265   **6.** 0.241

Round to the nearest tenth, p. 44

1. 0.3   **4.** 0.7
2. 0.9   **5.** 58.4
3. 2.4   **6.** 8.1

Round to the nearest hundredth, p. 44

1. 2.56   **4.** 3.92
2. 4.28   **5.** 6.53
3. 0.28   **6.** 2.99

Round to the nearest thousandth, p. 44

1. 27.863   **4.** 0.849
2. 5.925   **5.** 321.087
3. 2.157   **6.** 455.768

Division, pp. 44–45

1. 1.17   **4.** 400   **7.** 82.6   **9.** 0.48
2. 4140   **5.** 0.02   **8.** 4.53   **10.** 2.52
3. 7.8   **6.** 0.13

Divide by 10, p. 45

1. 0.6   **4.** 0.005
2. 0.02   **5.** 0.0375
3. 0.98   **6.** 0.099

Divide by 100, p. 45

1. 0.007   **4.** 0.0019
2. 0.0811   **5.** 0.12
3. 7   **6.** 0.302

Divide by 1000, p. 45

1. 0.0018   **4.** 0.0546
2. 0.36   **5.** 0.0075
3. 0.00025   **6.** 7.14

Divide by 0.1, p. 45

1. 28   **4.** 9.87
2. 1   **5.** 150
3. 6.5   **6.** 82.5

Divide by 0.01, p. 45

1. 3600   **4.** 959
2. 16   **5.** 80
3. 48   **6.** 9.7

Divide by 0.001, p. 45

1. 6200   **4.** 860
2. 839,000   **5.** 13,800
3. 5000   **6.** 15.6

Decimal fractions to proper fractions, p. 46

1. $3/50$ **4.** $1/400$ **7.** $16/25$ **9.** $1/100$
2. $4/5$ **5.** $5/8$ **8.** $1/200$ **10.** $11/250$
3. $17/25$ **6.** $1/4$

Proper fractions to decimal fractions, p. 46

1. 0.125   **4.** 0.6   **7.** 0.8   **9.** 0.005
2. 0.67   **5.** 0.04   **8.** 0.875   **10.** 0.83
3. 0.64   **6.** 0.33

Chapter 2 Decimals—Posttest 1, pp. 47–48

1. Six hundred thirty-four and eighteen hundredths
2. Nine tenths
3. Sixty-four and two hundred thirty-one thousandths

4. 0.15
5. 0.6666
6. 54.66
7. 8.89
8. 6.352
9. 6.104
10. 2152.626
11. 0.339
12. 1.4532
13. 323.08
14. 43.6077

15. 0.211
16. 702.4472
17. 0.13904
18. 162
19. 44.278
20. 0.585
21. 16.8
22. 1481.67
23. 627
24. 1.41
25. 55.19

26. $^9/_{100}$
27. $^1/_{400}$
28. $^3/_8$
29. $^2/_5$
30. $^3/_{500}$
31. 0.71
32. 0.01
33. 0.004
34. 0.125
35. 0.09

Chapter 2 Decimals—Posttest 2, pp. 49–50

1. Five hundred sixteen thousandths
2. Four and two ten thousandths
3. One hundred twenty-three and sixty-nine hundredths

4. 0.86
5. 1.222
6. 456.8191
7. 16.055
8. 33.209
9. 47.725
10. 339
11. 612.969
12. 0.587
13. 2.766
14. 2.513

15. 1.085
16. 167.04
17. 104,552
18. 1.01574
19. 83.2
20. 161.975
21. 1.11
22. 5
23. 15,500
24. 0.30
25. 2.47

26. $^1/_{200}$
27. $^7/_{20}$
28. $^1/_8$
29. $^{17}/_{20}$
30. $^3/_5$
31. 0.17
32. 0.003
33. 0.875
34. 0.007
35. 0.008

Chapter 3 Percents—Pretest, pp. 51–53

Fractions to percents, p. 51

1. $1^2/_3$%, 1.6666%
2. $71^3/_7$%, 71.4285%
3. $12^1/_2$%, 12.5%
4. 30%
5. $133^1/_3$%, 133.3333%

Decimals to percents, p. 51

6. 0.6%
7. 35%
8. 42.7%
9. 382.1%
10. 70%

Percents to fractions, p. 52

11. $^1/_{200}$
12. $^3/_4$
13. $^{19}/_{200}$
14. $^{31}/_{125}$
15. $^3/_{800}$

Percents to decimals, p. 52

16. 0.0116
17. 0.075
18. 0.133
19. 0.0088
20. 0.63

What percent of, pp. 52–53

21. 375%
22. $16^2/_3$%, 16.6666%
23. 65%
24. $^1/_5$%, 0.2%
25. $33^1/_3$%, 33.333%
26. $12^{32}/_{189}$%, 12.1693%
27. $43^7/_{26}$%, 43.2692%
28. 10%
29. $7^1/_7$%, 7.1428%
30. $1^{209}/_{291}$%, 1.7182%

What is, p. 53

31. 1.8
32. 0.15
33. 2.565
34. 0.68
35. 3.08
36. 4.278
37. 0.06
38. 19.36
39. 11.856
40. 15

Chapter 3 Percents—Work Sheet, pp. 61–63

Fractions to percents, p. 61

1. 75%	**4.** 32%	**7.** 2¼% or 2.25%	**10.** 68¾% or 68.75%
2. 37½%	**5.** ³⁄₁₀% or 0.3%	**8.** 15%	**11.** 83⅓% or 81.3%
3. 80%	**6.** 3½%	**9.** 6%	**12.** ¾% or 0.75%

Decimals to percents, p. 61

1. 40.2%	**4.** 98%	**7.** 70%	**10.** 67.3%
2. 3.67%	**5.** 30%	**8.** 42%	**11.** 37.12%
3. 16.3%	**6.** 14.5%	**9.** 15.9%	**12.** 220%

Percents to fractions, p. 62

1. $^7/_{200}$	**4.** $^1/_{10}$	**7.** $^3/_{25}$	**10.** $^1/_{16}$
2. $^3/_{400}$	**5.** $^1/_{150}$	**8.** $^1/_{400}$	**11.** $^{21}/_{1000}$
3. $^1/_{800}$	**6.** $^{101}/_{500}$	**9.** $^{19}/_{800}$	**12.** $^2/_3$

Percents to decimals, p. 62

1. 0.375	**4.** 0.0042	**7.** 0.0023	**10.** 0.003125
2. 0.03	**5.** 0.0025	**8.** 0.726	**11.** 0.005
3. 0.0675	**6.** 0.025	**9.** 0.16	**12.** 0.0058

What percent of, p. 63

1. 55%	**4.** 12%	**7.** 20%	**10.** 1%
2. 7⅞%, 7.875%	**5.** 5%	**8.** 10%	**11.** 2²⁄₂₅%, 2.08%
3. 2%	**6.** 15%	**9.** 45%	**12.** 20%

What is, p. 63

1. 119.5	**4.** 0.14	**7.** 0.585	**10.** 0.17
2. 3.4	**5.** 999.9 or 1000	**8.** 0.12	**11.** 11.07
3. 14.28	**6.** 0.13	**9.** 540.02	**12.** 10.752

Chapter 3 Percents—Posttest 1, pp. 65–66

Fractions to percents, p. 65

1. 87½%, 87.5%	**3.** ³⁄₁₀%, 0.3%
2. 55%	

Decimals to percents, p. 65

4. 25.6%	**6.** 90%
5. 0.4%	

Percents to fractions, p. 65

7. $^{17}/_{20}$	**9.** $^7/_{200}$
8. $^3/_{1000}$	

Percents to decimals, p. 65

10. 0.863	**12.** 0.0036
11. 0.04625	

What percent of, pp. 65–66

13. 10%	**18.** 20%
14. 5%	**19.** 50%
15. ⅓%, 0.33%	**20.** 7½%, 7.5%
16. 12%	**21.** 8%
17. 42⁶⁄₇%, 42.8571%	

What is, p. 66

22. 520	**27.** 292.5
23. 36	**28.** 0.15
24. 0.09	**29.** 2.408
25. 170	**30.** 0.4576
26. 42.3	

Chapter 3 Percents—Posttest 2, pp. 67–68

Fractions to percents, p. 67

1. 12½%, 12.5%
2. 40%
3. 16⅔%, 16.6666%

Decimals to percents, p. 67

4. 6.5%　　**6.** 20%
5. 0.5%

Percents to fractions, p. 67

7. ³/₁₀₀₀　　**9.** ¹/₄₀₀
8. ³³/₂₀₀

Percents to decimals, p. 67

10. 0.0375　　**12.** 0.0555
11. 0.07

What percent of, pp. 67–68

13. 22²/₉%, 22.2222%　**18.** 10%
14. 50%　　　　　　　**19.** 41⁷/₂₃%, 41.3043%
15. 2²/₅%, 2.4%　　　　**20.** 12½%, 12.5%
16. 80%　　　　　　　**21.** 126⁶²/₆₃%, 126.9841%
17. 7½%, 7.5%

What is, p. 68

22. 227.5　　**27.** 19.575
23. 0.29　　　**28.** 10.9215
24. 42.3　　　**29.** 0.56
25. 9.68　　　**30.** 97.232
26. 14.4

Chapter 4 Ratios—Pretest, p. 69

1. ⅓, 0.3333, 33.33%　　**5.** ¹/₂₀, 0.05, 5%　　　　　　　　**8.** 5 : 7, ⁵/₇, 0.714
2. 143 : 200, ¹⁴³/₂₀₀, 71.5%　**6.** 5 : 32, 0.15625, 15.625%　**9.** 13 : 80, ¹³/₈₀, 0.1625
3. 2 : 5, 0.4, 40%　　　　**7.** 143 : 500, ¹⁴³/₅₀₀, 28.6%　**10.** 231 : 500, ²³¹/₅₀₀, 46.2%
4. 1 : 8, ⅛, 0.125

Chapter 4 Ratios—Work Sheet, pp. 75–78

Fractions to ratios, p. 75

1. 3 : 4　　**4.** 14 : 25　　**7.** 5 : 8　　**10.** 10 : 1
2. 2 : 3　　**5.** 2 : 5　　　**8.** 1 : 4　　**11.** 7 : 30
3. 1 : 2　　**6.** 31 : 100　　**9.** 16 : 27　**12.** 1 : 1

Decimals to ratios, pp. 75–76

1. 112 : 125　　**5.** 252 : 625　　**9.** 123 : 250
2. 24 : 25　　　**6.** 37 : 50　　　**10.** 19 : 20
3. 3 : 50　　　**7.** 83 : 500　　　**11.** 47 : 200
4. 3 : 5　　　**8.** 13 : 50　　　　**12.** 43 : 250

Percents to ratios, p. 76

1. 1 : 10　　**4.** 27 : 1000　　**7.** 31 : 400　　**10.** 1 : 100
2. 1 : 3　　　**5.** 11 : 25　　　**8.** 11 : 2500　　**11.** 3 : 500
3. 3 : 800　　**6.** 157 : 1000　　**9.** 39 : 500　　**12.** 6 : 175

Ratios to fractions, p. 77

1. ¹/₁₆　　**4.** 1½　　**7.** 3⅕　　**10.** 1⁶/₁₁
2. ¹/₂₀₀　　**5.** 1　　　**8.** ½　　　**11.** ³⁷/₆₇
3. ¹/₅₀　　**6.** ⅓　　　**9.** ⁸/₄₅　　**12.** ⁸²/₁₂₇

Ratios to decimal numbers, pp. 77–78

1. 0.5　　**4.** 0.3333　　**7.** 1.5　　**10.** 0.9
2. 0.25　　**5.** 6.25　　　**8.** 0.1　　**11.** 0.027
3. 0.375　　**6.** 0.5　　　**9.** 0.4　　**12.** 3.5

Ratios to percents, p. 78

1. 50%
2. 3$\frac{1}{33}$%, 3.0303%
3. 10%
4. 20%

5. 37$\frac{1}{27}$%, 37.037%
6. $\frac{1}{10}$%, 0.1%
7. 25%
8. 52$\frac{1}{12}$%, 52.0833%

9. $\frac{1}{5}$%, 0.2%
10. 66$\frac{2}{3}$%, 66.6666%
11. 55$\frac{5}{9}$%, 55.5555%
12. 2133$\frac{1}{3}$%, 2133.3333%

Chapter 4 Ratios—Posttest 1, p. 79

1. $\frac{7}{8}$, 0.875, 87.5%
2. 1 : 250, $\frac{1}{250}$, 0.4%
3. 13 : 20, 0.65, 65%
4. 9 : 400, $\frac{9}{400}$, 0.0225

5. 7 : 20, $\frac{7}{20}$, 35%
6. 6 : 25, 0.24, 24%
7. $\frac{27}{40}$, 0.675, 67.5%

8. 3 : 1000, $\frac{3}{1000}$, 0.003
9. 41 : 200, $\frac{41}{200}$, 20.5%
10. 4 : 11, 0.3636, 36.36%

Chapter 4 Ratios—Posttest 2, p. 81

1. $\frac{7}{10}$, 0.7, 70%
2. 5 : 16, 0.3125, 31.25%
3. 3 : 40, $\frac{3}{40}$, 7.5%
4. 3 : 50, $\frac{3}{50}$, 0.06

5. 3 : 800, $\frac{3}{800}$, 0.00375
6. 1 : 150, 0.0066, 0.66%
7. 7 : 1000, $\frac{7}{1000}$, 0.7%

8. $\frac{2}{7}$, 0.2857, 28.57%
9. 161 : 500, $\frac{161}{500}$, 32.2%
10. 91 : 500, $\frac{91}{500}$, 0.182

Chapter 5 Proportions—Pretest, pp. 83–84

1. 100
2. 7$\frac{1}{2}$ or 7.5
3. $\frac{1}{600}$
4. 3.2
5. 128

6. 4
7. 400 or 399.9
8. $\frac{1}{2}$
9. $\frac{3}{7}$
10. 8

11. 80
12. $\frac{1}{6}$
13. 14
14. 48
15. $\frac{3}{10}$

16. 80
17. 10
18. 126
19. $\frac{1}{150}$
20. 16$\frac{1}{4}$ or 16.25

Chapter 5 Proportions—Work Sheet, pp. 89–92

1. 84
2. 28.125
3. 1$\frac{1}{5}$
4. 52$\frac{1}{2}$
5. 1$\frac{1}{2}$ or 1.5
6. $\frac{3}{4}$
7. 1
8. 4$\frac{4}{5}$
9. 1$\frac{1}{2}$ or 1.5
10. 2000
11. 1
12. 80

13. 600
14. 40
15. 0.032
16. 0.2
17. 960
18. 25
19. 20
20. $\frac{1}{2}$ or 0.5
21. 1.2
22. 1.17
23. 3
24. 15

25. 48
26. 0.9
27. 16
28. 6
29. 1$\frac{1}{3}$
30. 3.6
31. 450
32. $\frac{657}{1100}$ or 0.597
33. $\frac{3}{5}$ or 0.6
34. 2$\frac{7}{10}$
35. 171.43

36. 500
37. 10
38. 12$\frac{1}{2}$ or 12.5
39. 240
40. 18$\frac{3}{4}$ or 18.75
41. 6
42. 180
43. 12$\frac{1}{2}$ or 12.5
44. 80
45. $\frac{1}{32}$, 0.03125
46. 1620

Chapter 5 Proportions—Posttest 1, pp. 93–94

1. 2
2. $\frac{35}{48}$
3. 6
4. 6.25
5. 32

6. $\frac{1}{2}$
7. 2$\frac{1}{2}$ or 2.5
8. 2
9. $\frac{5}{9}$
10. 36

11. 4
12. 4
13. 8
14. 1500
15. 42

16. $\frac{4}{9}$
17. 4
18. 100
19. 1
20. 3.2

Chapter 5 Proportions—Posttest 2, pp. 95–96

1. 225
2. $1^{7}/_{25}$, 1.28
3. 120
4. 6.84
5. $13^{1}/_{3}$
6. 56
7. 1
8. 3.8
9. $^{3}/_{20}$
10. 40
11. 3.6
12. 105
13. $2^{7}/_{10}$
14. $^{35}/_{72}$
15. 10
16. 360
17. 15
18. 72
19. $1^{2}/_{25}$ or 1.08
20. 150

Review of Mathematics Posttest, pp. 97–101

1. mixed
   whole
2. $^{7}/_{6}$
   $^{6}/_{3}$
   $^{9}/_{9}$
3. fraction
4. $^{1}/_{2}/4$
   $^{3}/_{7}/^{4}/_{2}$
   $21/^{2}/_{3}$
5. relationship
6. two
7. 4 : 12 or 1 : 3
8. 24 : 100 or 6 : 25
9. 3 : 100
10. 13 : 8
11. 22 : 1000 or 2.2 : 100
    (same value)
12. 124 : 100
13. denominator
14. 2 / ③
15. 4 ÷ ⑧
16. 10 : ⑤
17. ④)‾12‾
18. 14 / ⑧
19. 6 ÷ ㉔
20. ㊷)‾7‾
21. 7 : ⑩
22. numerator
23. 10
24. 10
25. $^{436}/_{1000}$
26. $^{51}/_{1000}$
27. $1^{42}/_{10,000}$
28. $^{9684}/_{10,000}$
29. $^{19}/_{10,000}$
30. $1^{2064}/_{100,000}$
31. $1^{28}/_{45}$
32. $7^{1}/_{12}$
33. $5^{5}/_{6}$
34. $5^{1}/_{2}$
35. 8.52
36. 46.29
37. 234.93
38. 459.56
39. $^{1}/_{6}$
40. $1^{13}/_{21}$
41. $^{41}/_{45}$
42. $5^{11}/_{18}$
43. 23.9
44. 0.1
45. 4.1
46. 1.0
47. $5^{5}/_{8}$
48. $^{2}/_{3}$
49. $8^{26}/_{27}$
50. $26^{3}/_{5}$
51. 1.93
52. 1.97
53. 4.48
54. 181.79
55. $1^{31}/_{32}$
56. $^{18}/_{35}$
57. $^{1}/_{225}$
58. $^{473}/_{576}$
59. 5.654
60. 0.001
61. 80,000
62. 17.349
63. 0.014, 0.048, 0.407, 0.45, 1.46, 2.401
64. 0.015, 0.15, 0.155, 1.0015, 1.015, 1.15
65. 0.090, 0.90, 0.99, 9.009, 9.09, 90.90
66. 0.24, 0.4, 0.44, 0.52, 0.6, 0.7
67. 0.021, 0.1091, 0.191, 0.2, 0.201, 0.21
68. 0.83
69. 0.56
70. 0.56
71. 0.01
72. $^{9}/_{40}$
73. $^{93}/_{200}$
74. $^{3}/_{50}$
75. $^{93}/_{250}$
76. 27.5%
77. 37.5%
78. $^{21}/_{50}$
79. 62 : 10,000 or 31 : 5000
80. 12.5%
81. 25%
82. 15%
83. 0.24
84. 54.6
85. 149.5
86. 2 : 9
87. 3 : 8
88. 73 : 125
89. 2 : 3
90. 12 : 25
91. 270
92. 1.68
93. 13.04
94. 1.13
95. 150
96. 484
97. 198.33
98. $533^{1}/_{3}$ or 533.33
99. 27
100. 3.75

PART II UNITS AND MEASUREMENTS FOR THE CALCULATION OF DRUG DOSAGES

Chapter 6 Metric and Household Measurements—Pretest, pp. 105–106

1. 0.8 g
2. 3000 mcg
3. 0.255 g
4. 46,000 mcg
5. 3 mg
6. 680 mg
7. 0.326 L
8. 72.6 lb or 72⅗ lb
9. 2100 mg
10. 3 kg
11. 100 mL
12. 116.6 lb or 116⅗ lb
13. 5 mcg
14. 800 g
15. 0.25 mg
16. 300 mL
17. 10,000 g
18. 630 mL
19. 0.733 kg
20. 1,250,000 mcg
21. 0.06 g
22. 250 mcg
23. 250 mL
24. 20.45 kg
25. 0.01 g
26. 1200 g
27. 25 mL
28. 710 mg
29. 0.48 L
30. 1⁴³/₁₀₀ lb or 1.43 lb

Chapter 6 Metric and Household Measurements—Work Sheet, pp. 113–116

1. 0.00023 g
2. 5000 mcg
3. 2,500,000 mcg
4. 4 mg
5. 330 mg
6. 6000 g
7. 0.725 L
8. 0.002 g
9. 30 mm
10. 0.62 kg
11. 360 mcg
12. 0.46 L
13. 660 mcg
14. 500,000 mcg
15. 45 cm
16. 0.35 g
17. 0.025 g
18. 1460 mL
19. 2500 g
20. 12,000 mcg
21. 3400 g
22. 0.00092 g
23. 2.5 cm
24. 0.3 mg
25. 160 mL
26. 10 mg
27. 0.5 mg
28. 0.36 g
29. 1700 mL
30. 450 mg
31. 0.24 L
32. 0.01 mg
33. 7.5 cm
34. 540 mL
35. 10 mL
36. 45 mL
37. 360 mL
38. 17⅗ lb or 17.6 lb
39. 8.415 lb, 8⁸³/₂₀₀ lb, or 8.41 lb
40. 17.5 cm
41. 1.36 kg
42. 26⅖ lb or 26.4 lb
43. 3²/₂₅ lb or 3.08 lb
44. 30 inches
45. 68.18 kg

Chapter 6 Metric and Household Measurements—Posttest 1, pp. 117–118

1. 0.005 g
2. 10,000 mcg
3. 810 mL
4. 0.035 g
5. 30 inches
6. 120,000 mcg
7. 35⅕ lb or 35.2 lb
8. 0.28 L
9. 400 g
10. 3½ feet
11. 12727.27 g
12. 10 cm
13. 0.5 g
14. 0.037 L
15. ⅔ oz
16. 320 mL
17. 2500 mg
18. 0.35 g
19. 6.7 kg
20. 300 mL
21. 4000 mcg
22. 5¹⁸/₂₅ lb or 5.72 lb
23. 7.5 mL
24. 200 mL
25. 0.533 L
26. 1,500,000 mcg
27. 0.62 g
28. 2300 g
29. 1¼ feet
30. 3.18 kg

Chapter 6 Metric and Household Measurements—Posttest 2, pp. 119–120

1. 4 mg	**11.** 100 mL	**21.** 0.037 mg
2. 0.15 kg	**12.** 32,000 mcg	**22.** 1400 mL
3. 600 mL	**13.** 0.618 L	**23.** 780 mg
4. 1¹⁹⁄₂₅ lb or 1.76 lb	**14.** 0.1 g	**24.** 0.225 mg
5. 96⁴⁄₅ lb or 96.8 lb	**15.** 2⅓ feet	**25.** 4.5 kg
6. 0.76 g	**16.** 0.714 L	**26.** 200 mL
7. 550 mL	**17.** 0.35 g	**27.** 40 inches
8. 3.5 cm	**18.** 0.25 g	**28.** 0.42 g
9. 60 mL	**19.** 870 mg	**29.** 2,600,000 mcg
10. 965.909 g	**20.** 7000 mcg	**30.** 33.18 kg

Chapter 7 Apothecary and Household Measurements—Pretest, p. 121

1-2. 1¼ pt, ⅝ qt	**8.** 2 pt
3-4. 80 fl oz, 2½ qt	**9.** 12 fl oz
5-6. 1¾ gal, 14 pt	**10.** 20 fl oz
7. 24 fl oz	

Chapter 7 Apothecary and Household Measurements—Work Sheet, pp. 127–128

Arabic to Roman numerals, p. 127

1. xxii	**3.** iii	**5.** xiv	**7.** xv
2. ix	**4.** xxx	**6.** vi	**8.** xii

Roman to Arabic numerals, p. 127

1. 29	**3.** 20	**5.** 16	**7.** 25
2. 7	**4.** 6	**6.** 4	**8.** 240

Equivalents within the apothecary system, p. 127

1. ⁵⁄₃₂ pt	**5.** 4 qt, 1 gal
2. ¹⁵⁄₁₆ pt	**6.** 8 fl oz
3. 64 fl oz, 2 qt	**7.** ¾ gal, 6 pt
4. 40 fl oz	**8.** 20 pt, 2½ gal

Household measures to equivalents in the apothecary system, p. 128

1. 16 fl oz	**3.** 26 fl oz
2. 4 fl oz	**4.** 14 fl oz

Chapter 7 Apothecary and Household Measurements—Posttest 1, p. 129

1-2. ¾ qt, 1½ pt	**7-8.** 7 qt, 224 fl oz
3-4. 3 pt, 1½ qt	**9-10.** 12 fl oz, ¾ pt
5-6. 1¼ gal, 10 pt	**11.** 6 fl oz

Chapter 7 Apothecary and Household Measurements—Posttest 2, p. 131

1-2. 3 pt, 1½ qt	**7-8.** 10 qt, 20 pt
3-4. 72 fl oz, 2¼ qt	**9-10.** 18 fl oz, 1⅛ pt
5-6. 1½ gal, 192 fl oz	**11.** 4 fl oz

Chapter 8 Equivalents between Apothecary and Metric Measurements—Pretest, pp. 133–134

1. 50 kg
2. $\frac{1}{2}$ qt
3. $79\frac{1}{5}$ lb or 79.2 lb
4. 5250 mL
5. 3 fl oz
6. 1.75 L
7. 6 g
8. $18\frac{1}{25}$ lb or 18.04 lb
9. 3909.0909 g
10. 1125 mL
11. 210 mL
12. 0.6666 g
13. $5\frac{1}{2}$ qt
14. $3\frac{13}{25}$ lb or 3.52 lb
15. 240 mg
16. 12 fl oz
17. $1\frac{1}{5}$ pt
18. $12\frac{1}{10}$ lb or 12.1 lb
19. $\frac{2}{3}$ fl oz
20. $\frac{1}{5}$ gr
21. 0.2 mg
22. 38.6363 kg
23. $\frac{1}{150}$ gr
24. 5.57 kg
25. $4\frac{1}{5}$ qt
26. 45 mL
27. 12 mg
28. 69 gr
29. 37.1° C
30. 105.8° F
31. 36.4° C
32. 101.3° F
33. 37.7° C
34. 103.3° F
35. 39.2° C
36. 104.4° F

Chapter 8 Equivalents between Apothecary and Metric Measurements—Work Sheet, pp. 139–141

1. $3\frac{1}{3}$ gr
2. 10 kg
3. 9 g
4. 1750 mL
5. 7 fl oz
6. 22 lb
7. $3\frac{1}{2}$ pt
8. 15 mL
9. 270 mg
10. $9\frac{6}{25}$ lb or 9.24 lb
11. 7 gr
12. 3000 mL
13. $3\frac{1}{2}$ qt
14. 300 mg
15. 5 fl oz
16. 7.26 lb
17. 3090.909 g
18. 11.25 mL
19. 165 mg
20. 2.2727 kg
21. $5\frac{2}{5}$ pt
22. $5\frac{2}{3}$ gr
23. 2.5 L
24. $8\frac{3}{100}$ lb or 8.03 lb
25. 120 mL
26. 5454.5454 g
27. 34.0909 kg
28. 2125 mL
29. $1\frac{2}{3}$ gr
30. $3\frac{1}{2}$ qt
31. 90 mg
32. 55 lb
33. 37.6° C
34. 38.8° C
35. 40.1° C
36. 36.3° C
37. 104.7° F
38. 95.7° F
39. 98.2° F
40. 102.6° F
41. 91.4° F
42. 36.9° C
43. 106.2° F
44. 39.8° C
45. 105.1° F
46. 39° C
47. 99.3° F
48. 38° C

Chapter 8 Equivalents between Apothecary and Metric Measurements—Posttest 1, pp. 143–144

1. 180 mg
2. 4.5 g
3. 90 mL
4. 750 mL
5. $\frac{1}{4}$ gr
6. $1\frac{1}{2}$ qt
7. 3409.0909 g
8. $1\frac{7}{10}$ qt
9. 0.3333 g
10. 9.0909 kg
11. 10 mg
12. 2 pt
13. $\frac{1}{200}$ gr
14. 50 gr
15. 2 fl oz
16. $5\frac{47}{50}$ lb or 5.94 lb
17. 150 mL
18. $70\frac{2}{5}$ lb or 70.4 lb
19. $\frac{1}{120}$ gr
20. 4.8 g
21. 2.75 L
22. 18 fl oz
23. 35.2° C
24. 96.1° F
25. 39.6° C
26. 105.4° F
27. 40.1° C
28. 99° F
29. 37.4° C
30. 92.8° F

Chapter 8 Equivalents between Apothecary and Metric Measurements—Posttest 2, pp. 145–146

1. 27.2727 kg
2. 2½ qt
3. 625 mL
4. 15 mg
5. 1¼ qt
6. ⅓ gr
7. 9.09 kg
8. 375 mL
9. 2375 mL
10. 10 gr

11. 0.5 mg
12. 0.42 g
13. 3.5 L
14. 3 pt
15. 2¹⁶⁄₂₅ lb or 2.64 lb
16. ¹⁄₇₅ gr
17. 92²⁄₅ lb or 92.4 lb
18. 3 mg
19. 1515.1515 g
20. 15²⁄₅ lb or 15.4 lb

21. 21²⁄₃ gr
22. 1590.909 g
23. 35.7° C
24. 100.8° F
25. 98.2° F
26. 36.6° C
27. 104.7° F
28. 38.2° C
29. 106.5° F
30. 39.6° C

PART III PREPARATION FOR CALCULATION OF DRUG DOSAGES

Chapter 9 Safety in Medication Administration—Posttest, p. 153

1. False
2. False
3. True
4. True
5. True
6. True
7. True
8. False

Chapter 10 Interpretation of the Physician's Orders—Posttest, p. 161

1 1/12	Cefuroxime						
	1 g dose	IV route	q8 h interval	08	16	24	
2 1/12	Lasix						
	40 mg dose	po route	twice daily interval		09	21	
3 1/12	Slow-K						
	10 mEq dose	po route	twice daily interval		09	21	

Chapter 11 How to Read Drug Labels—Posttest 1, pp. 167–168

1. Glucophage
   metformin hydrochloride
   500 mg
   tablets
   500 tablets

2. Diabinese
   chlorpropamide
   250 mg
   tablets
   250 tablets

3. Robinul
   glycopyrrolate
   0.4 mg/2 mL or 0.2 mg/mL
   milliliters
   IM or IV

4. Cefobid
   cefoperazone sodium
   10 g
   milliliters
   IM or IV

Chapter 11 How to Read Drug Labels—Posttest 2, pp. 169–170

1. Furadantin
nitrofurantoin
5 mg/mL
suspension
oral
60 mL

2. Decadron
dexamethasone
1.5 mg
tablets

3. Biaxin
clarithromycin
250 mg
tablet
60 tablets

4. Kefzol
cefazolin sodium
225 mg/mL
milliliters after reconstitution
IM or IV

Chapter 12 Dimensional Analysis and the Calculation of Drug Dosages— Work Sheet, pp. 183–188

1. $x \text{ tab} = \dfrac{1 \text{ tab}}{5 \text{ mg}} \times 10 \text{ mg}$

$x = \dfrac{1 \times 10}{5}$

$x = 2 \text{ tablets}$

2. $x \text{ mL} = \dfrac{5 \text{ mL}}{25 \text{ mg}} \times 60 \text{ mg}$

$x = \dfrac{5 \times 60}{25}$

$x = 12 \text{ mL}$

3. $x \text{ tab} = \dfrac{1 \text{ tab}}{50 \text{ mg}} \times \dfrac{1000 \text{ mg}}{1 \text{ g}} \times 0.025 \text{ g}$

$x = \dfrac{1 \times 1000 \times 0.025}{50 \times 1}$

$x = \dfrac{25}{50}$

$x = \frac{1}{2} \text{ tablet}$

4. $x \text{ tab} = \dfrac{1 \text{ tab}}{30 \text{ mg}} \times 30 \text{ mg}$

$x = \dfrac{1 \times 30}{30}$

$x = \dfrac{30}{30}$

$x = 1 \text{ tablet}$

5. $x \text{ cap} = \dfrac{1 \text{ cap}}{250 \text{ mg}} \times \dfrac{1000 \text{ mg}}{1 \text{ g}} \times 0.5 \text{ g}$

$x = \dfrac{1 \times 1000 \times 0.5}{250}$

$x = \dfrac{500}{250}$

$x = 2 \text{ capsules}$

6. $x \text{ mL} = \dfrac{1 \text{ mL}}{4 \text{ mg}} \times 3 \text{ mg}$

$x = \dfrac{1 \times 3}{4}$

$x = \dfrac{3}{4} \text{ or } 0.75 \text{ mL}$

7. $x \text{ mL} = \dfrac{1 \text{ mL}}{0.05 \text{ mg}} \times \dfrac{1 \text{ mg}}{1000 \text{ mcg}} \times 40 \text{ mcg}$

$x = \dfrac{1 \times 1 \times 40}{0.05 \times 1000}$

$x = \dfrac{40}{50}$

$x = 0.8 \text{ mL}$

8. $x \text{ mL} = \dfrac{1 \text{ mL}}{2 \text{ mg}} \times 1 \text{ mg}$

$x = \dfrac{1}{2}$

$x = 0.5 \text{ mL}$

9. $x \text{ mL} = \dfrac{1 \text{ mL}}{5000 \text{ units}} \times 2500 \text{ units}$

$x = \dfrac{1 \times 2500}{5000}$

$x = \dfrac{2500}{5000} \text{ or } 0.5 \text{ mL}$

10. $x \text{ tab} = \dfrac{1 \text{ tab}}{500 \text{ mg}} \times \dfrac{1000 \text{ mg}}{1 \text{ g}} \times 2 \text{ g}$

$x = \dfrac{1 \times 1000 \times 2}{500 \times 1}$

$x = \dfrac{2000}{500}$

$x = 4 \text{ tablets}$

11. $x \text{ gtt/min} = \dfrac{20 \text{ gtt} \times 100 \text{ mL} \times 1 \text{ h}}{1 \text{ mL} \times 1 \text{ h} \times 60 \text{ min}}$

$x = \dfrac{2000}{60}$

$x = 33.3 \text{ or } 33 \text{ gtt/min}$

12. $x \text{ gtt/min} = \dfrac{10 \text{ gtt} \times 500 \text{ mL} \times 1 \text{ h}}{1 \text{ mL} \times 2 \text{ h} \times 60 \text{ min}}$

$x = \dfrac{5000}{120}$

$x = 41.6 \text{ or } 42 \text{ gtt/min}$

13. $x \text{ mL/h} = \dfrac{250 \text{ mL} \times 1400 \text{ units}}{25,000 \text{ units} \times 1 \text{ h}}$

$x = \dfrac{350,000}{25,000}$

$x = 14 \text{ mL/h}$

14. $x \text{ mL/h} = \dfrac{100 \text{ mL} \times 8 \text{ units}}{50 \text{ units} \times 1 \text{ h}}$

$x = \dfrac{800}{50}$

$x = 16 \text{ mL/h}$

15. *Bolus*

$x \text{ units} = \dfrac{70 \text{ units}}{1 \text{ kg}} \times \dfrac{1 \text{ kg}}{2.2 \text{ lb}} \times \dfrac{132 \text{ lb}}{1}$

$x = \dfrac{70 \times 1 \times 132}{1 \times 2.2 \times 1}$

$x = \dfrac{9240}{2.2} = 4200 \text{ units IV bolus}$

IV infusion

$x \text{ mL} = \dfrac{1 \text{ mL}}{100 \text{ units}} \times \dfrac{17 \text{ units}}{1 \text{ kg}} \times \dfrac{1 \text{ kg}}{2.2 \text{ lb}} \times \dfrac{132 \text{ lb}}{1}$

$x = \dfrac{1 \times 17 \times 1 \times 132}{100 \times 1 \times 2.2 \times 1}$

$x = \dfrac{2244}{220} = 10.2 \text{ mL}$

16. $x \text{ mL/h} = \dfrac{250 \text{ mL}}{1 \text{ g}} \times \dfrac{1 \text{ g}}{1,000,000 \text{ mcg}} \times \dfrac{12 \text{ mcg/kg}}{1 \text{ min}} \times \dfrac{60 \text{ min}}{1 \text{ h}} \times \dfrac{75 \text{ kg}}{1}$

$x = \dfrac{250 \times 1 \times 12 \times 60 \times 75}{1 \times 1,000,000 \times 1 \times 1 \times 1}$

$x = \dfrac{13,500,000}{1,000,000} = 13.5 \text{ mL/h}$

17. $x \text{ mL/h} = \dfrac{500 \text{ mL}}{100 \text{ mg}} \times \dfrac{1 \text{ mg}}{1000 \text{ mcg}} \times \dfrac{10 \text{ mcg}}{1 \text{ min}} \times \dfrac{60 \text{ min}}{1 \text{ h}}$

$x = \dfrac{500 \times 1 \times 10 \times 60}{100 \times 1000 \times 1 \times 1}$

$x = \dfrac{300,000}{100,000} = 3 \text{ mL/h}$

18. x mL/h $= \dfrac{500 \text{ mL}}{900 \text{ mg}} \times \dfrac{0.5 \text{ mg}}{1 \text{ min}} \times \dfrac{60 \text{ min}}{1 \text{ h}}$

$x = \dfrac{500 \times 0.5 \times 60}{900 \times 1 \times 1}$

$x = \dfrac{15{,}000}{900} = 16.66$ or 16.7 mL/h

19. a. $\dfrac{10 \text{ to } 15 \text{ mg} \mid 14.5 \text{ kg}}{\text{kg/dose} \mid} = 145$ to 217.5 mg/dose

b. $\dfrac{145 \text{ to } 217.5 \text{ mg} \mid 5 \text{ mL}}{\mid 160 \text{ mg}} = 4.5$ to 6.8 mL

20. $\dfrac{20 \text{ mcg} \mid 1 \text{ mg} \mid 1 \text{ mL}}{\mid 1000 \text{ mcg} \mid 0.1 \text{ mg}} = 0.2$ mL

21. $\dfrac{20 \text{ to } 50 \text{ mg} \mid 50 \text{ kg}}{\text{kg/day (24 h)} \mid} = \dfrac{1250 \text{ to } 2500 \text{ mg}}{\text{day (24 h)}}$

$\dfrac{1250 \text{ to } 2500 \text{ mg} \mid 1 \text{ day}}{\text{day (24 h)} \mid 4 \text{ doses}} = \dfrac{312.5 \text{ to } 625 \text{ mg}}{\text{dose}} = 312.5$ to 625 mg/dose

22. $\dfrac{7.5 \text{ mg} \mid 1 \text{ mL}}{\mid 4 \text{ mg}} = 1.88$ mL

Chapter 13 Oral Dosages—Work Sheet, pp. 205–235

Proportion

1. 1 mg : 1 cap :: 2 mg : x cap
1 : 1 :: 2 : x
$x = 2$ capsules

2. 20 mg : 5 mL :: 30 mg : x mL
20 : 5 :: 30 : x
$20x = 150$
$x = \dfrac{150}{20}$
$x = 7.5$ mL

Formula

$\dfrac{2 \text{ mg}}{1 \text{ mg}} \times 1 \text{ cap} = 2$ capsules

$\dfrac{30 \text{ mg}}{20 \text{ mg}} \times 5 \text{ mL} =$

$\dfrac{30}{\underset{4}{20}} \times \dfrac{\overset{1}{5}}{1} = \dfrac{30}{4}$

$\dfrac{30}{4} = 7.5$ mL

Proportion	Formula

3. 0.05 mg : 1 tab :: 0.2 mg : x tab

$\quad$ 0.05 : 1 :: 0.2 : x

$\quad$ 0.05x = 0.2

$\qquad x = \dfrac{0.2}{0.05}$

$\qquad x$ = 4 tablets

$\dfrac{0.2 \text{ mg}}{0.05 \text{ mg}} \times 1 \text{ tab} =$

$\qquad \dfrac{0.2}{0.05} = 4 \text{ tablets}$

$\quad$ 0.05 mg : 1 tab :: 0.15 mg : x tab

$\quad$ 0.05 : 1 :: 0.15 : x

$\quad$ 0.05x = 0.15

$\qquad x = \dfrac{0.15}{0.05}$

$\qquad x$ = 3 tablets

$\dfrac{0.15 \text{ mg}}{0.05 \text{ mg}} \times 1 \text{ tab} =$

$\qquad \dfrac{0.15}{0.05} = 3 \text{ tablets}$

---

4. 250 mg : 1 tab :: 500 mg : x tab

$\quad$ 250 : 1 :: 500 : x

$\quad$ 250x = 500

$\qquad x = \dfrac{500}{250}$

$\qquad x$ = 2 tablets

$\dfrac{500}{250} \times 1 \text{ tab} =$

$\qquad \dfrac{\cancel{500}^{2}}{\cancel{250}_{1}} =$

$\qquad \dfrac{2}{1} = 2 \text{ tablets}$

---

5. 5 mg : 5 mL :: 2.5 mg : x mL

$\quad$ 5 : 5 :: 2.5 : x

$\quad$ 5x = 12.5

$\qquad x = \dfrac{12.5}{5}$

$\qquad x$ = 2.5 mL

$\dfrac{2.5 \text{ mg}}{5 \text{ mg}} \times 5 \text{ mL} =$

$\qquad \dfrac{2.5}{\cancel{5}} \times \dfrac{\cancel{5}^{1}}{1} = \dfrac{2.5}{1} = 2.5 \text{ mL}$

6. 1 mg : 1 tab :: 2 mg : x tab

$\quad$ 1 : 1 :: 2 : x

$\qquad x$ = 2 tablets

$\dfrac{2 \text{ mg}}{1 \text{ mg}} \times 1 \text{ tab} =$

$\qquad \dfrac{2}{1} = 2 \text{ tablets}$

---

7. 10 mg : 1 tab :: 20 mg : x tab

$\quad$ 10 : 1 :: 20 : x

$\quad$ 10x = 20

$\qquad x = \dfrac{20}{10}$

$\qquad x$ = 2 tablets

$\dfrac{20}{10} \times 1 \text{ tab} =$

$\qquad \dfrac{\cancel{20}^{2}}{\cancel{10}_{1}} = 2 \text{ tablets}$

Proportion	Formula

8. 0.5 g : 1 tab :: 1 g : x tab
0.5 : 1 :: 1 : x
0.5x = 1
$x = \dfrac{1}{0.5}$
x = 2 tablets

$\dfrac{1\ \text{g}}{0.5\ \text{g}} \times 1\ \text{tab} =$

$\dfrac{1}{0.5} = 2$ tablets

9. 20 mg : 5 mL :: 40 mg : x mL
20 : 5 :: 40 : x
20x = 200
$x = \dfrac{200}{20}$
x = 10 mL

$\dfrac{40}{20} \times 5\ \text{mL} =$

$\dfrac{\overset{10}{\cancel{40}}}{\underset{\cancel{4}}{\cancel{20}}} \times \dfrac{\overset{1}{\cancel{5}}}{1} =$

$\dfrac{10}{1} = 10\ \text{mL}$

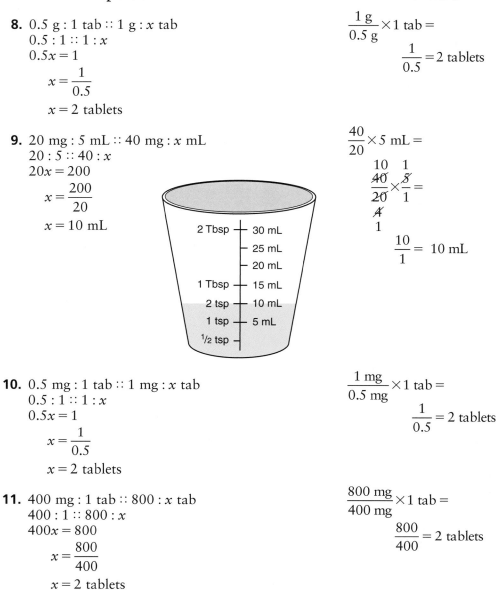

10. 0.5 mg : 1 tab :: 1 mg : x tab
0.5 : 1 :: 1 : x
0.5x = 1
$x = \dfrac{1}{0.5}$
x = 2 tablets

$\dfrac{1\ \text{mg}}{0.5\ \text{mg}} \times 1\ \text{tab} =$

$\dfrac{1}{0.5} = 2$ tablets

11. 400 mg : 1 tab :: 800 : x tab
400 : 1 :: 800 : x
400x = 800
$x = \dfrac{800}{400}$
x = 2 tablets

$\dfrac{800\ \text{mg}}{400\ \text{mg}} \times 1\ \text{tab} =$

$\dfrac{800}{400} = 2$ tablets

Proportion	Formula

12. 1000 mg : 1 g : x mg : 0.6 g
1000 : 1 :: x : 0.6
$x = 600$ mg

300 mg : 1 tab :: 600 mg : x tab
300 : 1 :: 600 : x
$300x = 600$
$x = \dfrac{600}{300}$
$x = 2$ tablets

$\dfrac{600 \text{ mg}}{300 \text{ mg}} \times 1 \text{ tab} =$
$\dfrac{600}{300} = 2$ tablets

600 mg : 1 dose :: x mg : 2 dose
600 : 1 :: x : 2
$x = 1200$ mg

13. 10 mg : 1 tablet :: 30 mg : x tablets
$10x = 30$
$x = \dfrac{30}{10}$
$x = 3$ tablets

$\dfrac{30 \text{ mg}}{10 \text{ mg}} \times 1 \text{ tab} =$
$\dfrac{30}{10} = 3$ tablets

14. 1 g : 1000 mg :: 0.75 g : x mg
1 : 1000 :: 0.75 : x
$x = 750$ mg

750 mg : 1 tab :: 750 mg : x tab
750 : 1 :: 750 : x
$750x = 750$
$x = \dfrac{750}{750}$
$x = 1$ tablet

$\dfrac{750 \text{ mg}}{750 \text{ mg}} \times 1 \text{ tab} =$
$\dfrac{750}{750} = 1$ tablet

15. 1000 mg : 1 g :: x mg : 0.324 g
$x = 324$ mg

324 mg : 1 tab :: 324 mg : x tab
324 : 1 :: 324 : x
$324x = 324$
$x = 1$ tablet

$\dfrac{324 \text{ mg}}{324 \text{ mg}} \times 1 \text{ tab} = 1$ tablet

Proportion	Formula

Proportion

16. $0.5 \text{ g} : 1 \text{ tab} :: 4 \text{ g} : x \text{ tab}$
$0.5 : 1 :: 4 : x$
$0.5x = 4$
$\quad x = \dfrac{4}{0.5}$
$\quad x = 8 \text{ tablets}$

$0.5 \text{ g} : 1 \text{ tab} :: 2 \text{ g} : x \text{ tab}$
$0.5 : 1 :: 2 : x$
$0.5x = 2$
$\quad x = \dfrac{2}{0.5}$
$\quad x = 4 \text{ tablets}$

17. $400 \text{ mg} : 1 \text{ tab} :: 800 \text{ mg} : x \text{ tab}$
$400 : 1 :: 800 : x$
$400x = 800$
$\quad x = \dfrac{800}{400}$
$\quad x = 2 \text{ tablets}$

18. $30 \text{ mL} = 1 \text{ fl oz each dose}$
$4 \text{ fl oz given each day}$

19. $12.5 \text{ mg} : 5 \text{ mL} :: 30 \text{ mg} : x \text{ mL}$
$12.5 : 5 :: 30 : x$
$12.5x = 150$
$\quad x = \dfrac{150}{12.5}$
$\quad x = 12 \text{ mL}$

20. $30 \text{ mg} : 1 \text{ tab} :: 60 \text{ mg} : x \text{ tab}$
$30 : 1 :: 60 : x$
$30x = 60$
$\quad x = \dfrac{60}{30}$
$\quad x = 2 \text{ tablets}$

Formula

$\dfrac{4 \text{ g}}{0.5 \text{ g}} \times 1 \text{ tab} =$
$\dfrac{4}{0.5} = 8 \text{ tablets}$

$\dfrac{2 \text{ g}}{0.5 \text{ g}} \times 1 \text{ tab} =$
$\dfrac{2}{0.5} = 4 \text{ tablets}$

$\dfrac{800 \text{ mg}}{400 \text{ mg}} \times 1 \text{ tab} =$
$\dfrac{\overset{2}{\cancel{800}}}{\underset{1}{\cancel{400}}} = 2 \text{ tablets}$

$\dfrac{30 \text{ mg}}{12.5 \text{ mg}} \times \dfrac{5 \text{ mL}}{1} =$
$\dfrac{30}{12.5} \times \dfrac{5}{1} =$
$\dfrac{150}{12.5} = 12 \text{ mL}$

$\dfrac{60 \text{ mg}}{30 \text{ mg}} \times 1 \text{ tab} =$
$\dfrac{60}{30} = 2 \text{ tablets}$

<table>
<tr><td align="center">**Proportion**</td><td align="center">**Formula**</td></tr>
</table>

21. 125 mg : 5 mL :: x mg : 5.5 mL
125 : 5 :: x : 5.5
$5x = 687.5$
$x = \dfrac{687.5}{5}$
$x = 137.5$ mg

$\dfrac{x \text{ mg}}{125 \text{ mg}} \times 5 \text{ mL} = 5.5 \text{ mL}$

$\dfrac{x}{\overset{}{\underset{25}{\cancel{125}}}} \times \dfrac{\overset{1}{\cancel{5}}}{1} = 5.5$

$\dfrac{x}{25} = 5.5$

$\dfrac{\overset{1}{\cancel{25}}}{1} \times \dfrac{x}{\underset{1}{\cancel{25}}} = 5.5 \times 25$

$x = 137.5$ mg

22. 40 mg : 1 tab :: 80 mg : x tab
40 : 1 :: 80 : x
$40x = 80$
$x = \dfrac{80}{40}$
$x = 2$ tablets

$\dfrac{80 \text{ mg}}{40 \text{ mg}} \times 1 \text{ tab} =$

$\dfrac{80}{40} = 2$ tablets

23. 0.4 mg : 1 tab :: x mg : 2 tab
0.4 : 1 :: x : 2
$x = 0.8$ mg

$\dfrac{x \text{ mg}}{0.4 \text{ mg}} \times 1 \text{ tab} = 2$ tablets

$\dfrac{x}{0.4} = 2$
$x = 2 \times 0.4$
$x = 0.8$ mg

24. 0.5 mg : 5 mL :: 1.5 mg : x mL
0.5 : 5 :: 1.5 : x
$0.5x = 7.5$
$x = \dfrac{7.5}{0.5}$
$x = 15$ mL

$\dfrac{1.5 \text{ mg}}{0.5 \text{ mg}} \times \dfrac{5 \text{ mL}}{1} =$

$\dfrac{1.5}{0.5} \times \dfrac{5}{1} = \dfrac{7.5}{0.5}$

$\dfrac{7.5}{0.5} = 15$ mL

30 mL : 1 fl oz :: 15 mL : x fl oz
30 : 1 :: 15 : x
$30x = 15$
$x = \dfrac{15}{30}$
$x = \frac{1}{2}$ fl oz

25. 375 mg : 5 mL :: 500 mg : x mL
375 : 5 :: 500 : x
$375x = 2500$
$x = \dfrac{2500}{375}$
$x = 6.6666$ mL or 6.7 mL

$\dfrac{500 \text{ mg}}{375 \text{ mg}} \times 5 \text{ mL} =$

$\dfrac{500}{\underset{75}{\cancel{375}}} \times \dfrac{\overset{1}{\cancel{5}}}{1} =$

$\dfrac{500}{75} = 6.67$ mL

	Proportion	Formula

26. 50 mg : 1 tab :: 25 mg : x tab
50 : 1 :: 25 : x
$50x = 25$
$x = \dfrac{25}{50}$
$x = \frac{1}{2}$ tablet

$\dfrac{25 \text{ mg}}{50 \text{ mg}} \times 1 \text{ tab} =$
$\dfrac{25}{50} = \frac{1}{2}$ tablet

27. Supplied in 12-oz bottle
1 fl oz : 1 dose :: 12 fl oz : x dose
1 : 1 :: 12 : x
$x = 12$ doses

30 mL = 1 fl oz
Order is for 1 fl oz

28. 0.125 mg : 1 tab :: 0.25 mg : x tab
0.125 : 1 :: 0.25 : x
$0.125x = 0.25$
$x = \dfrac{0.25}{0.125}$
$x = 2$ tablets

$\dfrac{0.25 \text{ mg}}{0.125 \text{ mg}} \times 1 \text{ tab} =$
$\dfrac{0.25}{0.125} = 2$ tablets

29. 30 mg : 1 tab :: 15 mg : x tab
30 : 1 :: 15 : x
$30x = 15$
$x = \dfrac{15}{30}$
$x = \frac{1}{2}$ tablet

$\dfrac{15 \text{ mg}}{30 \text{ mg}} \times 1 \text{ tab} =$
$\dfrac{15}{30} = \frac{1}{2}$ tablet

30. 250 mg : 5 mL :: 125 mg : x mL
250 : 5 :: 125 : x
$250x = 625$
$x = \dfrac{625}{250}$
$x = 2.5$ mL

$\dfrac{125 \text{ mg}}{250 \text{ mg}} \times 5 \text{ mL} =$
$\dfrac{\overset{1}{\cancel{125}}}{\underset{2}{\cancel{250}}} \times \dfrac{5}{1} = \dfrac{5}{2}$
$\dfrac{5}{2} = 2.5$ mL

31. 50 mg : 1 tab :: 25 mg : x tab
50 : 1 :: 25 : x
$50x = 25$
$x = \dfrac{25}{50}$
$x = \frac{1}{2}$ tablet

$\dfrac{25 \text{ mg}}{50 \text{ mg}} \times 1 \text{ tab} =$
$\dfrac{25}{50} = \frac{1}{2}$ tablet

Proportion   **Formula**

32. 1000 mg : 1 g :: x mg : 0.6 g
1000 : 1 :: x : 0.6
$x = 600$ mg

200 mg : 1 tab :: 600 mg : x tab
200 : 1 :: 600 : x
$200x = 600$
$x = \dfrac{600}{200}$
$x = 3$ tablets

$\dfrac{600 \text{ mg}}{200 \text{ mg}} \times 1 \text{ tab} =$

$\dfrac{600}{200} = 3$ tablets

3 tablets : 1 dose :: x tab : 6 doses
3 : 1 :: x : 6
$x = 18$ tablets

33. 6.25 mg : 5 mL :: 12.5 mg : x mL
6.25 : 5 :: 12.5 : x
$6.25x = 62.5$
$x = \dfrac{62.5}{6.25}$
$x = 10$ mL

$\dfrac{12.5 \text{ mg}}{6.25 \text{ mg}} \times 5 \text{ mL} =$

$\dfrac{\cancel{12.5}^{\,2}}{\cancel{6.25}_{\,1}} \times \dfrac{5}{1} =$

$\dfrac{2 \times 5}{1} = 10$ mL

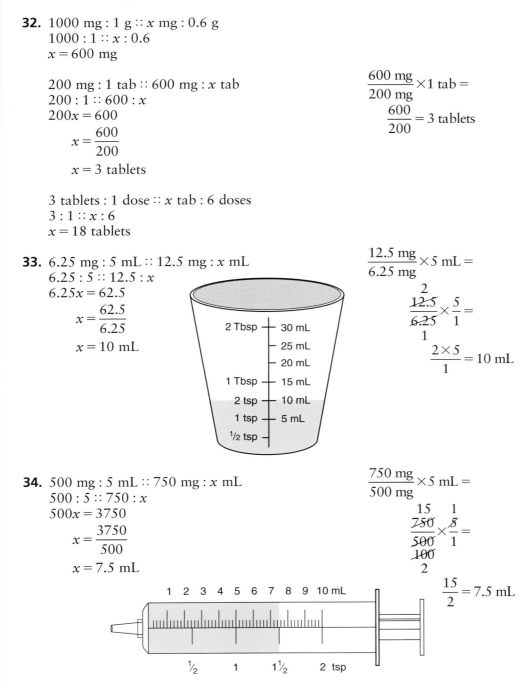

34. 500 mg : 5 mL :: 750 mg : x mL
500 : 5 :: 750 : x
$500x = 3750$
$x = \dfrac{3750}{500}$
$x = 7.5$ mL

$\dfrac{750 \text{ mg}}{500 \text{ mg}} \times 5 \text{ mL} =$

$\dfrac{\cancel{750}^{\,15}}{\cancel{500}_{\,100}^{\,}} \times \dfrac{\cancel{5}^{\,1}}{1} =$

$\dfrac{15}{2} = 7.5$ mL

Proportion	Formula

35. 20 mg : 5 mL :: 100 mg : x mL

20 : 5 :: 100 : x

$20x = 500$

$x = \dfrac{500}{20}$

$x = 25$ mL

$$\dfrac{100 \text{ mg}}{20 \text{ mg}} \times 5 \text{ mL} =$$

$$\dfrac{100}{\underset{4}{20}} \times \dfrac{\overset{1}{5}}{1} =$$

$$\dfrac{100}{4} = 25 \text{ mL}$$

36. 500 mg : 1 tab :: 1000 mg : x tab

500 : 1 :: 1000 : x

$500x = 1000$

$x = \dfrac{1000}{500}$

$x = 2$ tablets

$$\dfrac{1000 \text{ mg}}{500 \text{ mg}} \times 1 \text{ tab} =$$

$$\dfrac{1000}{500} = 2 \text{ tablets}$$

37. 2.5 mg : 1 tab :: 7.5 mg : x tab

2.5 : 1 :: 7.5 : x

$2.5x = 7.5$

$x = \dfrac{7.5}{2.5}$

$x = 3$ tablets

$$\dfrac{7.5 \text{ mg}}{2.5 \text{ mg}} \times 1 \text{ tab} =$$

$$\dfrac{7.5}{2.5} = 3 \text{ tablets}$$

38. 1000 mg : 1 g :: x mg : 0.2 g

1000 : 1 :: x : 0.2

$x = 200$ mg

100 mg : 1 tab :: 200 mg : x tab

100 : 1 :: 200 : x

$100x = 200$

$x = \dfrac{200}{100}$

$x = 2$ tablets

$$\dfrac{200 \text{ mg}}{100 \text{ mg}} \times 1 \text{ tab} =$$

$$\dfrac{200}{100} = 2 \text{ tablets}$$

39. 1 tablet

500 mg acetaminophen in each tablet

40. 0.25 mg : 1 tab :: 0.5 mg : x tab

0.25 : 1 :: 0.5 : x

$0.25x = 0.5$

$x = \dfrac{0.5}{0.25}$

$x = 2$ tablets

$$\dfrac{0.5 \text{ mg}}{0.25 \text{ mg}} \times 1 \text{ tab} =$$

$$\dfrac{0.5}{0.25} = 2 \text{ tablets}$$

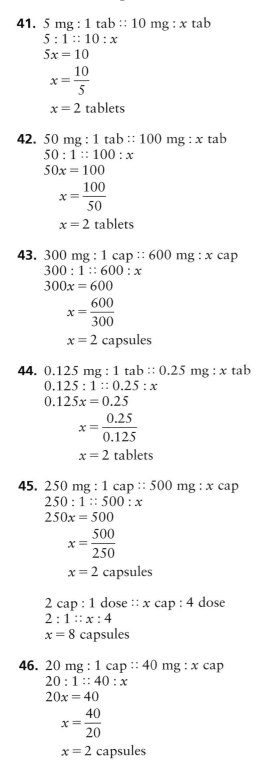

Proportion	Formula

41. 5 mg : 1 tab :: 10 mg : x tab

    5 : 1 :: 10 : x

    $5x = 10$

    $x = \dfrac{10}{5}$

    $x = 2$ tablets

$\dfrac{10\text{ mg}}{5\text{ mg}} \times 1$ tab $=$

    $\dfrac{10}{5} = 2$ tablets

42. 50 mg : 1 tab :: 100 mg : x tab

    50 : 1 :: 100 : x

    $50x = 100$

    $x = \dfrac{100}{50}$

    $x = 2$ tablets

$\dfrac{100\text{ mg}}{50\text{ mg}} \times 1$ tab $=$

    $\dfrac{100}{50} = 2$ tablets

43. 300 mg : 1 cap :: 600 mg : x cap

    300 : 1 :: 600 : x

    $300x = 600$

    $x = \dfrac{600}{300}$

    $x = 2$ capsules

$\dfrac{600\text{ mg}}{300\text{ mg}} \times 1$ cap $=$

    $\dfrac{600}{300} = 2$ capsules

44. 0.125 mg : 1 tab :: 0.25 mg : x tab

    0.125 : 1 :: 0.25 : x

    $0.125x = 0.25$

    $x = \dfrac{0.25}{0.125}$

    $x = 2$ tablets

$\dfrac{0.25\text{ mg}}{0.125\text{ mg}} \times 1$ tab $=$

    $\dfrac{0.25}{0.125} = 2$ tablets

45. 250 mg : 1 cap :: 500 mg : x cap

    250 : 1 :: 500 : x

    $250x = 500$

    $x = \dfrac{500}{250}$

    $x = 2$ capsules

$\dfrac{500\text{ mg}}{250\text{ mg}} \times 1$ cap $=$

    $\dfrac{500}{250} = 2$ capsules

    2 cap : 1 dose :: x cap : 4 dose

    2 : 1 :: x : 4

    $x = 8$ capsules

46. 20 mg : 1 cap :: 40 mg : x cap

    20 : 1 :: 40 : x

    $20x = 40$

    $x = \dfrac{40}{20}$

    $x = 2$ capsules

$\dfrac{40\text{ mg}}{20\text{ mg}} \times 1$ cap $=$

    $\dfrac{40}{20} = 2$ capsules

	Proportion	Formula

47. 60 mg : 1 gr :: x mg : 1½ gr
60 : 1 :: x : 1½

$$x = \dfrac{\overset{30}{\cancel{60}}}{1} \times \dfrac{3}{\underset{1}{\cancel{2}}}$$

$x = 90$ mg

30 mg : 1 tab :: 90 mg : x tab
30 : 1 :: 90 : x
$30x = 90$

$$x = \frac{90}{30}$$

$x = 3$ tablets

$$\frac{90 \text{ mg}}{30 \text{ mg}} \times 1 \text{ tab} =$$

$$\frac{90}{30} = 3 \text{ tablets}$$

48. 75 mg : 1 tab :: 150 mg : x tab
75 : 1 :: 150 : x
$75x = 150$

$$x = \frac{150}{75}$$

$x = 2$ tablets

$$\frac{150 \text{ mg}}{75 \text{ mg}} \times 1 \text{ tab} =$$

$$\frac{150}{75} = 2 \text{ tablets}$$

49. 65 mg : 1 gr :: x mg : 10 gr
65 : 1 :: x : 10
$x = 650$ mg

325 mg : 1 tab :: 650 mg : x tab
325 : 1 :: 650 : x
$325x = 650$

$$x = \frac{650}{325}$$

$x = 2$ tablets

$$\frac{650 \text{ mg}}{325 \text{ mg}} \times 1 \text{ tab} =$$

$$\frac{650}{325} = 2 \text{ tablets}$$

50. 15 mg : 1 mL :: 150 mg : x mL
15 : 1 :: 150 : x
$15x = 150$

$$x = \frac{150}{15}$$

$x = 10$ mL

$$\frac{150 \text{ mg}}{15 \text{ mg}} \times 1 \text{ mL} =$$

$$\frac{\overset{10}{\cancel{150}}}{\underset{1}{\cancel{15}}} = 10 \text{ mL}$$

51. 250 mg : 1 tab :: 500 mg : x tab
250 : 1 :: 500 : x
$250x = 500$

$$x = \frac{500}{250}$$

$x = 2$ tablets

$$\frac{500 \text{ mg}}{250 \text{ mg}} \times 1 \text{ tab} =$$

$$\frac{500}{250} = 2 \text{ tablets}$$

Proportion	Formula

52. 60 mg : 1 gr :: x mg : 5 gr
60 : 1 :: x : 5
$x = 300$ mg
0.3 g = 300 mg

324 mg : 1 tab :: 300 mg : x tab
324 : 1 :: 300 : x
$324x = 300$
$x = \dfrac{300}{324} = 0.93$
$x = 1$ tablet

$\dfrac{300 \text{ mg}}{324 \text{ mg}} \times 1 \text{ tab} =$

$\dfrac{300}{324} = 0.93$; give 1 tablet

53. 10 mg : 1 cap :: 20 mg : x cap
10 : 1 :: 20 : x
$10x = 20$
$x = \dfrac{20}{10}$
$x = 2$ capsules

$\dfrac{20 \text{ mg}}{10 \text{ mg}} \times 1 \text{ cap} =$

$\dfrac{20}{10} = 2$ capsules

54. 10 mg : 5 mL :: 30 mg : x mL
10 : 5 :: 30 : x
$10x = 150$
$x = \dfrac{150}{10}$
$x = 15$ mL

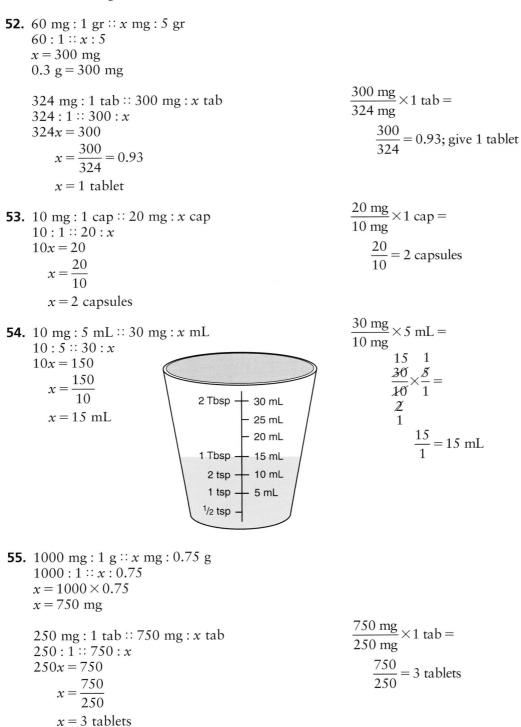

$\dfrac{30 \text{ mg}}{10 \text{ mg}} \times 5 \text{ mL} =$

$\dfrac{\overset{15}{\cancel{30}}}{\underset{2}{\cancel{10}}} \times \dfrac{\overset{1}{\cancel{5}}}{1} =$

$\dfrac{15}{1} = 15$ mL

55. 1000 mg : 1 g :: x mg : 0.75 g
1000 : 1 :: x : 0.75
$x = 1000 \times 0.75$
$x = 750$ mg

250 mg : 1 tab :: 750 mg : x tab
250 : 1 :: 750 : x
$250x = 750$
$x = \dfrac{750}{250}$
$x = 3$ tablets

$\dfrac{750 \text{ mg}}{250 \text{ mg}} \times 1 \text{ tab} =$

$\dfrac{750}{250} = 3$ tablets

Proportion	Formula

56. $4 \text{ mg} : 1 \text{ tab} :: 8 \text{ mg} : x \text{ tab}$
$4 : 1 :: 8 : x$
$4x = 8$
$x = \dfrac{8}{4}$
$x = 2 \text{ tablets}$

$\dfrac{8 \text{ mg}}{4 \text{ mg}} \times 1 \text{ tab} =$

$\dfrac{8}{4} = 2 \text{ tablets}$

57. $25 \text{ mg} : 5 \text{ mL} :: 15 \text{ mg} : x \text{ mL}$
$25 : 5 :: 15 : x$
$25x = 75$
$x = \dfrac{75}{25}$
$x = 3 \text{ mL}$

$\dfrac{15 \text{ mg}}{25 \text{ mg}} \times 5 \text{ mL} =$

$\dfrac{15}{\underset{5}{\cancel{25}}} \times \dfrac{\overset{1}{\cancel{5}}}{1} = \dfrac{15}{5}$

$\dfrac{15}{5} = 3 \text{ mL}$

58. $50 \text{ mg} : 1 \text{ tab} :: 100 \text{ mg} : x \text{ tab}$
$50 : 1 :: 100 : x$
$50x = 100$
$x = \dfrac{100}{50}$
$x = 2 \text{ tablets}$

$\dfrac{100 \text{ mg}}{50 \text{ mg}} \times 1 \text{ tab} =$

$\dfrac{\overset{2}{\cancel{100}}}{\underset{1}{\cancel{50}}} = \dfrac{2}{1}$

$\dfrac{2}{1} = 2 \text{ tablets}$

59. $500 \text{ mg} : 1 \text{ tab} :: 1000 \text{ mg} : x \text{ tab}$
$500 : 1 :: 1000 : x$
$500x = 1000$
$x = \dfrac{1000}{500}$
$x = 2 \text{ tablets}$

$\dfrac{1000 \text{ mg}}{500 \text{ mg}} \times 1 \text{ tab} =$

$\dfrac{1000}{500} = 2 \text{ tablets}$

60. $150 \text{ mg} : 5 \text{ mL} :: 250 \text{ mg} : x \text{ mL}$
$150 : 5 :: 250 : x$
$150x = 1250$
$x = \dfrac{1250}{150}$
$x = 8.33 \text{ mL}$

$\dfrac{250 \text{ mg}}{150 \text{ mg}} \times 5 \text{ mL} =$

$\dfrac{250}{\underset{30}{\cancel{150}}} \times \dfrac{\overset{1}{\cancel{5}}}{1} = \dfrac{250}{30}$

$\dfrac{250}{30} = 8.33 \text{ mL}$

Proportion	Formula

61. $50 \text{ mg} : 5 \text{ mL} :: 100 \text{ mg} : x \text{ mL}$
$50 : 5 :: 100 : x$
$50x = 500$
$x = \dfrac{500}{50}$
$x = 10 \text{ mL}$

$$\dfrac{100 \text{ mg}}{50 \text{ mg}} \times 5 \text{ mL} =$$

$$\dfrac{100}{\cancel{50}_{10}} \times \dfrac{\cancel{5}^{1}}{1} =$$

$$\dfrac{100}{10} = 10 \text{ mL}$$

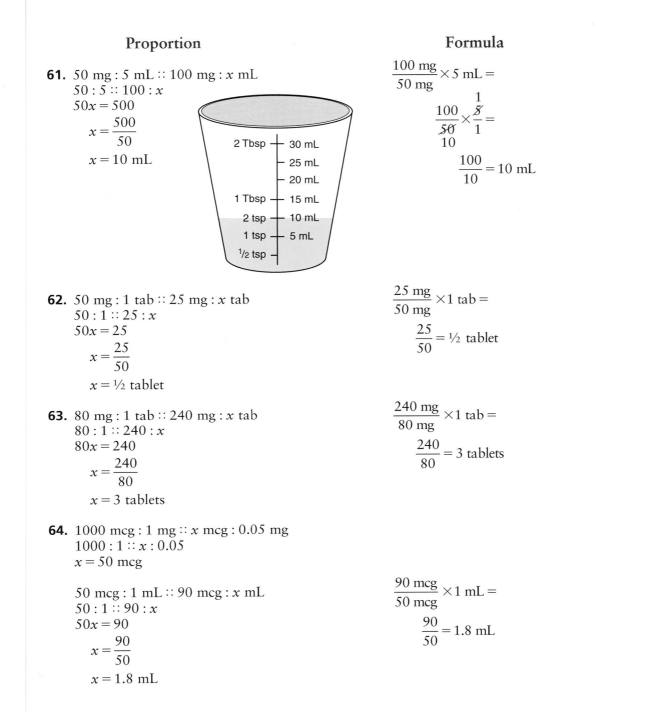

62. $50 \text{ mg} : 1 \text{ tab} :: 25 \text{ mg} : x \text{ tab}$
$50 : 1 :: 25 : x$
$50x = 25$
$x = \dfrac{25}{50}$
$x = \text{½ tablet}$

$$\dfrac{25 \text{ mg}}{50 \text{ mg}} \times 1 \text{ tab} =$$

$$\dfrac{25}{50} = \text{½ tablet}$$

63. $80 \text{ mg} : 1 \text{ tab} :: 240 \text{ mg} : x \text{ tab}$
$80 : 1 :: 240 : x$
$80x = 240$
$x = \dfrac{240}{80}$
$x = 3 \text{ tablets}$

$$\dfrac{240 \text{ mg}}{80 \text{ mg}} \times 1 \text{ tab} =$$

$$\dfrac{240}{80} = 3 \text{ tablets}$$

64. $1000 \text{ mcg} : 1 \text{ mg} :: x \text{ mcg} : 0.05 \text{ mg}$
$1000 : 1 :: x : 0.05$
$x = 50 \text{ mcg}$

$50 \text{ mcg} : 1 \text{ mL} :: 90 \text{ mcg} : x \text{ mL}$
$50 : 1 :: 90 : x$
$50x = 90$
$x = \dfrac{90}{50}$
$x = 1.8 \text{ mL}$

$$\dfrac{90 \text{ mcg}}{50 \text{ mcg}} \times 1 \text{ mL} =$$

$$\dfrac{90}{50} = 1.8 \text{ mL}$$

Proportion

65. $12.5 \text{ mg} : 5 \text{ mL} :: x \text{ mg} : 10 \text{ mL}$

$12.5 : 5 :: x : 10$

$5x = 125$

$x = \dfrac{125}{5}$

$x = 25 \text{ mg}$

66. $25 \text{ mg} : 1 \text{ cap} :: 50 \text{ mg} : x \text{ cap}$

$25 : 1 :: 50 : x$

$25x = 50$

$x = \dfrac{50}{25}$

$x = 2 \text{ capsules}$

67. $60 \text{ mg} : 1 \text{ gr} :: x \text{ mg} : 1.5 \text{ gr}$

$60 : 1 :: x : 1.5$

$x = 90 \text{ mg}$

$30 \text{ mg} : 1 \text{ cap} :: 90 \text{ mg} : x \text{ cap}$

$30 : 1 :: 90 : x$

$30x = 90$

$x = \dfrac{90}{30}$

$x = 3 \text{ capsules}$

68. $40 \text{ mg} : 1 \text{ tab} :: 40 \text{ mg} : x \text{ tab}$

$40 : 1 :: 40 : x$

$40x = 40$

$x = \dfrac{40}{40}$

$x = 1 \text{ tablet}$

Formula

$\dfrac{x \text{ mg}}{12.5 \text{ mg}} \times 5 \text{ mL} = 10 \text{ mL}$

$\dfrac{x}{12.5} \times \dfrac{5}{1} = 10$

$\dfrac{\cancel{12.5}^{\,1}}{1} \times \dfrac{x}{\cancel{12.5}_{\,1}} \times \dfrac{5}{1} = \dfrac{10}{1} \times 12.5$

$5x = 125$

$x = \dfrac{125}{5}$

$x = 25 \text{ mg}$

$\dfrac{50 \text{ mg}}{25 \text{ mg}} \times 1 \text{ cap} =$

$\dfrac{50}{25} = 2 \text{ capsules}$

$\dfrac{90 \text{ mg}}{30 \text{ mg}} \times 1 \text{ cap} =$

$\dfrac{90}{30} = 3 \text{ capsules}$

The other strengths of the medication would require swallowing more pills.

Proportion

Formula

69. 20 mEq : 15 mL :: 10 mEq : x mL

20 : 15 :: 10 : x

20x = 150

$x = \dfrac{150}{20}$

$x = 7.5$ mL

$\dfrac{10 \text{ mEq}}{20 \text{ mEq}} \times \dfrac{15 \text{mL}}{1} =$

$\dfrac{10}{\overset{}{\underset{4}{20}}} \times \dfrac{\overset{3}{15}}{1} = \dfrac{30}{4}$

$\dfrac{30}{4} = 7.5$ mL

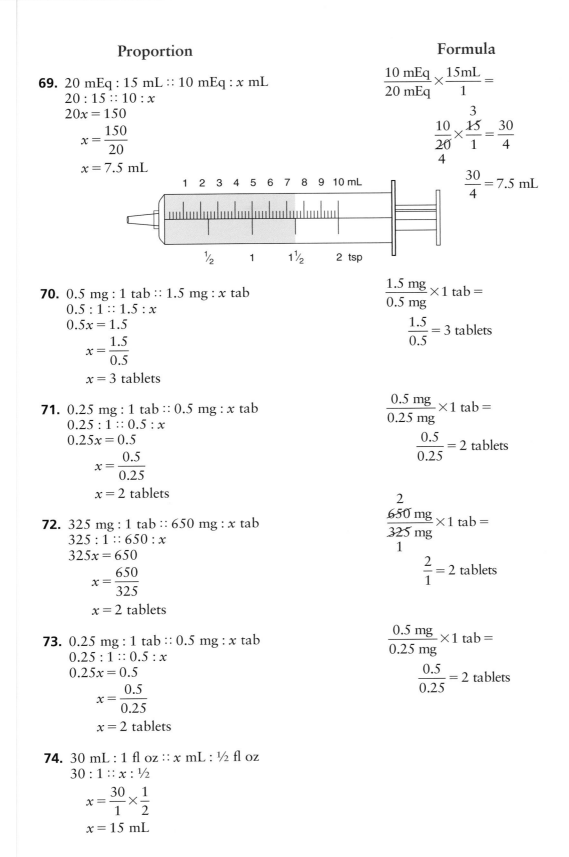

1 2 3 4 5 6 7 8 9 10 mL

½   1   1½   2 tsp

70. 0.5 mg : 1 tab :: 1.5 mg : x tab

0.5 : 1 :: 1.5 : x

0.5x = 1.5

$x = \dfrac{1.5}{0.5}$

$x = 3$ tablets

$\dfrac{1.5 \text{ mg}}{0.5 \text{ mg}} \times 1 \text{ tab} =$

$\dfrac{1.5}{0.5} = 3$ tablets

71. 0.25 mg : 1 tab :: 0.5 mg : x tab

0.25 : 1 :: 0.5 : x

0.25x = 0.5

$x = \dfrac{0.5}{0.25}$

$x = 2$ tablets

$\dfrac{0.5 \text{ mg}}{0.25 \text{ mg}} \times 1 \text{ tab} =$

$\dfrac{0.5}{0.25} = 2$ tablets

72. 325 mg : 1 tab :: 650 mg : x tab

325 : 1 :: 650 : x

325x = 650

$x = \dfrac{650}{325}$

$x = 2$ tablets

$\dfrac{\overset{2}{650} \text{ mg}}{\underset{1}{325} \text{ mg}} \times 1 \text{ tab} =$

$\dfrac{2}{1} = 2$ tablets

73. 0.25 mg : 1 tab :: 0.5 mg : x tab

0.25 : 1 :: 0.5 : x

0.25x = 0.5

$x = \dfrac{0.5}{0.25}$

$x = 2$ tablets

$\dfrac{0.5 \text{ mg}}{0.25 \text{ mg}} \times 1 \text{ tab} =$

$\dfrac{0.5}{0.25} = 2$ tablets

74. 30 mL : 1 fl oz :: x mL : ½ fl oz

30 : 1 :: x : ½

$x = \dfrac{30}{1} \times \dfrac{1}{2}$

$x = 15$ mL

Proportion

Formula

75. $50 \text{ mg} : 5 \text{ mL} :: 30 \text{ mg} : x \text{ mL}$
$50 : 5 :: 30 : x$
$50x = 150$
$x = \dfrac{150}{50}$
$x = 3 \text{ mL}$

$$\dfrac{30 \text{ mg}}{50 \text{ mg}} \times 5 \text{ mL} =$$

$$\dfrac{30}{\cancel{50}} \times \dfrac{\cancel{5}^{\,1}}{1} = \dfrac{30}{10}$$
$$\dfrac{30}{10} = 3 \text{ mL}$$

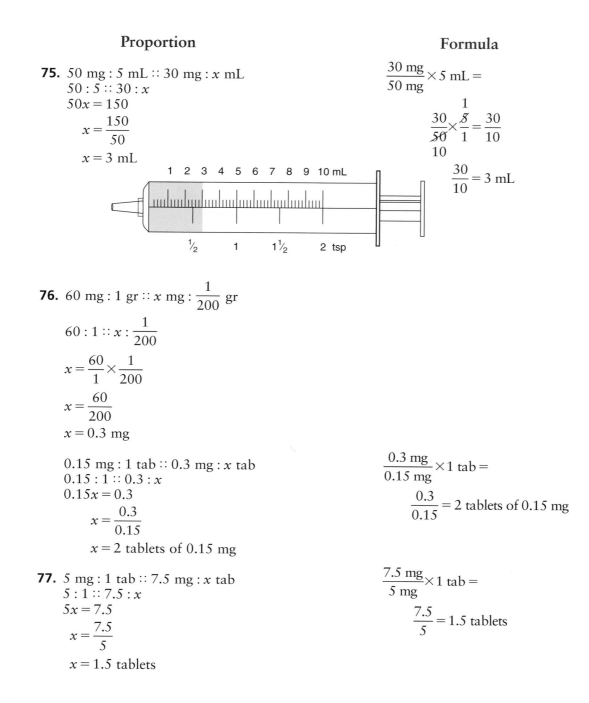

76. $60 \text{ mg} : 1 \text{ gr} :: x \text{ mg} : \dfrac{1}{200} \text{ gr}$

$60 : 1 :: x : \dfrac{1}{200}$

$x = \dfrac{60}{1} \times \dfrac{1}{200}$

$x = \dfrac{60}{200}$

$x = 0.3 \text{ mg}$

$0.15 \text{ mg} : 1 \text{ tab} :: 0.3 \text{ mg} : x \text{ tab}$
$0.15 : 1 :: 0.3 : x$
$0.15x = 0.3$
$x = \dfrac{0.3}{0.15}$
$x = 2 \text{ tablets of } 0.15 \text{ mg}$

$$\dfrac{0.3 \text{ mg}}{0.15 \text{ mg}} \times 1 \text{ tab} =$$

$$\dfrac{0.3}{0.15} = 2 \text{ tablets of } 0.15 \text{ mg}$$

77. $5 \text{ mg} : 1 \text{ tab} :: 7.5 \text{ mg} : x \text{ tab}$
$5 : 1 :: 7.5 : x$
$5x = 7.5$
$x = \dfrac{7.5}{5}$
$x = 1.5 \text{ tablets}$

$$\dfrac{7.5 \text{ mg}}{5 \text{ mg}} \times 1 \text{ tab} =$$

$$\dfrac{7.5}{5} = 1.5 \text{ tablets}$$

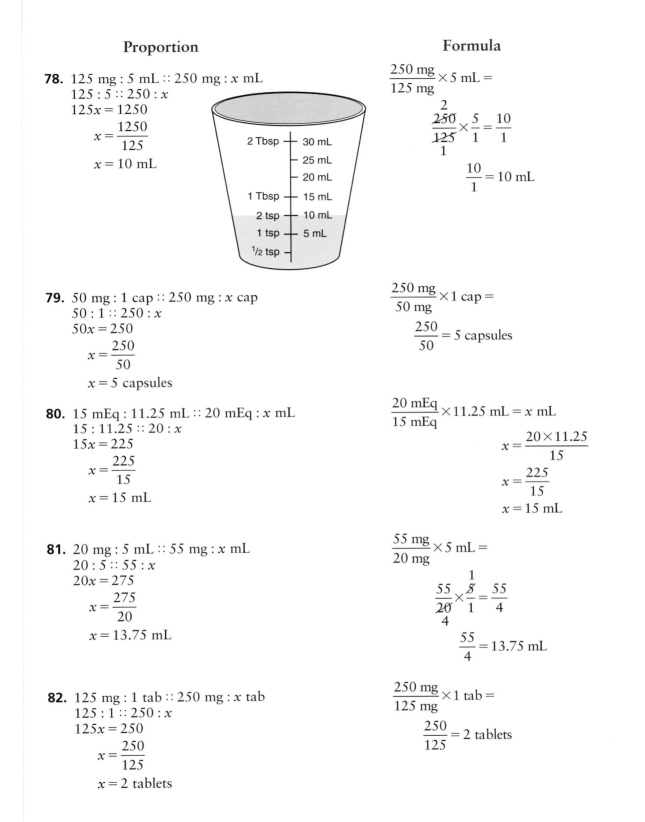

Proportion

Formula

78. 125 mg : 5 mL :: 250 mg : x mL
125 : 5 :: 250 : x
$125x = 1250$
$x = \dfrac{1250}{125}$
$x = 10$ mL

$\dfrac{250 \text{ mg}}{125 \text{ mg}} \times 5 \text{ mL} =$

$\dfrac{\overset{2}{\cancel{250}}}{\underset{1}{\cancel{125}}} \times \dfrac{5}{1} = \dfrac{10}{1}$

$\dfrac{10}{1} = 10$ mL

2 Tbsp — 30 mL
— 25 mL
— 20 mL
1 Tbsp — 15 mL
2 tsp — 10 mL
1 tsp — 5 mL
1/2 tsp —

79. 50 mg : 1 cap :: 250 mg : x cap
50 : 1 :: 250 : x
$50x = 250$
$x = \dfrac{250}{50}$
$x = 5$ capsules

$\dfrac{250 \text{ mg}}{50 \text{ mg}} \times 1 \text{ cap} =$

$\dfrac{250}{50} = 5$ capsules

80. 15 mEq : 11.25 mL :: 20 mEq : x mL
15 : 11.25 :: 20 : x
$15x = 225$
$x = \dfrac{225}{15}$
$x = 15$ mL

$\dfrac{20 \text{ mEq}}{15 \text{ mEq}} \times 11.25 \text{ mL} = x \text{ mL}$

$x = \dfrac{20 \times 11.25}{15}$

$x = \dfrac{225}{15}$

$x = 15$ mL

81. 20 mg : 5 mL :: 55 mg : x mL
20 : 5 :: 55 : x
$20x = 275$
$x = \dfrac{275}{20}$
$x = 13.75$ mL

$\dfrac{55 \text{ mg}}{20 \text{ mg}} \times 5 \text{ mL} =$

$\dfrac{55}{\underset{4}{\cancel{20}}} \times \dfrac{\overset{1}{\cancel{5}}}{1} = \dfrac{55}{4}$

$\dfrac{55}{4} = 13.75$ mL

82. 125 mg : 1 tab :: 250 mg : x tab
125 : 1 :: 250 : x
$125x = 250$
$x = \dfrac{250}{125}$
$x = 2$ tablets

$\dfrac{250 \text{ mg}}{125 \text{ mg}} \times 1 \text{ tab} =$

$\dfrac{250}{125} = 2$ tablets

Proportion	Formula

83. $0.05 \text{ mg} : 1 \text{ tab} :: 0.05 \text{ mg} : x \text{ tab}$
$0.05 : 1 :: 0.05 : x$
$0.05x = 0.05$
$x = \dfrac{0.05}{0.05}$
$x = 1 \text{ tablet}$

$\dfrac{0.05 \text{ mg}}{0.05 \text{ mg}} \times 1 \text{ tab} =$
$\dfrac{0.05}{0.05} = 1 \text{ tablet}$

84. $1000 \text{ mg} : 1 \text{ g} :: x \text{ mg} : 0.2 \text{ g}$
$1000 : 1 :: x : 0.2$
$x = 200 \text{ mg}$
Give 1 tablet of 200 mg

$200 \text{ mg} : 1 \text{ dose} :: x \text{ mg} : 3 \text{ doses}$
$x = 600 \text{ mg}$ will be given per day

$\dfrac{200 \text{ mg}}{200 \text{ mg}} \times 1 \text{ tab} =$
$\dfrac{200}{200} = 1 \text{ tablet}$

85. $5 \text{ mg} : 1 \text{ tab} :: 15 \text{ mg} : x \text{ tab}$
$5 : 1 :: 15 : x$
$5x = 15$
$x = \dfrac{15}{5}$
$x = 3 \text{ tablets}$

$\dfrac{15 \text{ mg}}{5 \text{ mg}} \times 1 \text{ tab} =$
$\dfrac{15}{5} = 3 \text{ tablets}$

86. $400 \text{ mg} : 1 \text{ tab} :: 800 \text{ mg} : x \text{ tab}$
$400 : 1 :: 800 : x$
$400x = 800$
$x = \dfrac{800}{400}$
$x = 2 \text{ tablets}$

$\dfrac{800 \text{ mg}}{400 \text{ mg}} \times 1 \text{ tab} =$
$\dfrac{800}{400} = 2 \text{ tablets}$

87. $15 \text{ mg} : 1 \text{ cap} :: 30 \text{ mg} : x \text{ cap}$
$15 : 1 :: 30 : x$
$15x = 30$
$x = \dfrac{30}{15}$
$x = 2 \text{ capsules}$

$\dfrac{30 \text{ mg}}{15 \text{ mg}} \times 1 \text{ cap} =$
$\dfrac{30}{15} = 2 \text{ capsules}$

88. $25 \text{ mg} : 1 \text{ tab} :: 50 \text{ mg} : x \text{ tab}$
$25 : 1 :: 50 : x$
$25x = 50$
$x = \dfrac{50}{25}$
$x = 2 \text{ tablets}$

$\dfrac{50 \text{ mg}}{25 \text{ mg}} \times 1 \text{ tab} =$
$\dfrac{50}{25} = 2 \text{ tablets}$

89. $10 \text{ mg} : 1 \text{ tab} :: 30 \text{ mg} : x \text{ tab}$
$10 : 1 :: 30 : x$
$10x = 30$
$x = \dfrac{30}{10}$
$x = 3 \text{ tablets}$

$\dfrac{30 \text{ mg}}{10 \text{ mg}} \times 1 \text{ tab} =$
$\dfrac{30}{10} = 3 \text{ tablets}$

	Proportion	Formula

Proportion

90. 10 mg : 1 mL : 6 mg : x mL
10 : 1 :: 6 : x
$10x = 6$
$x = \dfrac{6}{10}$
$x = 0.6$ mL

91. 75 mg : 1 cap :: 150 mg : x cap
75 : 1 :: 150 : x
$75x = 150$
$x = \dfrac{150}{75}$
$x = 2$ capsules

92. 100 mg : 1 cap :: 200 mg : x cap
100 : 1 :: 200 : x
$100x = 200$
$x = \dfrac{200}{100}$
$x = 2$ capsules

93. 2.5 mg : 1 tab :: 10 mg : x tab
2.5 : 1 :: 10 : x
$2.5x = 10$
$x = \dfrac{10}{2.5}$
$x = 4$ tablets

94. 1000 mg : 1 g :: x mg : 0.25 g
1000 : 1 :: x : 0.25
$x = 250$ mg

250 mg : 1 tab :: 250 mg : x tab
250 : 1 :: 250 : x
$250x = 250$
$x = 1$ tablet

Formula

$\dfrac{6 \text{ mg}}{10 \text{ mg}} \times 1 \text{ mL} =$
$x = \dfrac{6}{10}$
$x = 0.06$ mL

$\dfrac{150 \text{ mg}}{75 \text{ mg}} \times 1 \text{ cap} =$
$\dfrac{150}{75} = 2$ capsules

$\dfrac{200 \text{ mg}}{100 \text{ mg}} \times 1 \text{ cap} =$
$\dfrac{200}{100} = 2$ capsules

$\dfrac{10 \text{ mg}}{2.5 \text{ mg}} \times 1 \text{ tab} =$
$\dfrac{10}{2.5} = 4$ tablets

$\dfrac{250 \text{ mg}}{250 \text{ mg}} \times 1 \text{ tab} =$
$\dfrac{250}{250} = 1$ tablet

	Proportion	Formula

95. 60 mg : 1 gr :: x mg : ⅙ gr
60 : 1 :: x : ⅙

$$x = \frac{\overset{10}{\cancel{60}}}{1} \times \frac{1}{\underset{1}{\cancel{6}}}$$

$x = 10$ mg

10 mg : 1 tab :: 25 mg : x tab
10 : 1 :: 25 : x
$10x = 25$

$$x = \frac{25}{10}$$

$x = 2.5$ tablets

$$\frac{25 \text{ mg}}{10 \text{ mg}} \times 1 \text{ tab} =$$

$$\frac{25}{10} = 2.5 \text{ tablets}$$

96. 10 mg : 1 tab :: 30 mg : x tab
10 : 1 :: 30 : x
$10x = 30$

$$x = \frac{30}{10}$$

$x = 3$ tablets

$$\frac{30 \text{ mg}}{10 \text{ mg}} \times 1 \text{ tab} =$$

$$\frac{\overset{3}{\cancel{30}}}{\underset{1}{\cancel{10}}} = 3 \text{ tablets}$$

97. 5 mg : 1 tab :: 15 mg : x tab
5 : 1 :: 15 : x
$5x = 15$

$$x = \frac{15}{5}$$

$x = 3$ tablets

$$\frac{15 \text{ mg}}{5 \text{ mg}} \times 1 \text{ tab} =$$

$$\frac{15}{5} = 3 \text{ tablets}$$

98. 1000 mg : 1 g :: x mg : 0.015 g
1000 : 1 :: x : 0.015
$x = 15$ mg

15 mg : 1 cap :: 15 mg : x cap
15 : 1 :: 15 : x
$15x = 15$

$$x = \frac{15}{15}$$

$x = 1$ capsule

$$\frac{15 \text{ mg}}{15 \text{ mg}} \times 1 \text{ cap} =$$

$$\frac{15}{15} = 1 \text{ capsule}$$

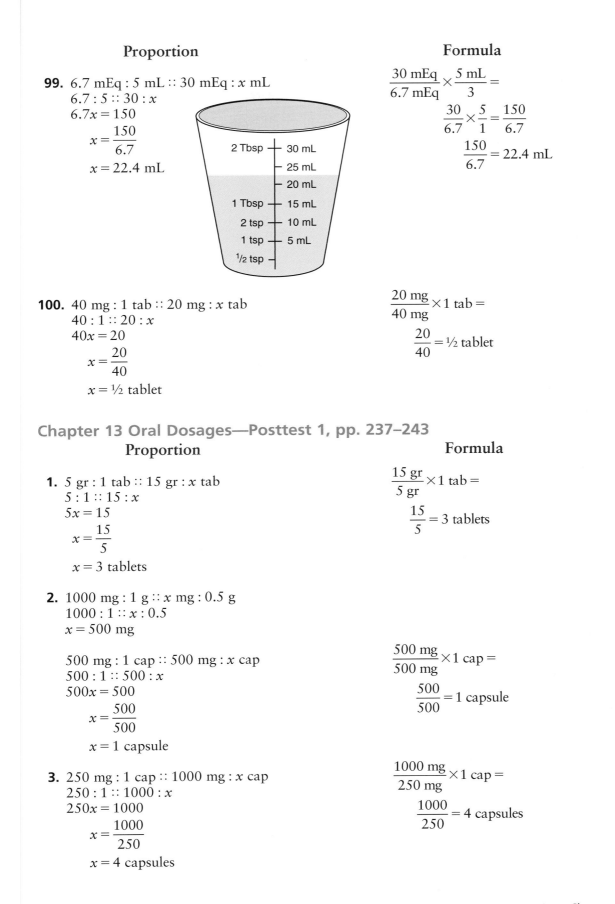

Proportion

99. 6.7 mEq : 5 mL :: 30 mEq : x mL
6.7 : 5 :: 30 : x
6.7x = 150
$x = \dfrac{150}{6.7}$
x = 22.4 mL

Formula

$\dfrac{30\text{ mEq}}{6.7\text{ mEq}} \times \dfrac{5\text{ mL}}{3} =$

$\dfrac{30}{6.7} \times \dfrac{5}{1} = \dfrac{150}{6.7}$

$\dfrac{150}{6.7} = 22.4$ mL

2 Tbsp — 30 mL
— 25 mL
— 20 mL
1 Tbsp — 15 mL
2 tsp — 10 mL
1 tsp — 5 mL
½ tsp

100. 40 mg : 1 tab :: 20 mg : x tab
40 : 1 :: 20 : x
40x = 20
$x = \dfrac{20}{40}$
x = ½ tablet

$\dfrac{20\text{ mg}}{40\text{ mg}} \times 1$ tab =

$\dfrac{20}{40} = ½$ tablet

Chapter 13 Oral Dosages—Posttest 1, pp. 237–243

Proportion

1. 5 gr : 1 tab :: 15 gr : x tab
5 : 1 :: 15 : x
5x = 15
$x = \dfrac{15}{5}$
x = 3 tablets

Formula

$\dfrac{15\text{ gr}}{5\text{ gr}} \times 1$ tab =

$\dfrac{15}{5} = 3$ tablets

2. 1000 mg : 1 g :: x mg : 0.5 g
1000 : 1 :: x : 0.5
x = 500 mg

500 mg : 1 cap :: 500 mg : x cap
500 : 1 :: 500 : x
500x = 500
$x = \dfrac{500}{500}$
x = 1 capsule

$\dfrac{500\text{ mg}}{500\text{ mg}} \times 1$ cap =

$\dfrac{500}{500} = 1$ capsule

3. 250 mg : 1 cap :: 1000 mg : x cap
250 : 1 :: 1000 : x
250x = 1000
$x = \dfrac{1000}{250}$
x = 4 capsules

$\dfrac{1000\text{ mg}}{250\text{ mg}} \times 1$ cap =

$\dfrac{1000}{250} = 4$ capsules

Proportion	Formula

4. $30 \text{ mg} : 1 \text{ tab} :: 60 \text{ mg} : x \text{ tab}$
$30 : 1 :: 60 : x$
$30x = 60$
$$x = \dfrac{\overset{2}{\cancel{60}}}{\underset{1}{\cancel{30}}}$$
$x = 2 \text{ tablets}$

$$\dfrac{60 \text{ mg}}{30 \text{ mg}} \times 1 \text{ tab} =$$
$$\dfrac{\overset{2}{\cancel{60}}}{\underset{1}{\cancel{30}}} = 2 \text{ tablets}$$

5. $100 \text{ mcg} = 0.1 \text{ mg}$
$0.05 \text{ mg} : 1 \text{ tab} :: 0.1 : x \text{ tab}$
$0.05 : 1 :: 0.1 : x$
$0.05x = 0.1$
$$x = \dfrac{0.1}{0.05}$$
$x = 2 \text{ tablets}$

$$\dfrac{0.1 \text{ mg}}{0.05 \text{ mg}} \times 1 \text{ tab} =$$
$$\dfrac{0.1}{0.05} = 2 \text{ tablets}$$

6. $10 \text{ mg} : 5 \text{ mL} :: 25 \text{ mg} : x \text{ mL}$
$10 : 5 :: 25 : x$
$10x = 125$
$$x = \dfrac{125}{10}$$
$x = 12.5 \text{ mL}$

$$\dfrac{25 \text{ mg}}{10 \text{ mg}} \times 5 \text{ mL} =$$
$$\dfrac{25}{\underset{2}{\cancel{10}}} \times \dfrac{\overset{1}{\cancel{5}}}{1} = \dfrac{25}{2}$$
$$\dfrac{25}{2} = 12.5 \text{ mL}$$

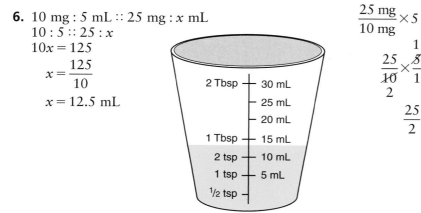

7. $120 \text{ mg} : 1 \text{ tab} :: 60 \text{ mg} : x \text{ tab}$
$120 : 1 :: 60 : x$
$120x = 60$
$$x = \dfrac{60}{120}$$
$x = \frac{1}{2} \text{ tablet}$

$$\dfrac{60 \text{ mg}}{120 \text{ mg}} \times 1 \text{ tab} =$$
$$\dfrac{\overset{1}{\cancel{60}}}{\underset{2}{\cancel{120}}} = \frac{1}{2} \text{ tablet}$$

8. $30 \text{ mg} : 1 \text{ tab} :: 30 \text{ mg} : x \text{ tab}$
$30 : 1 :: 30 : x$
$30x = 30$
$$x = \dfrac{30}{30}$$
$x = 1 \text{ tablet}$

$$\dfrac{30 \text{ mg}}{30 \text{ mg}} \times 1 \text{ tab} =$$
$$\dfrac{30}{30} = 1 \text{ tablet}$$

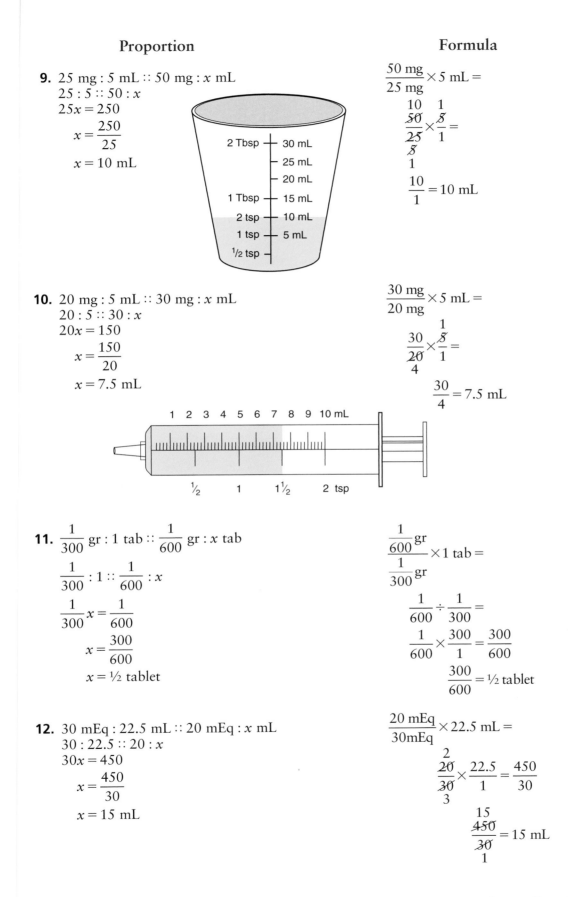

Proportion

9. 25 mg : 5 mL :: 50 mg : x mL

25 : 5 :: 50 : x

$25x = 250$

$x = \dfrac{250}{25}$

$x = 10$ mL

10. 20 mg : 5 mL :: 30 mg : x mL

20 : 5 :: 30 : x

$20x = 150$

$x = \dfrac{150}{20}$

$x = 7.5$ mL

11. $\dfrac{1}{300}$ gr : 1 tab :: $\dfrac{1}{600}$ gr : x tab

$\dfrac{1}{300}$: 1 :: $\dfrac{1}{600}$: x

$\dfrac{1}{300}x = \dfrac{1}{600}$

$x = \dfrac{300}{600}$

$x = \frac{1}{2}$ tablet

12. 30 mEq : 22.5 mL :: 20 mEq : x mL

30 : 22.5 :: 20 : x

$30x = 450$

$x = \dfrac{450}{30}$

$x = 15$ mL

Formula

$\dfrac{50 \text{ mg}}{25 \text{ mg}} \times 5 \text{ mL} =$

$\dfrac{\overset{10}{\cancel{50}}}{\underset{5}{\cancel{25}}} \times \dfrac{\overset{1}{\cancel{5}}}{1} =$

$\dfrac{10}{1} = 10$ mL

$\dfrac{30 \text{ mg}}{20 \text{ mg}} \times 5 \text{ mL} =$

$\dfrac{30}{\underset{4}{\cancel{20}}} \times \dfrac{\overset{1}{\cancel{5}}}{1} =$

$\dfrac{30}{4} = 7.5$ mL

$\dfrac{\dfrac{1}{600} \text{ gr}}{\dfrac{1}{300} \text{ gr}} \times 1 \text{ tab} =$

$\dfrac{1}{600} \div \dfrac{1}{300} =$

$\dfrac{1}{600} \times \dfrac{300}{1} = \dfrac{300}{600}$

$\dfrac{300}{600} = \frac{1}{2}$ tablet

$\dfrac{20 \text{ mEq}}{30 \text{mEq}} \times 22.5 \text{ mL} =$

$\dfrac{\overset{2}{\cancel{20}}}{\underset{3}{\cancel{30}}} \times \dfrac{22.5}{1} = \dfrac{450}{30}$

$\dfrac{\overset{15}{\cancel{450}}}{\underset{1}{\cancel{30}}} = 15$ mL

Proportion	Formula

13. 20 mg : 1 tab :: 40 mg : x tab

20 : 1 :: 40 : x

20x = 40

$x = \dfrac{40}{20}$

x = 2 tablets

$\dfrac{40 \text{ mg}}{20 \text{ mg}} \times 1 \text{ tab} =$

$\dfrac{40}{20} = 2 \text{ tablets}$

14. 50 mg : 1 cap :: 100 mg : x cap

50 : 1 :: 100 : x

50x = 100

$x = \dfrac{100}{50}$

x = 2 capsules

$\dfrac{100 \text{ mg}}{50 \text{ mg}} \times 1 \text{ cap} =$

$\dfrac{100}{50} = 2 \text{ capsules}$

15. 10 mg : 1 mL :: 38 mg : x mL

10 : 1 :: 38 : x

10x = 38

$x = \dfrac{38}{10}$

x = 3.8 mL

$\dfrac{38 \text{ mg}}{10 \text{ mg}} \times 1 \text{ mL} =$

$\dfrac{38}{10} = 3.8 \text{ mL}$

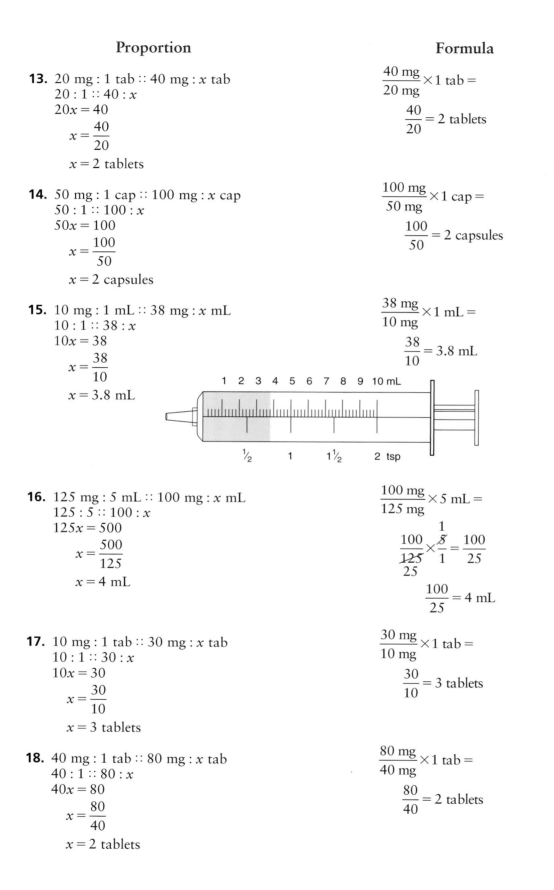

16. 125 mg : 5 mL :: 100 mg : x mL

125 : 5 :: 100 : x

125x = 500

$x = \dfrac{500}{125}$

x = 4 mL

$\dfrac{100 \text{ mg}}{125 \text{ mg}} \times 5 \text{ mL} =$

$\dfrac{100}{\underset{25}{\cancel{125}}} \times \dfrac{\overset{1}{\cancel{5}}}{1} = \dfrac{100}{25}$

$\dfrac{100}{25} = 4 \text{ mL}$

17. 10 mg : 1 tab :: 30 mg : x tab

10 : 1 :: 30 : x

10x = 30

$x = \dfrac{30}{10}$

x = 3 tablets

$\dfrac{30 \text{ mg}}{10 \text{ mg}} \times 1 \text{ tab} =$

$\dfrac{30}{10} = 3 \text{ tablets}$

18. 40 mg : 1 tab :: 80 mg : x tab

40 : 1 :: 80 : x

40x = 80

$x = \dfrac{80}{40}$

x = 2 tablets

$\dfrac{80 \text{ mg}}{40 \text{ mg}} \times 1 \text{ tab} =$

$\dfrac{80}{40} = 2 \text{ tablets}$

Proportion	Formula

19. 10 mg : 1 tab :: 20 mg : x tab
10 : 1 :: 20 : x
$10x = 20$
$x = \dfrac{20}{10}$
$x = 2$ tablets

$\dfrac{20 \text{ mg}}{10 \text{ mg}} \times 1 \text{ tab} =$
$\dfrac{20}{10} = 2$ tablets

20. 60 mg : 1 gr :: x mg : 1½ gr
60 : 1 :: x : ³⁄₂
$x = \dfrac{\overset{30}{\cancel{60}}}{1} \times \dfrac{3}{\underset{1}{\cancel{2}}}$
$x = 90$ mg

60 mg : 1 tab :: 90 mg : x tab
60 : 1 :: 90 : x
$60x = 90$
$x = \dfrac{90}{60}$
$x = 1½$ tablets per dose

$\dfrac{90 \text{ mg}}{60 \text{ mg}} \times 1 \text{ tab} =$
$\dfrac{90}{60} = 1½$ tablets per dose

1½ tab : 1 dose :: x tab : 3 doses
³⁄₂ : 1 :: x : 3
$x = \dfrac{3}{2} \times \dfrac{3}{1}$
$x = \dfrac{9}{2}$
$x = 4½$ tablets/day

21. 0.25 mg : 1 tab :: 0.5 mg : x tab
0.25 : 1 :: 0.5 : x
$0.25x = 0.5$
$x = \dfrac{0.5}{0.25}$
$x = 2$ tablets

$\dfrac{0.5 \text{ mg}}{0.25 \text{ mg}} \times 1 \text{ tab} =$
$\dfrac{0.5}{0.25} = 2$ tablets

22. 5 mg : 1 tab :: 10 mg : x tab
5 : 1 :: 10 : x
$5x = 10$
$x = \dfrac{10}{5}$
$x = 2$ tablets

$\dfrac{10 \text{ mg}}{5 \text{ mg}} \times 1 \text{ tab} =$
$\dfrac{10}{5} = 2$ tablets

Proportion	Formula

23. $100 \text{ mg} : 1 \text{ tab} :: 150 \text{ mg} : x \text{ tab}$
$100 : 1 :: 150 : x$
$100x = 150$
$x = \dfrac{150}{100}$
$x = 1\frac{1}{2} \text{ tablets}$

$\dfrac{150 \text{ mg}}{100 \text{ mg}} \times 1 \text{ tab} =$
$\dfrac{150}{100} = 1\frac{1}{2} \text{ tablets}$

24. $10 \text{ mg} : 1 \text{ tab} :: 30 \text{ mg} : x \text{ tab}$
$10 : 1 :: 30 : x$
$10x = 30$
$x = \dfrac{30}{10}$
$x = 3 \text{ tablets}$

$\dfrac{30 \text{ mg}}{10 \text{ mg}} \times 1 \text{ tab} =$
$\dfrac{30}{10} = 3 \text{ tablets}$

25. $30 \text{ mg} : 1 \text{ tab} :: 60 \text{ mg} : x \text{ tab}$
$30 : 1 :: 60 : x$
$30x = 60$
$x = \dfrac{60}{30}$
$x = 2 \text{ tablets}$

$\dfrac{60 \text{ mg}}{30 \text{ mg}} \times 1 \text{ tab} =$
$\dfrac{60}{30} = 2 \text{ tablets}$

Chapter 13 Oral Dosages—Posttest 2, pp. 245–253

Proportion	Formula

1. $10 \text{ mg} : 1 \text{ cap} :: 20 \text{ mg} : x \text{ cap}$
$10 : 1 :: 20 : x$
$10x = 20$
$x = \dfrac{20}{10}$
$x = 2 \text{ capsules}$

$\dfrac{20 \text{ mg}}{10 \text{ mg}} \times 1 \text{ cap} =$
$\dfrac{20}{10} = 2 \text{ capsules}$

2. $4 \text{ mg} : 5 \text{ mL} :: 8 \text{ mg} : x \text{ mL}$
$4 : 5 :: 8 : x$
$4x = 40$
$x = \dfrac{40}{4}$
$x = 10 \text{ mL}$

$\dfrac{8 \text{ mg}}{4 \text{ mg}} \times 5 \text{ mL} =$
$\dfrac{\overset{2}{\cancel{8}}}{\underset{1}{\cancel{4}}} \times \dfrac{5}{1} = \dfrac{10}{1} = 10 \text{ mL}$

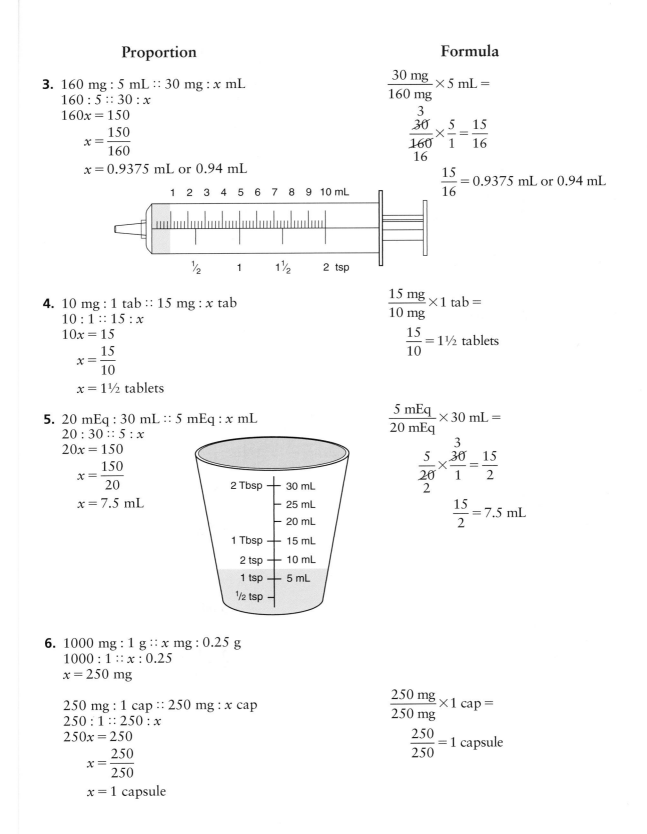

Proportion

3. 160 mg : 5 mL :: 30 mg : x mL
160 : 5 :: 30 : x
$160x = 150$
$x = \dfrac{150}{160}$
$x = 0.9375$ mL or 0.94 mL

4. 10 mg : 1 tab :: 15 mg : x tab
10 : 1 :: 15 : x
$10x = 15$
$x = \dfrac{15}{10}$
$x = 1\frac{1}{2}$ tablets

5. 20 mEq : 30 mL :: 5 mEq : x mL
20 : 30 :: 5 : x
$20x = 150$
$x = \dfrac{150}{20}$
$x = 7.5$ mL

6. 1000 mg : 1 g :: x mg : 0.25 g
1000 : 1 :: x : 0.25
$x = 250$ mg

250 mg : 1 cap :: 250 mg : x cap
250 : 1 :: 250 : x
$250x = 250$
$x = \dfrac{250}{250}$
$x = 1$ capsule

Formula

$\dfrac{30 \text{ mg}}{160 \text{ mg}} \times 5 \text{ mL} =$

$\dfrac{\overset{3}{\cancel{30}}}{\underset{16}{\cancel{160}}} \times \dfrac{5}{1} = \dfrac{15}{16}$

$\dfrac{15}{16} = 0.9375$ mL or 0.94 mL

$\dfrac{15 \text{ mg}}{10 \text{ mg}} \times 1 \text{ tab} =$

$\dfrac{15}{10} = 1\frac{1}{2}$ tablets

$\dfrac{5 \text{ mEq}}{20 \text{ mEq}} \times 30 \text{ mL} =$

$\dfrac{5}{\underset{2}{\cancel{20}}} \times \dfrac{\overset{3}{\cancel{30}}}{1} = \dfrac{15}{2}$

$\dfrac{15}{2} = 7.5$ mL

$\dfrac{250 \text{ mg}}{250 \text{ mg}} \times 1 \text{ cap} =$

$\dfrac{250}{250} = 1$ capsule

Proportion	**Formula**

7. 2.5 mg : 1 tab :: 7.5 mg : x tab

  2.5 : 1 :: 7.5 : x

  $2.5x = 7.5$

  $x = \dfrac{7.5}{2.5}$

  $x = 3$ tablets

$\dfrac{7.5\ \text{mg}}{2.5\ \text{mg}} \times 1\ \text{cap} =$

$\dfrac{7.5}{2.5} = 3$ tablets

8. 0.05 mg : 1 mL :: 0.05 mg : x mL

  0.05 : 1 :: 0.05 : x

  $0.05x = 0.05$

  $x = \dfrac{0.05}{0.05}$

  $x = 1$ mL

$\dfrac{0.05\ \text{mg}}{0.05\ \text{mg}} \times 1\ \text{mL} =$

$\dfrac{0.5}{0.5} = 1$ mL

9. 1000 mg : 1 g :: x mg : 0.1 g

  1000 : 1 :: x : 0.1

  $x = 100$ mg

  50 mg : 1 cap :: 100 mg : x cap

  50 : 1 :: 100 : x

  $50x = 100$

  $x = \dfrac{100}{50}$

  $x = 2$ capsules

$\dfrac{100\ \text{mg}}{50\ \text{mg}} \times 1\ \text{cap} =$

$\dfrac{100}{50} = 2$ capsules

10. 325 mg : 1 tab :: 650 mg : x tab

  325 : 1 :: 650 : x

  $325x = 650$

  $x = \dfrac{650}{325}$

  $x = 2$ tablets

$\dfrac{650\ \text{mg}}{325\ \text{mg}} \times 1\ \text{tab} =$

$\dfrac{650}{325} = 2$ tablets

11. 50 mg : 1 tab :: 100 mg : x tab

  50 : 1 :: 100 : x

  $50x = 100$

  $x = \dfrac{100}{50}$

  $x = 2$ tablets

$\dfrac{100\ \text{mg}}{50\ \text{mg}} \times 1\ \text{tab} =$

$\dfrac{100}{50} = 2$ tablets

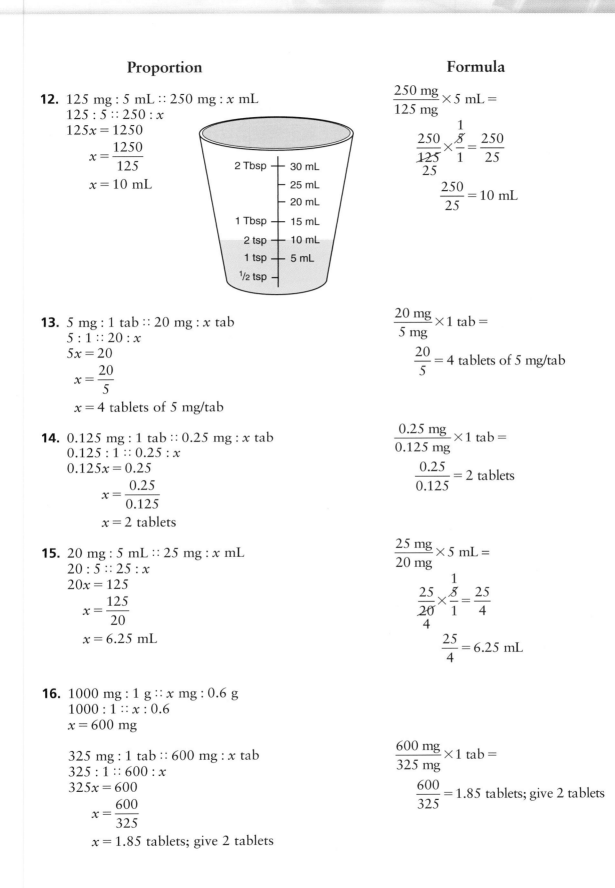

Proportion

Formula

12. 125 mg : 5 mL :: 250 mg : x mL
125 : 5 :: 250 : x
$125x = 1250$
$x = \dfrac{1250}{125}$
$x = 10$ mL

$\dfrac{250 \text{ mg}}{125 \text{ mg}} \times 5 \text{ mL} =$

$\dfrac{250}{\underset{25}{\cancel{125}}} \times \dfrac{\overset{1}{\cancel{5}}}{1} = \dfrac{250}{25}$

$\dfrac{250}{25} = 10$ mL

13. 5 mg : 1 tab :: 20 mg : x tab
5 : 1 :: 20 : x
$5x = 20$
$x = \dfrac{20}{5}$
$x = 4$ tablets of 5 mg/tab

$\dfrac{20 \text{ mg}}{5 \text{ mg}} \times 1 \text{ tab} =$

$\dfrac{20}{5} = 4$ tablets of 5 mg/tab

14. 0.125 mg : 1 tab :: 0.25 mg : x tab
0.125 : 1 :: 0.25 : x
$0.125x = 0.25$
$x = \dfrac{0.25}{0.125}$
$x = 2$ tablets

$\dfrac{0.25 \text{ mg}}{0.125 \text{ mg}} \times 1 \text{ tab} =$

$\dfrac{0.25}{0.125} = 2$ tablets

15. 20 mg : 5 mL :: 25 mg : x mL
20 : 5 :: 25 : x
$20x = 125$
$x = \dfrac{125}{20}$
$x = 6.25$ mL

$\dfrac{25 \text{ mg}}{20 \text{ mg}} \times 5 \text{ mL} =$

$\dfrac{25}{\underset{4}{\cancel{20}}} \times \dfrac{\overset{1}{\cancel{5}}}{1} = \dfrac{25}{4}$

$\dfrac{25}{4} = 6.25$ mL

16. 1000 mg : 1 g :: x mg : 0.6 g
1000 : 1 :: x : 0.6
$x = 600$ mg

325 mg : 1 tab :: 600 mg : x tab
325 : 1 :: 600 : x
$325x = 600$
$x = \dfrac{600}{325}$
$x = 1.85$ tablets; give 2 tablets

$\dfrac{600 \text{ mg}}{325 \text{ mg}} \times 1 \text{ tab} =$

$\dfrac{600}{325} = 1.85$ tablets; give 2 tablets

Proportion	Formula

17. 40 mg : 1 tab :: 80 mg : x tab

40 : 1 :: 80 : x

$40x = 80$

$x = \dfrac{80}{40}$

$x = 2$ tablets

$\dfrac{80 \text{ mg}}{40 \text{ mg}} \times 1 \text{ tab} =$

$\dfrac{\overset{2}{\cancel{80}}}{\underset{1}{\cancel{40}}} = 2$ tablets

18. 7.5 mg : 1 tab :: 15 mg : x tab

7.5 : 1 :: 15 : x

$7.5x = 15$

$x = \dfrac{15}{7.5}$

$x = 2$ tablets

$\dfrac{15 \text{ mg}}{7.5 \text{ mg}} \times 1 \text{ tab} =$

$\dfrac{15}{7.5} = 2$ tablets

19. 15 mg : 1 tab :: 30 mg : x tab

15 : 1 :: 30 : x

$15x = 30$

$x = \dfrac{30}{15}$

$x = 2$ tablets

$\dfrac{30 \text{ mg}}{15 \text{ mg}} \times 1 \text{ tab} =$

$\dfrac{30}{15} = 2$ tablets

20. 250 mg : 1 tab :: 750 mg : x tab

250 : 1 :: 750 : x

$250x = 750$

$x = \dfrac{750}{250}$

$x = 3$ tablets

$\dfrac{750 \text{ mg}}{250 \text{ mg}} \times 1 \text{ tab} =$

$\dfrac{750}{250} = 3$ tablets

21. 5 mg : 1 tab :: 10 mg : x tab

5 : 1 :: 10 : x

$5x = 10$

$x = \dfrac{10}{5}$

$x = 2$ tablets

$\dfrac{10 \text{ mg}}{5 \text{ mg}} \times 1 \text{ tab} =$

$\dfrac{10}{5} = 2$ tablets

22. 75 mg : 1 tab :: 225 mg : x tab

75 : 1 :: 225 : x

$75x = 225$

$x = \dfrac{225}{75}$

$x = 3$ tablets

$\dfrac{225 \text{ mg}}{75 \text{ mg}} \times 1 \text{ tab} =$

$\dfrac{225}{75} = 3$ tablets

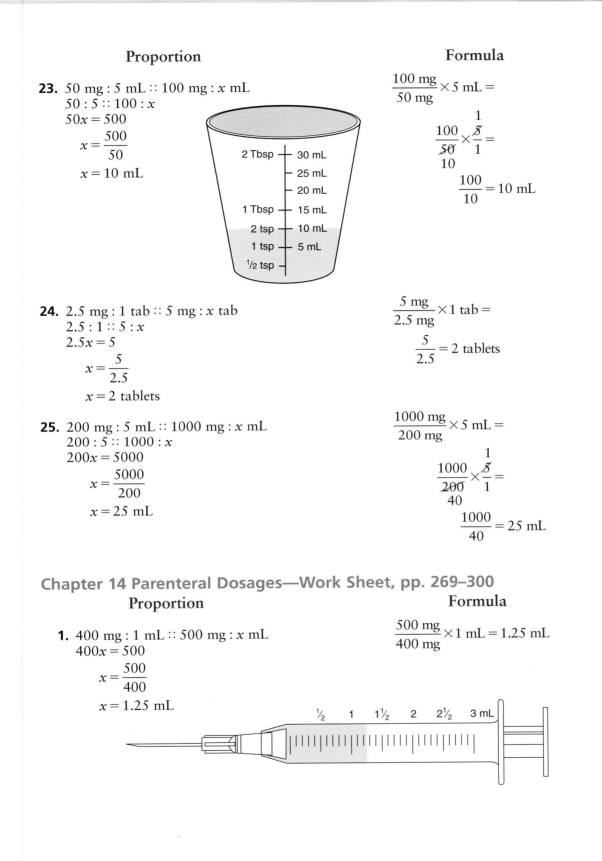

Proportion

23. 50 mg : 5 mL :: 100 mg : x mL
50 : 5 :: 100 : x
$50x = 500$
$x = \dfrac{500}{50}$
$x = 10$ mL

24. 2.5 mg : 1 tab :: 5 mg : x tab
2.5 : 1 :: 5 : x
$2.5x = 5$
$x = \dfrac{5}{2.5}$
$x = 2$ tablets

25. 200 mg : 5 mL :: 1000 mg : x mL
200 : 5 :: 1000 : x
$200x = 5000$
$x = \dfrac{5000}{200}$
$x = 25$ mL

Formula

$\dfrac{100 \text{ mg}}{50 \text{ mg}} \times 5 \text{ mL} =$

$\dfrac{100}{\cancelto{10}{50}} \times \dfrac{\cancelto{1}{5}}{1} =$

$\dfrac{100}{10} = 10$ mL

$\dfrac{5 \text{ mg}}{2.5 \text{ mg}} \times 1 \text{ tab} =$

$\dfrac{5}{2.5} = 2$ tablets

$\dfrac{1000 \text{ mg}}{200 \text{ mg}} \times 5 \text{ mL} =$

$\dfrac{1000}{\cancelto{40}{200}} \times \dfrac{\cancelto{1}{5}}{1} =$

$\dfrac{1000}{40} = 25$ mL

Chapter 14 Parenteral Dosages—Work Sheet, pp. 269–300

Proportion

1. 400 mg : 1 mL :: 500 mg : x mL
$400x = 500$
$x = \dfrac{500}{400}$
$x = 1.25$ mL

Formula

$\dfrac{500 \text{ mg}}{400 \text{ mg}} \times 1 \text{ mL} = 1.25$ mL

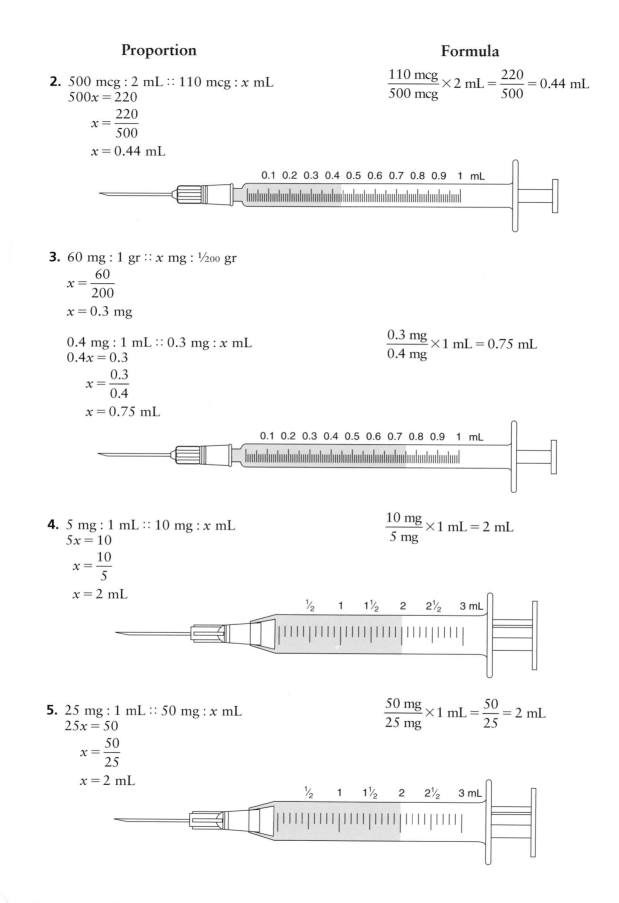

Proportion

Formula

2. 500 mcg : 2 mL :: 110 mcg : x mL
$500x = 220$
$x = \dfrac{220}{500}$
$x = 0.44$ mL

$\dfrac{110 \text{ mcg}}{500 \text{ mcg}} \times 2 \text{ mL} = \dfrac{220}{500} = 0.44 \text{ mL}$

3. 60 mg : 1 gr :: x mg : ¹⁄₂₀₀ gr
$x = \dfrac{60}{200}$
$x = 0.3$ mg

0.4 mg : 1 mL :: 0.3 mg : x mL
$0.4x = 0.3$
$x = \dfrac{0.3}{0.4}$
$x = 0.75$ mL

$\dfrac{0.3 \text{ mg}}{0.4 \text{ mg}} \times 1 \text{ mL} = 0.75 \text{ mL}$

4. 5 mg : 1 mL :: 10 mg : x mL
$5x = 10$
$x = \dfrac{10}{5}$
$x = 2$ mL

$\dfrac{10 \text{ mg}}{5 \text{ mg}} \times 1 \text{ mL} = 2 \text{ mL}$

5. 25 mg : 1 mL :: 50 mg : x mL
$25x = 50$
$x = \dfrac{50}{25}$
$x = 2$ mL

$\dfrac{50 \text{ mg}}{25 \text{ mg}} \times 1 \text{ mL} = \dfrac{50}{25} = 2 \text{ mL}$

Proportion	**Formula**

6. 1 g : 2.5 mL :: 3 g : x mL
  $x = 2.5 \times 3$
  $x = 7.5$ mL

$$\frac{3 \text{ g}}{1 \text{ g}} \times 2.5 \text{ mL} = 7.5 \text{ mL}$$

7. 10 mg : 1 mL :: 5 mg : x mL
  $10x = 5$
  $x = \dfrac{5}{10}$
  $x = 0.5$ mL

$$\frac{5 \text{ mg}}{10 \text{ mg}} \times 1 \text{ mL} = 0.5 \text{ mL}$$

8. 500 mg : 10 mL :: 500 mg : x mL
  $500x = 5000$
  $x = \dfrac{5000}{500}$
  $x = 10$ mL

$$\frac{500 \text{ mg}}{500 \text{ mg}} \times 10 \text{ mL} = \frac{5000}{500} = 10 \text{ mL}$$

9. 40 mg : 4 mL :: 30 mg : x mL
  $40x = 120$
  $x = \dfrac{120}{40}$
  $x = 3$ mL

$$\frac{30 \text{ mg}}{\overset{10}{\cancel{40}} \text{ mg}} \times \frac{\overset{1}{\cancel{4}} \text{ mL}}{1} = \frac{30}{10} = 3 \text{ mL}$$

10. 30 mg : 1 mL :: 15 mg : x mL
  $30x = 15$
  $x = \dfrac{15}{30}$
  $x = 0.5$ mL

$$\frac{\overset{1}{\cancel{15}} \text{ mg}}{\underset{2}{\cancel{30}} \text{ mg}} \times 1 \text{ mL} = \text{½ or } 0.5 \text{ mL}$$

11. 44.6 mEq : 50 mL :: 25.8 : x mL
  $44.6x = 1290$
  $x = \dfrac{1290}{44.6}$
  $x = 28.9$ mL or 29 mL

$$\frac{25.8 \text{ mEq}}{44.6 \text{ mEq}} \times 50 \text{ mL} =$$
$$0.58 \times 50 = 29 \text{ mL}$$

12. 25 mg : 1 mL :: 100 mg : x mL
  $25x = 100$
  $x = \dfrac{100}{25}$
  $x = 4$ mL

$$\frac{100 \text{ mg}}{25 \text{ mg}} \times 1 \text{ mL} = 4 \text{ mL}$$

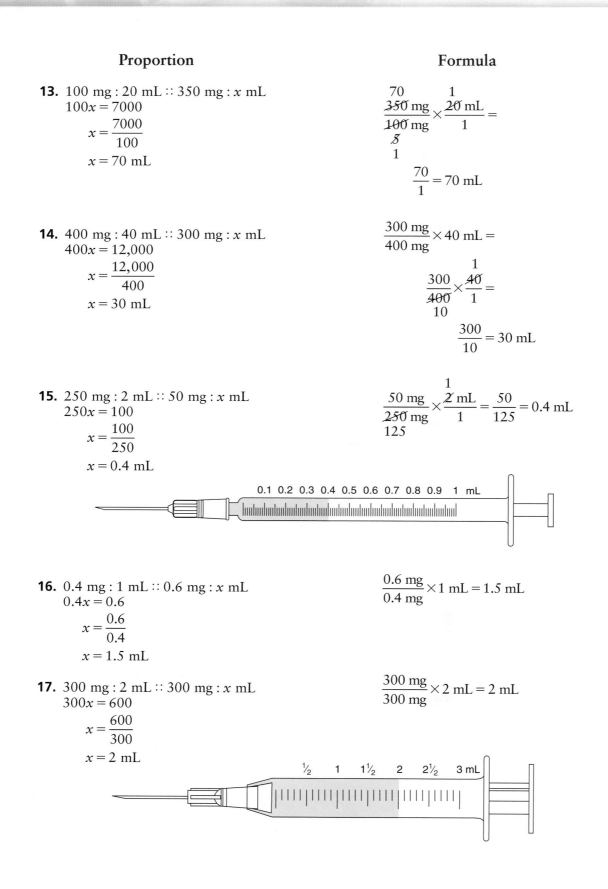

Proportion	Formula

13. $100 \text{ mg} : 20 \text{ mL} :: 350 \text{ mg} : x \text{ mL}$
$100x = 7000$
$x = \dfrac{7000}{100}$
$x = 70 \text{ mL}$

$$\dfrac{\overset{70}{\cancel{350}} \text{ mg}}{\underset{\underset{1}{\cancel{8}}}{\cancel{100}} \text{ mg}} \times \dfrac{\overset{1}{\cancel{20}} \text{ mL}}{1} =$$

$$\dfrac{70}{1} = 70 \text{ mL}$$

14. $400 \text{ mg} : 40 \text{ mL} :: 300 \text{ mg} : x \text{ mL}$
$400x = 12{,}000$
$x = \dfrac{12{,}000}{400}$
$x = 30 \text{ mL}$

$$\dfrac{300 \text{ mg}}{400 \text{ mg}} \times 40 \text{ mL} =$$

$$\dfrac{300}{\underset{10}{\cancel{400}}} \times \dfrac{\overset{1}{\cancel{40}}}{1} =$$

$$\dfrac{300}{10} = 30 \text{ mL}$$

15. $250 \text{ mg} : 2 \text{ mL} :: 50 \text{ mg} : x \text{ mL}$
$250x = 100$
$x = \dfrac{100}{250}$
$x = 0.4 \text{ mL}$

$$\dfrac{50 \text{ mg}}{\underset{125}{\cancel{250}} \text{ mg}} \times \dfrac{\overset{1}{\cancel{2}} \text{ mL}}{1} = \dfrac{50}{125} = 0.4 \text{ mL}$$

16. $0.4 \text{ mg} : 1 \text{ mL} :: 0.6 \text{ mg} : x \text{ mL}$
$0.4x = 0.6$
$x = \dfrac{0.6}{0.4}$
$x = 1.5 \text{ mL}$

$$\dfrac{0.6 \text{ mg}}{0.4 \text{ mg}} \times 1 \text{ mL} = 1.5 \text{ mL}$$

17. $300 \text{ mg} : 2 \text{ mL} :: 300 \text{ mg} : x \text{ mL}$
$300x = 600$
$x = \dfrac{600}{300}$
$x = 2 \text{ mL}$

$$\dfrac{300 \text{ mg}}{300 \text{ mg}} \times 2 \text{ mL} = 2 \text{ mL}$$

Proportion	**Formula**

18. 10 mg : 10 mL :: 6 mg : x mL

$10x = 60$

$x = \dfrac{60}{10}$

$x = 6$ mL

$$\dfrac{6 \text{ mg}}{10 \text{ mg}} \times 10 \text{ mL} =$$

$$\dfrac{6}{\overset{1}{\cancel{10}}} \times \dfrac{\overset{1}{\cancel{10}}}{1} = 6 \text{ mL}$$

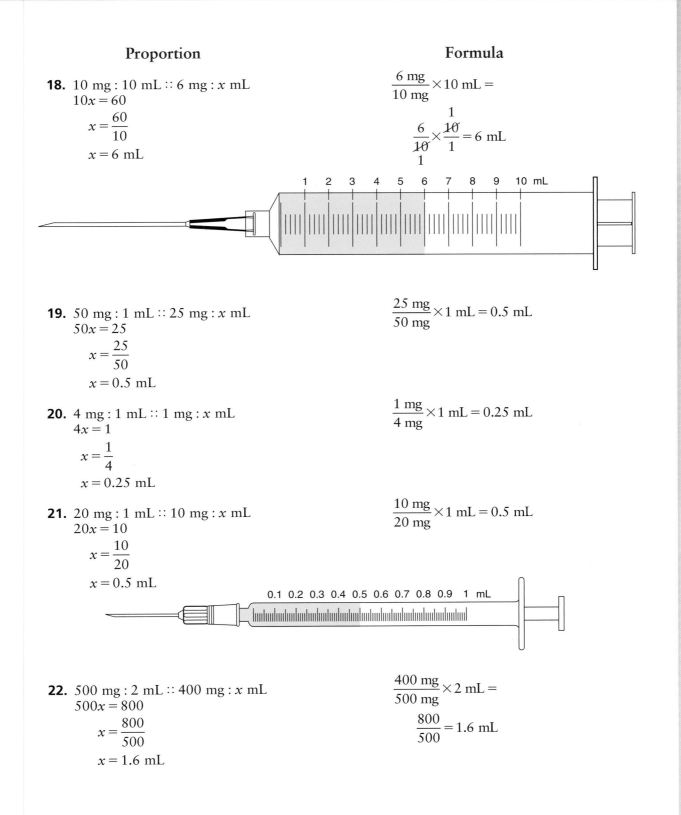

19. 50 mg : 1 mL :: 25 mg : x mL

$50x = 25$

$x = \dfrac{25}{50}$

$x = 0.5$ mL

$$\dfrac{25 \text{ mg}}{50 \text{ mg}} \times 1 \text{ mL} = 0.5 \text{ mL}$$

20. 4 mg : 1 mL :: 1 mg : x mL

$4x = 1$

$x = \dfrac{1}{4}$

$x = 0.25$ mL

$$\dfrac{1 \text{ mg}}{4 \text{ mg}} \times 1 \text{ mL} = 0.25 \text{ mL}$$

21. 20 mg : 1 mL :: 10 mg : x mL

$20x = 10$

$x = \dfrac{10}{20}$

$x = 0.5$ mL

$$\dfrac{10 \text{ mg}}{20 \text{ mg}} \times 1 \text{ mL} = 0.5 \text{ mL}$$

22. 500 mg : 2 mL :: 400 mg : x mL

$500x = 800$

$x = \dfrac{800}{500}$

$x = 1.6$ mL

$$\dfrac{400 \text{ mg}}{500 \text{ mg}} \times 2 \text{ mL} =$$

$$\dfrac{800}{500} = 1.6 \text{ mL}$$

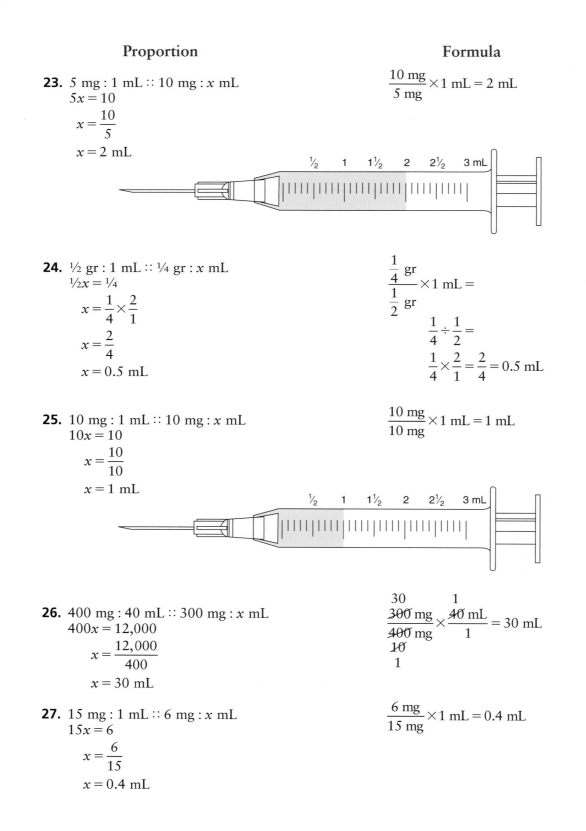

Proportion

Formula

23. 5 mg : 1 mL :: 10 mg : x mL

$5x = 10$

$x = \dfrac{10}{5}$

$x = 2$ mL

$$\dfrac{10 \text{ mg}}{5 \text{ mg}} \times 1 \text{ mL} = 2 \text{ mL}$$

24. ½ gr : 1 mL :: ¼ gr : x mL

$\tfrac{1}{2}x = \tfrac{1}{4}$

$x = \dfrac{1}{4} \times \dfrac{2}{1}$

$x = \dfrac{2}{4}$

$x = 0.5$ mL

$$\dfrac{\frac{1}{4} \text{ gr}}{\frac{1}{2} \text{ gr}} \times 1 \text{ mL} =$$

$$\dfrac{1}{4} \div \dfrac{1}{2} =$$

$$\dfrac{1}{4} \times \dfrac{2}{1} = \dfrac{2}{4} = 0.5 \text{ mL}$$

25. 10 mg : 1 mL :: 10 mg : x mL

$10x = 10$

$x = \dfrac{10}{10}$

$x = 1$ mL

$$\dfrac{10 \text{ mg}}{10 \text{ mg}} \times 1 \text{ mL} = 1 \text{ mL}$$

26. 400 mg : 40 mL :: 300 mg : x mL

$400x = 12{,}000$

$x = \dfrac{12{,}000}{400}$

$x = 30$ mL

$$\dfrac{\overset{30}{\cancel{300}} \text{ mg}}{\underset{1}{\underset{10}{\cancel{400}}} \text{ mg}} \times \dfrac{\overset{1}{\cancel{40}} \text{ mL}}{1} = 30 \text{ mL}$$

27. 15 mg : 1 mL :: 6 mg : x mL

$15x = 6$

$x = \dfrac{6}{15}$

$x = 0.4$ mL

$$\dfrac{6 \text{ mg}}{15 \text{ mg}} \times 1 \text{ mL} = 0.4 \text{ mL}$$

Proportion	Formula

28. $50 \text{ mg} : 1 \text{ mL} :: 100 \text{ mg} : x \text{ mL}$
$50x = 100$
$x = \dfrac{100}{50}$
$x = 2 \text{ mL}$

$\dfrac{100 \text{ mg}}{50 \text{ mg}} \times 1 \text{ mL} = 2 \text{ mL}$

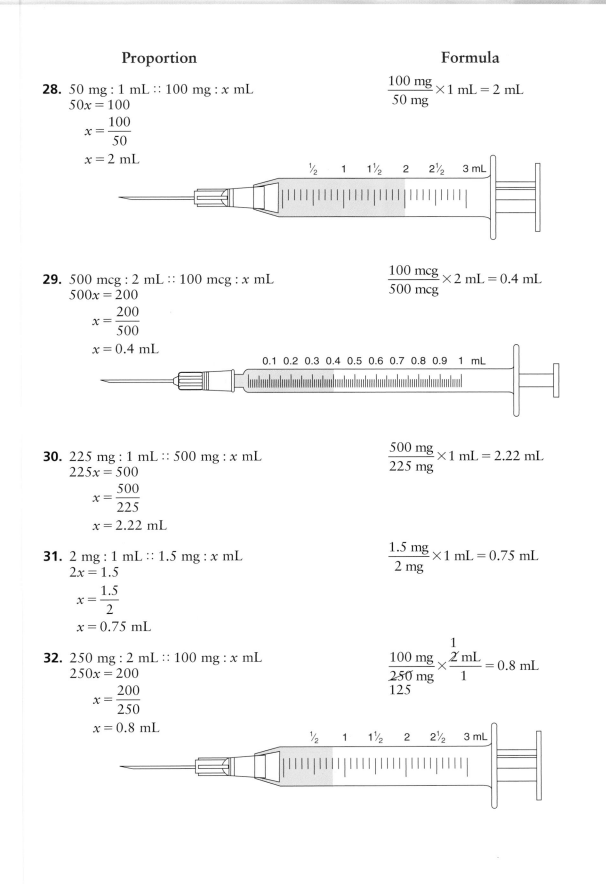

29. $500 \text{ mcg} : 2 \text{ mL} :: 100 \text{ mcg} : x \text{ mL}$
$500x = 200$
$x = \dfrac{200}{500}$
$x = 0.4 \text{ mL}$

$\dfrac{100 \text{ mcg}}{500 \text{ mcg}} \times 2 \text{ mL} = 0.4 \text{ mL}$

30. $225 \text{ mg} : 1 \text{ mL} :: 500 \text{ mg} : x \text{ mL}$
$225x = 500$
$x = \dfrac{500}{225}$
$x = 2.22 \text{ mL}$

$\dfrac{500 \text{ mg}}{225 \text{ mg}} \times 1 \text{ mL} = 2.22 \text{ mL}$

31. $2 \text{ mg} : 1 \text{ mL} :: 1.5 \text{ mg} : x \text{ mL}$
$2x = 1.5$
$x = \dfrac{1.5}{2}$
$x = 0.75 \text{ mL}$

$\dfrac{1.5 \text{ mg}}{2 \text{ mg}} \times 1 \text{ mL} = 0.75 \text{ mL}$

32. $250 \text{ mg} : 2 \text{ mL} :: 100 \text{ mg} : x \text{ mL}$
$250x = 200$
$x = \dfrac{200}{250}$
$x = 0.8 \text{ mL}$

$\dfrac{100 \text{ mg}}{\underset{125}{\cancel{250} \text{ mg}}} \times \dfrac{\overset{1}{\cancel{2} \text{ mL}}}{1} = 0.8 \text{ mL}$

Proportion	Formula

33. $2.5 \text{ mEq} : 1 \text{ mL} :: 7.5 \text{ mEq} : x \text{ mL}$
$2.5x = 7.5$
$x = \dfrac{7.5}{2.5}$
$x = 3 \text{ mL}$

$\dfrac{7.5 \text{ mEq}}{2.5 \text{ mEq}} \times 1 \text{ mL} = 3 \text{ mL}$

34. $50 \text{ mg} : 1 \text{ mL} :: 25 \text{ mg} : x \text{ mL}$
$50x = 25$
$x = \dfrac{25}{50}$
$x = 0.5 \text{ mL}$

$\dfrac{25 \text{ mg}}{50 \text{ mg}} \times 1 \text{ mL} = 0.5 \text{ mL}$

35. $\frac{1}{150} \text{ gr} : 1 \text{ mL} :: \frac{1}{100} \text{ gr} : x \text{ mL}$
$\dfrac{1}{150} x = \dfrac{1}{100}$
$x = \dfrac{150}{100}$
$x = 1.5 \text{ mL}$

$\dfrac{\dfrac{1}{100} \text{ gr}}{\dfrac{1}{150} \text{ gr}} \times 1 \text{ mL} =$

$\dfrac{1}{100} \div \dfrac{1}{150} =$

$\dfrac{1}{100} \times \dfrac{150}{1} = \dfrac{150}{100} = 1.5 \text{ mL}$

36. $100 \text{ mg} : 1 \text{ mL} :: 150 \text{ mg} : x \text{ mL}$
$100x = 150$
$x = \dfrac{150}{100}$
$x = 1.5 \text{ mL}$

$\dfrac{150 \text{ mg}}{100 \text{ mg}} \times 1 \text{ mL} = 1.5 \text{ mL}$

37. $0.25 \text{ mg} : 1 \text{ mL} :: 0.5 \text{ mg} : x \text{ mL}$
$0.25x = 0.5$
$x = \dfrac{0.5}{0.25}$
$x = 2 \text{ mL}$

$\dfrac{0.5 \text{ mg}}{0.25 \text{ mg}} \times 1 \text{ mL} = 2 \text{ mL}$

38. $25 \text{ mg} : 1 \text{ mL} :: 75 \text{ mg} : x \text{ mL}$
$25x = 75$
$x = \dfrac{75}{25}$
$x = 3 \text{ mL}$

$\dfrac{75 \text{ mg}}{25 \text{ mg}} \times 1 \text{ mL} = 3 \text{ mL}$

Proportion	Formula

39. $0.4 \text{ mg} : 1 \text{ mL} :: 0.6 \text{ mg} : x \text{ mL}$

$0.4x = 0.6$

$x = \dfrac{0.6}{0.4}$

$x = 1.5 \text{ mL}$

$\dfrac{0.6 \text{ mg}}{0.4 \text{ mg}} \times \dfrac{1 \text{ mL}}{1} = 1.5 \text{ mL}$

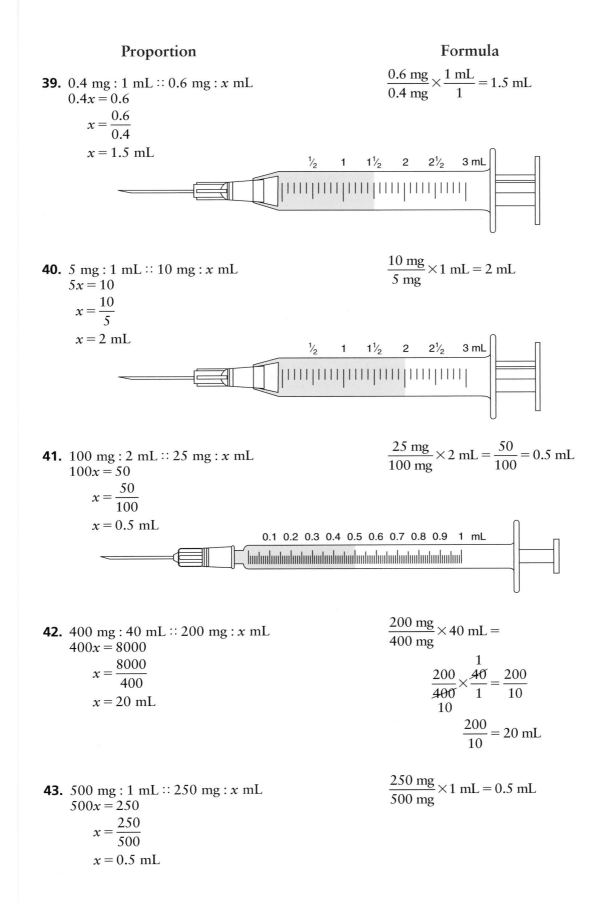

40. $5 \text{ mg} : 1 \text{ mL} :: 10 \text{ mg} : x \text{ mL}$

$5x = 10$

$x = \dfrac{10}{5}$

$x = 2 \text{ mL}$

$\dfrac{10 \text{ mg}}{5 \text{ mg}} \times 1 \text{ mL} = 2 \text{ mL}$

41. $100 \text{ mg} : 2 \text{ mL} :: 25 \text{ mg} : x \text{ mL}$

$100x = 50$

$x = \dfrac{50}{100}$

$x = 0.5 \text{ mL}$

$\dfrac{25 \text{ mg}}{100 \text{ mg}} \times 2 \text{ mL} = \dfrac{50}{100} = 0.5 \text{ mL}$

42. $400 \text{ mg} : 40 \text{ mL} :: 200 \text{ mg} : x \text{ mL}$

$400x = 8000$

$x = \dfrac{8000}{400}$

$x = 20 \text{ mL}$

$\dfrac{200 \text{ mg}}{400 \text{ mg}} \times 40 \text{ mL} =$

$\dfrac{200}{\underset{10}{\cancel{400}}} \times \dfrac{\overset{1}{\cancel{40}}}{1} = \dfrac{200}{10}$

$\dfrac{200}{10} = 20 \text{ mL}$

43. $500 \text{ mg} : 1 \text{ mL} :: 250 \text{ mg} : x \text{ mL}$

$500x = 250$

$x = \dfrac{250}{500}$

$x = 0.5 \text{ mL}$

$\dfrac{250 \text{ mg}}{500 \text{ mg}} \times 1 \text{ mL} = 0.5 \text{ mL}$

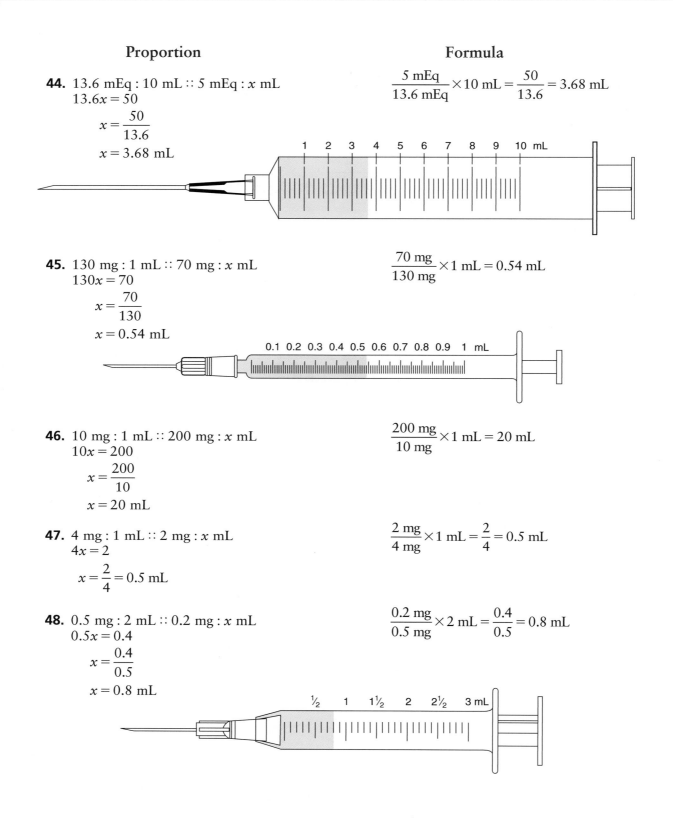

	Proportion	**Formula**

44. 13.6 mEq : 10 mL :: 5 mEq : x mL

13.6x = 50

$$x = \frac{50}{13.6}$$

x = 3.68 mL

$$\frac{5\ mEq}{13.6\ mEq} \times 10\ mL = \frac{50}{13.6} = 3.68\ mL$$

45. 130 mg : 1 mL :: 70 mg : x mL

130x = 70

$$x = \frac{70}{130}$$

x = 0.54 mL

$$\frac{70\ mg}{130\ mg} \times 1\ mL = 0.54\ mL$$

46. 10 mg : 1 mL :: 200 mg : x mL

10x = 200

$$x = \frac{200}{10}$$

x = 20 mL

$$\frac{200\ mg}{10\ mg} \times 1\ mL = 20\ mL$$

47. 4 mg : 1 mL :: 2 mg : x mL

4x = 2

$$x = \frac{2}{4} = 0.5\ mL$$

$$\frac{2\ mg}{4\ mg} \times 1\ mL = \frac{2}{4} = 0.5\ mL$$

48. 0.5 mg : 2 mL :: 0.2 mg : x mL

0.5x = 0.4

$$x = \frac{0.4}{0.5}$$

x = 0.8 mL

$$\frac{0.2\ mg}{0.5\ mg} \times 2\ mL = \frac{0.4}{0.5} = 0.8\ mL$$

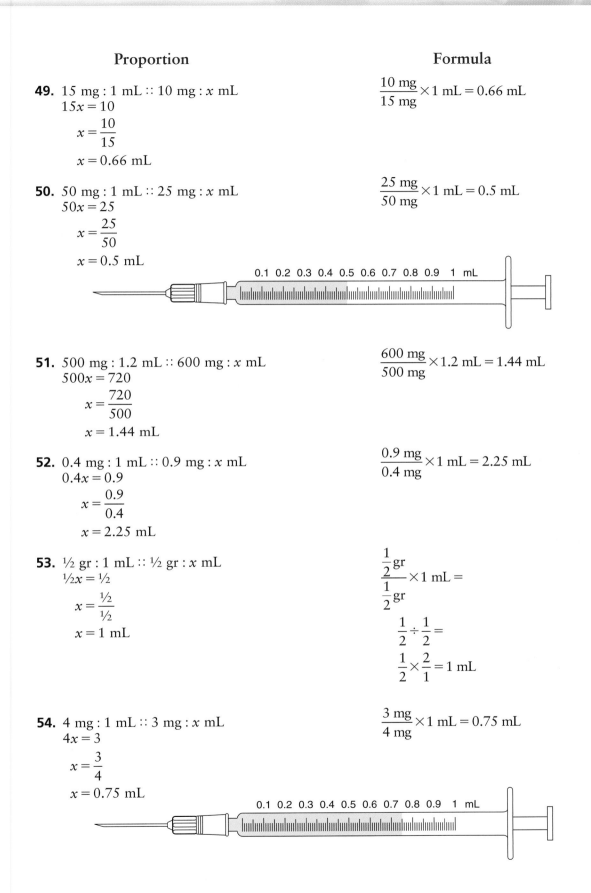

Proportion

49. 15 mg : 1 mL :: 10 mg : x mL
  15x = 10
  $x = \dfrac{10}{15}$
  x = 0.66 mL

50. 50 mg : 1 mL :: 25 mg : x mL
  50x = 25
  $x = \dfrac{25}{50}$
  x = 0.5 mL

51. 500 mg : 1.2 mL :: 600 mg : x mL
  500x = 720
  $x = \dfrac{720}{500}$
  x = 1.44 mL

52. 0.4 mg : 1 mL :: 0.9 mg : x mL
  0.4x = 0.9
  $x = \dfrac{0.9}{0.4}$
  x = 2.25 mL

53. ½ gr : 1 mL :: ½ gr : x mL
  ½x = ½
  $x = \dfrac{½}{½}$
  x = 1 mL

54. 4 mg : 1 mL :: 3 mg : x mL
  4x = 3
  $x = \dfrac{3}{4}$
  x = 0.75 mL

Formula

$\dfrac{10 \text{ mg}}{15 \text{ mg}} \times 1 \text{ mL} = 0.66 \text{ mL}$

$\dfrac{25 \text{ mg}}{50 \text{ mg}} \times 1 \text{ mL} = 0.5 \text{ mL}$

$\dfrac{600 \text{ mg}}{500 \text{ mg}} \times 1.2 \text{ mL} = 1.44 \text{ mL}$

$\dfrac{0.9 \text{ mg}}{0.4 \text{ mg}} \times 1 \text{ mL} = 2.25 \text{ mL}$

$\dfrac{\frac{1}{2}\text{ gr}}{\frac{1}{2}\text{ gr}} \times 1 \text{ mL} =$

$\dfrac{1}{2} \div \dfrac{1}{2} =$

$\dfrac{1}{2} \times \dfrac{2}{1} = 1 \text{ mL}$

$\dfrac{3 \text{ mg}}{4 \text{ mg}} \times 1 \text{ mL} = 0.75 \text{ mL}$

Proportion

Formula

55. $0.89 \text{ mEq} : 1 \text{ mL} :: 6 \text{ mEq} : x \text{ mL}$
$0.89x = 6$
$$x = \frac{6}{0.89}$$
$x = 6.74 \text{ mL}$

$$\frac{6 \text{ mEq}}{0.89 \text{ mEq}} \times 1 \text{ mL} = 6.74 \text{ mL}$$

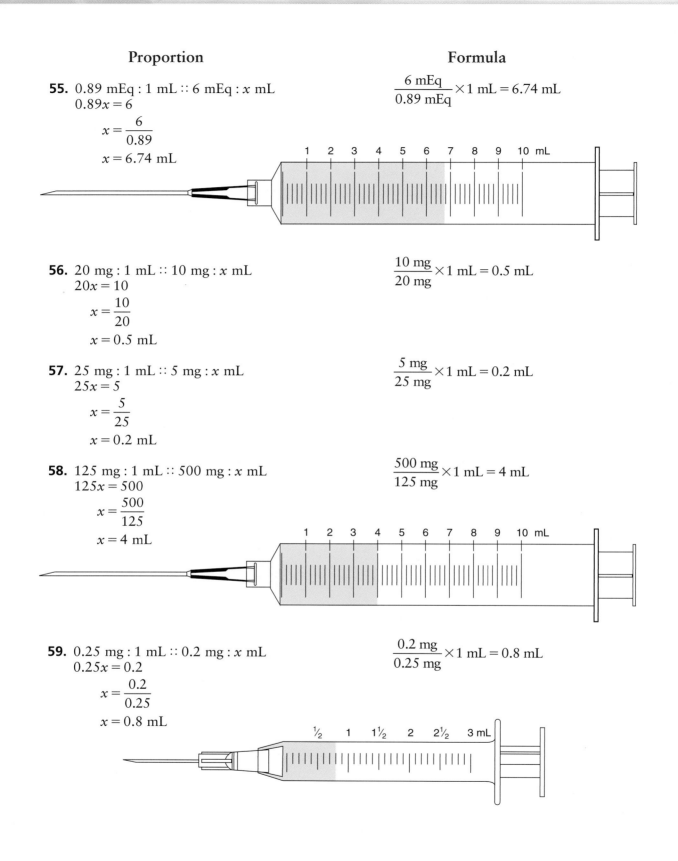

56. $20 \text{ mg} : 1 \text{ mL} :: 10 \text{ mg} : x \text{ mL}$
$20x = 10$
$$x = \frac{10}{20}$$
$x = 0.5 \text{ mL}$

$$\frac{10 \text{ mg}}{20 \text{ mg}} \times 1 \text{ mL} = 0.5 \text{ mL}$$

57. $25 \text{ mg} : 1 \text{ mL} :: 5 \text{ mg} : x \text{ mL}$
$25x = 5$
$$x = \frac{5}{25}$$
$x = 0.2 \text{ mL}$

$$\frac{5 \text{ mg}}{25 \text{ mg}} \times 1 \text{ mL} = 0.2 \text{ mL}$$

58. $125 \text{ mg} : 1 \text{ mL} :: 500 \text{ mg} : x \text{ mL}$
$125x = 500$
$$x = \frac{500}{125}$$
$x = 4 \text{ mL}$

$$\frac{500 \text{ mg}}{125 \text{ mg}} \times 1 \text{ mL} = 4 \text{ mL}$$

59. $0.25 \text{ mg} : 1 \text{ mL} :: 0.2 \text{ mg} : x \text{ mL}$
$0.25x = 0.2$
$$x = \frac{0.2}{0.25}$$
$x = 0.8 \text{ mL}$

$$\frac{0.2 \text{ mg}}{0.25 \text{ mg}} \times 1 \text{ mL} = 0.8 \text{ mL}$$

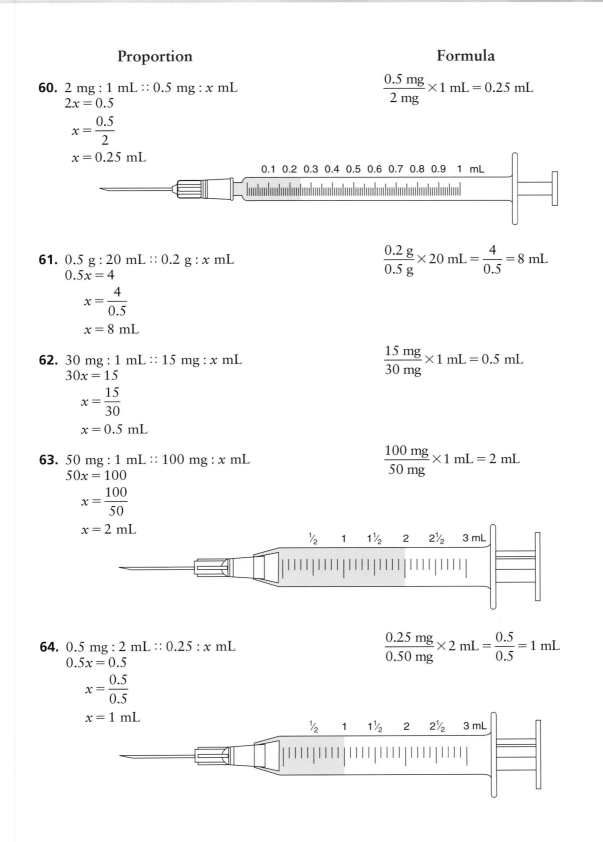

Proportion

60. 2 mg : 1 mL :: 0.5 mg : x mL
$2x = 0.5$

$x = \dfrac{0.5}{2}$

$x = 0.25$ mL

61. 0.5 g : 20 mL :: 0.2 g : x mL
$0.5x = 4$

$x = \dfrac{4}{0.5}$

$x = 8$ mL

62. 30 mg : 1 mL :: 15 mg : x mL
$30x = 15$

$x = \dfrac{15}{30}$

$x = 0.5$ mL

63. 50 mg : 1 mL :: 100 mg : x mL
$50x = 100$

$x = \dfrac{100}{50}$

$x = 2$ mL

64. 0.5 mg : 2 mL :: 0.25 : x mL
$0.5x = 0.5$

$x = \dfrac{0.5}{0.5}$

$x = 1$ mL

Formula

$$\dfrac{0.5 \text{ mg}}{2 \text{ mg}} \times 1 \text{ mL} = 0.25 \text{ mL}$$

$$\dfrac{0.2 \text{ g}}{0.5 \text{ g}} \times 20 \text{ mL} = \dfrac{4}{0.5} = 8 \text{ mL}$$

$$\dfrac{15 \text{ mg}}{30 \text{ mg}} \times 1 \text{ mL} = 0.5 \text{ mL}$$

$$\dfrac{100 \text{ mg}}{50 \text{ mg}} \times 1 \text{ mL} = 2 \text{ mL}$$

$$\dfrac{0.25 \text{ mg}}{0.50 \text{ mg}} \times 2 \text{ mL} = \dfrac{0.5}{0.5} = 1 \text{ mL}$$

Proportion

Formula

65. 1000 mcg : 1 mL :: 500 mcg : x mL
$$1000x = 500$$
$$x = \frac{500}{1000}$$
$$x = 0.5 \text{ mL}$$

$$\frac{500 \text{ mcg}}{1000 \text{ mcg}} \times 1 \text{ mL} = 0.5 \text{ mL}$$

66. 4.8 mEq : 10 mL :: 5 mEq : x mL
$$4.8x = 50$$
$$x = \frac{50}{4.8}$$
$$x = 10.42 \text{ mL}$$

$$\frac{5 \text{ mEq}}{4.8 \text{ mEq}} \times 10 \text{ mL} = \frac{50}{4.8} = 10.42 \text{ mL}$$

67. 150 mg : 1 mL :: 50 mg : x mL
$$150x = 50$$
$$x = \frac{50}{150}$$
$$x = 0.33 \text{ mL}$$

$$\frac{50 \text{ mg}}{150 \text{ mg}} \times 1 \text{ mL} = 0.33 \text{ mL}$$

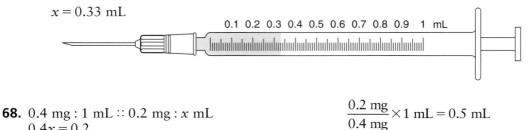

68. 0.4 mg : 1 mL :: 0.2 mg : x mL
$$0.4x = 0.2$$
$$x = \frac{0.2}{0.4}$$
$$x = 0.5 \text{ mL}$$

$$\frac{0.2 \text{ mg}}{0.4 \text{ mg}} \times 1 \text{ mL} = 0.5 \text{ mL}$$

69. 80 mg : 2 mL :: 55 mg : x mL
$$80x = 110$$
$$x = \frac{110}{80}$$
$$x = 1.38 \text{ mL}$$

$$\frac{55 \text{ mg}}{80 \text{ mg}} \times 2 \text{ mL} = \frac{110}{80} = 1.38 \text{ mL}$$

Proportion	Formula

70. $500 \text{ mg} : 2 \text{ mL} :: 600 \text{ mg} : x \text{ mL}$
$500x = 1200$
$x = \dfrac{1200}{500}$
$x = 2.4 \text{ mL}$

$\dfrac{600 \text{ mg}}{500 \text{ mg}} \times 2 \text{ mL} =$

$\dfrac{600}{\underset{250}{\cancel{500}}} \times \dfrac{\overset{1}{\cancel{2}}}{1} = \dfrac{600}{250}$

$x = 2.4 \text{ mL}$

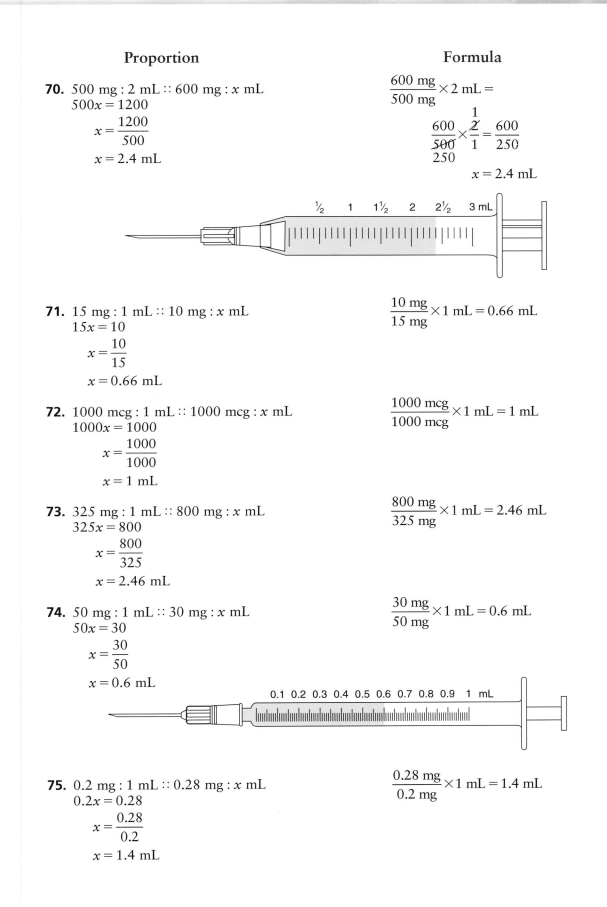

71. $15 \text{ mg} : 1 \text{ mL} :: 10 \text{ mg} : x \text{ mL}$
$15x = 10$
$x = \dfrac{10}{15}$
$x = 0.66 \text{ mL}$

$\dfrac{10 \text{ mg}}{15 \text{ mg}} \times 1 \text{ mL} = 0.66 \text{ mL}$

72. $1000 \text{ mcg} : 1 \text{ mL} :: 1000 \text{ mcg} : x \text{ mL}$
$1000x = 1000$
$x = \dfrac{1000}{1000}$
$x = 1 \text{ mL}$

$\dfrac{1000 \text{ mcg}}{1000 \text{ mcg}} \times 1 \text{ mL} = 1 \text{ mL}$

73. $325 \text{ mg} : 1 \text{ mL} :: 800 \text{ mg} : x \text{ mL}$
$325x = 800$
$x = \dfrac{800}{325}$
$x = 2.46 \text{ mL}$

$\dfrac{800 \text{ mg}}{325 \text{ mg}} \times 1 \text{ mL} = 2.46 \text{ mL}$

74. $50 \text{ mg} : 1 \text{ mL} :: 30 \text{ mg} : x \text{ mL}$
$50x = 30$
$x = \dfrac{30}{50}$
$x = 0.6 \text{ mL}$

$\dfrac{30 \text{ mg}}{50 \text{ mg}} \times 1 \text{ mL} = 0.6 \text{ mL}$

75. $0.2 \text{ mg} : 1 \text{ mL} :: 0.28 \text{ mg} : x \text{ mL}$
$0.2x = 0.28$
$x = \dfrac{0.28}{0.2}$
$x = 1.4 \text{ mL}$

$\dfrac{0.28 \text{ mg}}{0.2 \text{ mg}} \times 1 \text{ mL} = 1.4 \text{ mL}$

Proportion	Formula

76. 4 mg : 1 mL :: 3 mg : x mL

$4x = 3$

$x = \dfrac{3}{4}$

$x = 0.75$ mL

$\dfrac{3 \text{ mg}}{4 \text{ mg}} \times 1 \text{ mL} = 0.75 \text{ mL}$

77. 100 mEq : 40 mL :: 15 mEq : x mL

$100x = 600$

$x = \dfrac{600}{100}$

$x = 6$ mL

$\dfrac{15 \text{ mEq}}{100 \text{ mEq}} \times 40 \text{ mL} = \dfrac{600}{100} = 6 \text{ mL}$

78. 225 mg : 1 mL :: 250 mg : x mL

$225x = 250$

$x = \dfrac{250}{225}$

$x = 1.1$ mL

$\dfrac{250 \text{ mg}}{225 \text{ mg}} \times 1 \text{ mL} = 1.1 \text{ mL}$

79. 150 mg : 1 mL :: 300 mg : x mL

$150x = 300$

$x = \dfrac{300}{150}$

$x = 2$ mL

$\dfrac{300 \text{ mg}}{150 \text{ mg}} \times 1 \text{ mL} = 2 \text{ mL}$

80. 100 mg : 5 mL :: 75 mg : x mL

$100x = 375$

$x = \dfrac{375}{100}$

$x = 3.75$ mL

$\dfrac{75 \text{ mg}}{100 \text{ mg}} \times 5 \text{ mL} = \dfrac{375}{100} = 3.75 \text{ mL}$

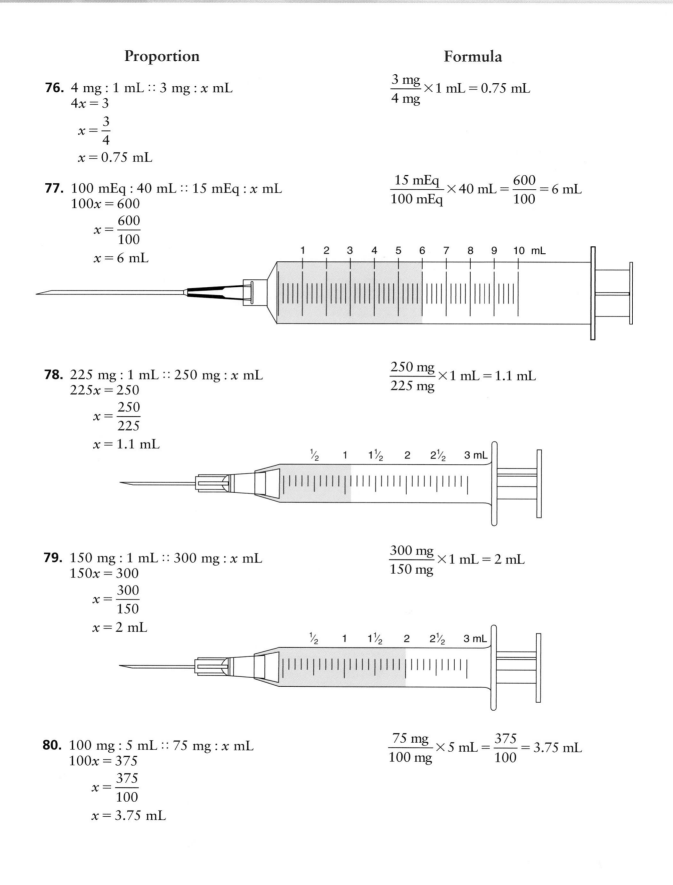

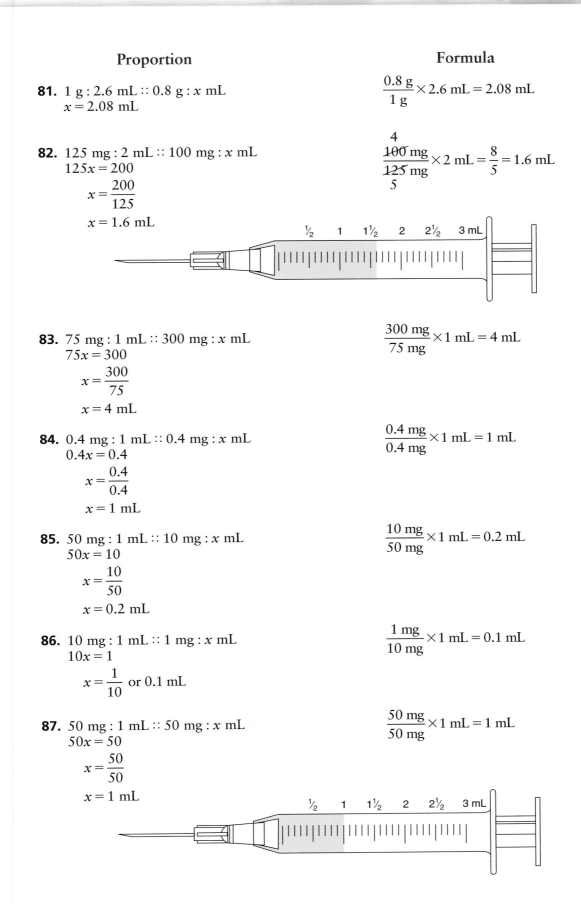

Proportion

81. $1 \text{ g} : 2.6 \text{ mL} :: 0.8 \text{ g} : x \text{ mL}$
$x = 2.08 \text{ mL}$

82. $125 \text{ mg} : 2 \text{ mL} :: 100 \text{ mg} : x \text{ mL}$
$125x = 200$
$x = \dfrac{200}{125}$
$x = 1.6 \text{ mL}$

83. $75 \text{ mg} : 1 \text{ mL} :: 300 \text{ mg} : x \text{ mL}$
$75x = 300$
$x = \dfrac{300}{75}$
$x = 4 \text{ mL}$

84. $0.4 \text{ mg} : 1 \text{ mL} :: 0.4 \text{ mg} : x \text{ mL}$
$0.4x = 0.4$
$x = \dfrac{0.4}{0.4}$
$x = 1 \text{ mL}$

85. $50 \text{ mg} : 1 \text{ mL} :: 10 \text{ mg} : x \text{ mL}$
$50x = 10$
$x = \dfrac{10}{50}$
$x = 0.2 \text{ mL}$

86. $10 \text{ mg} : 1 \text{ mL} :: 1 \text{ mg} : x \text{ mL}$
$10x = 1$
$x = \dfrac{1}{10} \text{ or } 0.1 \text{ mL}$

87. $50 \text{ mg} : 1 \text{ mL} :: 50 \text{ mg} : x \text{ mL}$
$50x = 50$
$x = \dfrac{50}{50}$
$x = 1 \text{ mL}$

Formula

$\dfrac{0.8 \text{ g}}{1 \text{ g}} \times 2.6 \text{ mL} = 2.08 \text{ mL}$

$\dfrac{\overset{4}{\cancel{100} \text{ mg}}}{\underset{5}{\cancel{125} \text{ mg}}} \times 2 \text{ mL} = \dfrac{8}{5} = 1.6 \text{ mL}$

$\dfrac{300 \text{ mg}}{75 \text{ mg}} \times 1 \text{ mL} = 4 \text{ mL}$

$\dfrac{0.4 \text{ mg}}{0.4 \text{ mg}} \times 1 \text{ mL} = 1 \text{ mL}$

$\dfrac{10 \text{ mg}}{50 \text{ mg}} \times 1 \text{ mL} = 0.2 \text{ mL}$

$\dfrac{1 \text{ mg}}{10 \text{ mg}} \times 1 \text{ mL} = 0.1 \text{ mL}$

$\dfrac{50 \text{ mg}}{50 \text{ mg}} \times 1 \text{ mL} = 1 \text{ mL}$

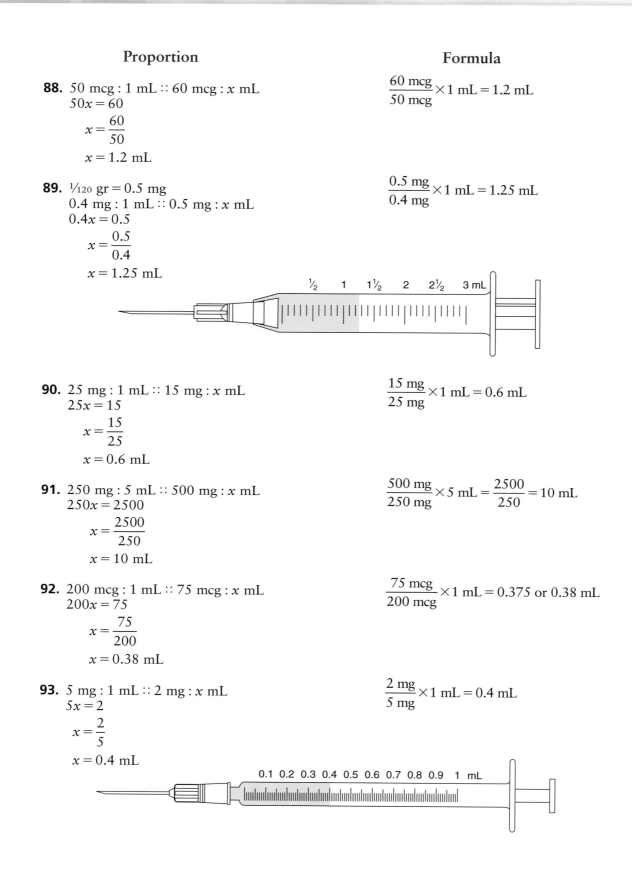

	Proportion		Formula

88. 50 mcg : 1 mL :: 60 mcg : x mL

$50x = 60$

$x = \dfrac{60}{50}$

$x = 1.2$ mL

$\dfrac{60 \text{ mcg}}{50 \text{ mcg}} \times 1 \text{ mL} = 1.2 \text{ mL}$

89. $^{1}\!/_{120}$ gr $= 0.5$ mg

0.4 mg : 1 mL :: 0.5 mg : x mL

$0.4x = 0.5$

$x = \dfrac{0.5}{0.4}$

$x = 1.25$ mL

$\dfrac{0.5 \text{ mg}}{0.4 \text{ mg}} \times 1 \text{ mL} = 1.25 \text{ mL}$

90. 25 mg : 1 mL :: 15 mg : x mL

$25x = 15$

$x = \dfrac{15}{25}$

$x = 0.6$ mL

$\dfrac{15 \text{ mg}}{25 \text{ mg}} \times 1 \text{ mL} = 0.6 \text{ mL}$

91. 250 mg : 5 mL :: 500 mg : x mL

$250x = 2500$

$x = \dfrac{2500}{250}$

$x = 10$ mL

$\dfrac{500 \text{ mg}}{250 \text{ mg}} \times 5 \text{ mL} = \dfrac{2500}{250} = 10 \text{ mL}$

92. 200 mcg : 1 mL :: 75 mcg : x mL

$200x = 75$

$x = \dfrac{75}{200}$

$x = 0.38$ mL

$\dfrac{75 \text{ mcg}}{200 \text{ mcg}} \times 1 \text{ mL} = 0.375 \text{ or } 0.38 \text{ mL}$

93. 5 mg : 1 mL :: 2 mg : x mL

$5x = 2$

$x = \dfrac{2}{5}$

$x = 0.4$ mL

$\dfrac{2 \text{ mg}}{5 \text{ mg}} \times 1 \text{ mL} = 0.4 \text{ mL}$

Proportion	Formula

94. $100 \text{ mg} : 1 \text{ mL} :: 500 \text{ mg} : x \text{ mL}$

$100x = 500$

$x = \dfrac{500}{100}$

$x = 5 \text{ mL}$

$\dfrac{500 \text{ mg}}{100 \text{ mg}} \times 1 \text{ mL} = 5 \text{ mL}$

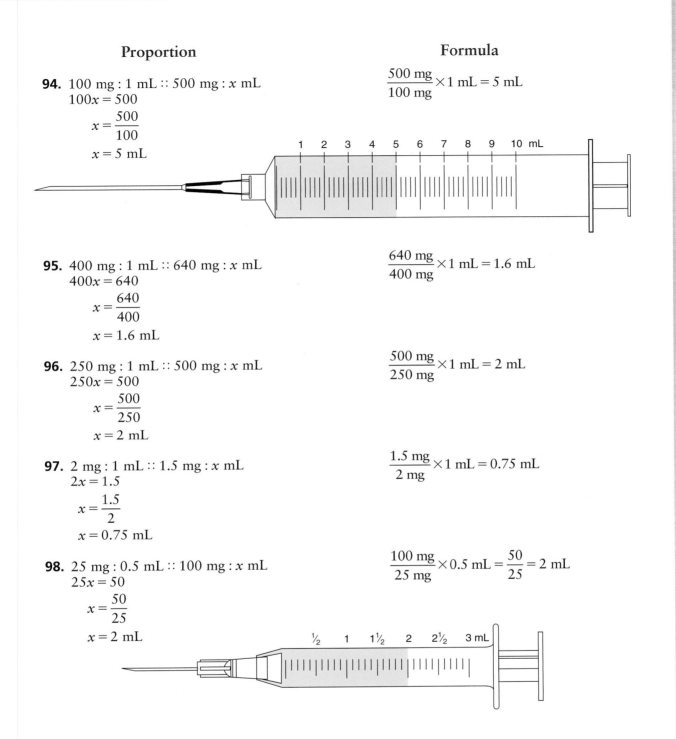

95. $400 \text{ mg} : 1 \text{ mL} :: 640 \text{ mg} : x \text{ mL}$

$400x = 640$

$x = \dfrac{640}{400}$

$x = 1.6 \text{ mL}$

$\dfrac{640 \text{ mg}}{400 \text{ mg}} \times 1 \text{ mL} = 1.6 \text{ mL}$

96. $250 \text{ mg} : 1 \text{ mL} :: 500 \text{ mg} : x \text{ mL}$

$250x = 500$

$x = \dfrac{500}{250}$

$x = 2 \text{ mL}$

$\dfrac{500 \text{ mg}}{250 \text{ mg}} \times 1 \text{ mL} = 2 \text{ mL}$

97. $2 \text{ mg} : 1 \text{ mL} :: 1.5 \text{ mg} : x \text{ mL}$

$2x = 1.5$

$x = \dfrac{1.5}{2}$

$x = 0.75 \text{ mL}$

$\dfrac{1.5 \text{ mg}}{2 \text{ mg}} \times 1 \text{ mL} = 0.75 \text{ mL}$

98. $25 \text{ mg} : 0.5 \text{ mL} :: 100 \text{ mg} : x \text{ mL}$

$25x = 50$

$x = \dfrac{50}{25}$

$x = 2 \text{ mL}$

$\dfrac{100 \text{ mg}}{25 \text{ mg}} \times 0.5 \text{ mL} = \dfrac{50}{25} = 2 \text{ mL}$

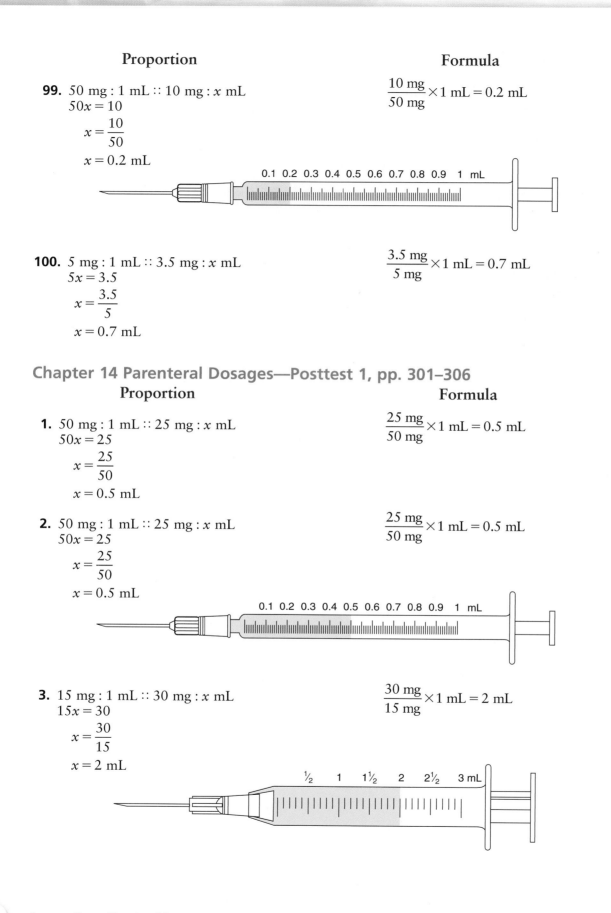

Proportion	Formula
99. 50 mg : 1 mL :: 10 mg : x mL $50x = 10$ $x = \dfrac{10}{50}$ $x = 0.2$ mL	$\dfrac{10 \text{ mg}}{50 \text{ mg}} \times 1 \text{ mL} = 0.2 \text{ mL}$

0.1 0.2 0.3 0.4 0.5 0.6 0.7 0.8 0.9   1   mL

| **100.** 5 mg : 1 mL :: 3.5 mg : x mL
$5x = 3.5$
$x = \dfrac{3.5}{5}$
$x = 0.7$ mL | $\dfrac{3.5 \text{ mg}}{5 \text{ mg}} \times 1 \text{ mL} = 0.7 \text{ mL}$ |

Chapter 14 Parenteral Dosages—Posttest 1, pp. 301–306

Proportion	Formula
1. 50 mg : 1 mL :: 25 mg : x mL $50x = 25$ $x = \dfrac{25}{50}$ $x = 0.5$ mL	$\dfrac{25 \text{ mg}}{50 \text{ mg}} \times 1 \text{ mL} = 0.5 \text{ mL}$
2. 50 mg : 1 mL :: 25 mg : x mL $50x = 25$ $x = \dfrac{25}{50}$ $x = 0.5$ mL	$\dfrac{25 \text{ mg}}{50 \text{ mg}} \times 1 \text{ mL} = 0.5 \text{ mL}$

0.1 0.2 0.3 0.4 0.5 0.6 0.7 0.8 0.9   1   mL

| **3.** 15 mg : 1 mL :: 30 mg : x mL
$15x = 30$
$x = \dfrac{30}{15}$
$x = 2$ mL | $\dfrac{30 \text{ mg}}{15 \text{ mg}} \times 1 \text{ mL} = 2 \text{ mL}$ |

½   1   1½   2   2½   3 mL

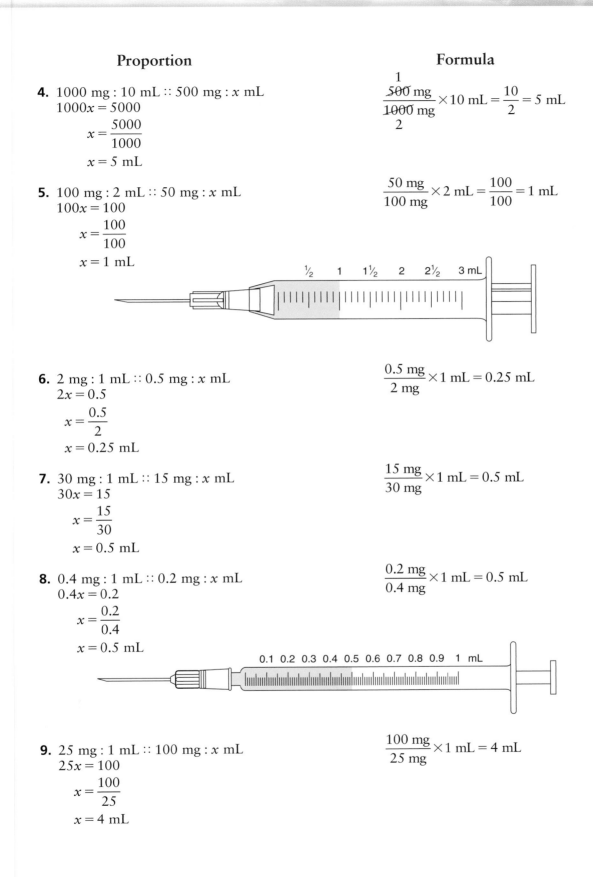

Proportion	**Formula**
4. 1000 mg : 10 mL :: 500 mg : x mL $1000x = 5000$ $x = \dfrac{5000}{1000}$ $x = 5$ mL	$\dfrac{\overset{1}{\cancel{500}}\text{ mg}}{\underset{2}{\cancel{1000}}\text{ mg}} \times 10\text{ mL} = \dfrac{10}{2} = 5\text{ mL}$
5. 100 mg : 2 mL :: 50 mg : x mL $100x = 100$ $x = \dfrac{100}{100}$ $x = 1$ mL	$\dfrac{50\text{ mg}}{100\text{ mg}} \times 2\text{ mL} = \dfrac{100}{100} = 1\text{ mL}$
6. 2 mg : 1 mL :: 0.5 mg : x mL $2x = 0.5$ $x = \dfrac{0.5}{2}$ $x = 0.25$ mL	$\dfrac{0.5\text{ mg}}{2\text{ mg}} \times 1\text{ mL} = 0.25\text{ mL}$
7. 30 mg : 1 mL :: 15 mg : x mL $30x = 15$ $x = \dfrac{15}{30}$ $x = 0.5$ mL	$\dfrac{15\text{ mg}}{30\text{ mg}} \times 1\text{ mL} = 0.5\text{ mL}$
8. 0.4 mg : 1 mL :: 0.2 mg : x mL $0.4x = 0.2$ $x = \dfrac{0.2}{0.4}$ $x = 0.5$ mL	$\dfrac{0.2\text{ mg}}{0.4\text{ mg}} \times 1\text{ mL} = 0.5\text{ mL}$
9. 25 mg : 1 mL :: 100 mg : x mL $25x = 100$ $x = \dfrac{100}{25}$ $x = 4$ mL	$\dfrac{100\text{ mg}}{25\text{ mg}} \times 1\text{ mL} = 4\text{ mL}$

	Proportion	Formula

10. 5 mg : 1 mL :: 2 mg : x mL

$5x = 2$

$x = \dfrac{2}{5}$

$x = 0.4$ mL

$\dfrac{2 \text{ mg}}{5 \text{ mg}} \times 1 \text{ mL} = 0.4 \text{ mL}$

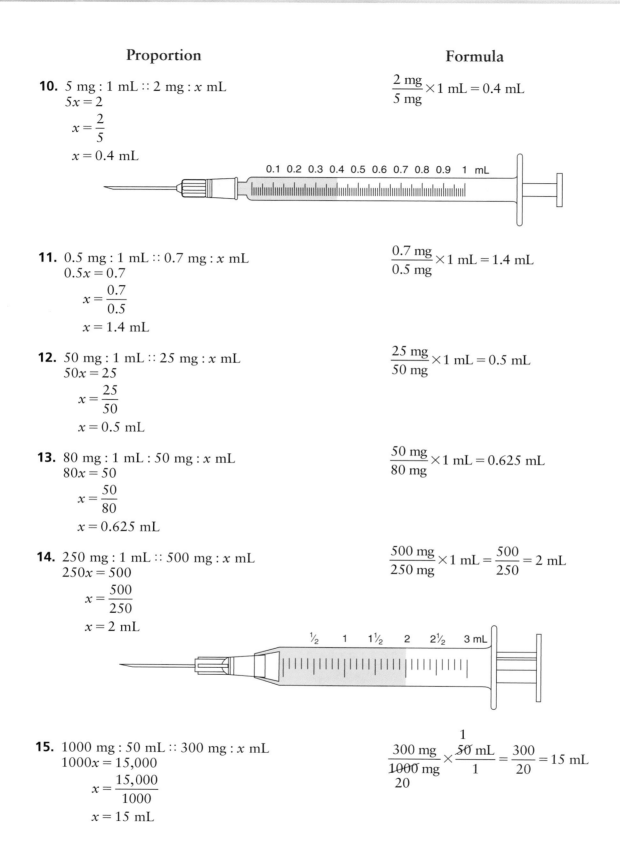

11. 0.5 mg : 1 mL :: 0.7 mg : x mL

$0.5x = 0.7$

$x = \dfrac{0.7}{0.5}$

$x = 1.4$ mL

$\dfrac{0.7 \text{ mg}}{0.5 \text{ mg}} \times 1 \text{ mL} = 1.4 \text{ mL}$

12. 50 mg : 1 mL :: 25 mg : x mL

$50x = 25$

$x = \dfrac{25}{50}$

$x = 0.5$ mL

$\dfrac{25 \text{ mg}}{50 \text{ mg}} \times 1 \text{ mL} = 0.5 \text{ mL}$

13. 80 mg : 1 mL : 50 mg : x mL

$80x = 50$

$x = \dfrac{50}{80}$

$x = 0.625$ mL

$\dfrac{50 \text{ mg}}{80 \text{ mg}} \times 1 \text{ mL} = 0.625 \text{ mL}$

14. 250 mg : 1 mL :: 500 mg : x mL

$250x = 500$

$x = \dfrac{500}{250}$

$x = 2$ mL

$\dfrac{500 \text{ mg}}{250 \text{ mg}} \times 1 \text{ mL} = \dfrac{500}{250} = 2 \text{ mL}$

15. 1000 mg : 50 mL :: 300 mg : x mL

$1000x = 15{,}000$

$x = \dfrac{15{,}000}{1000}$

$x = 15$ mL

$\dfrac{300 \text{ mg}}{\underset{20}{\cancel{1000} \text{ mg}}} \times \dfrac{\overset{1}{\cancel{50} \text{ mL}}}{1} = \dfrac{300}{20} = 15 \text{ mL}$

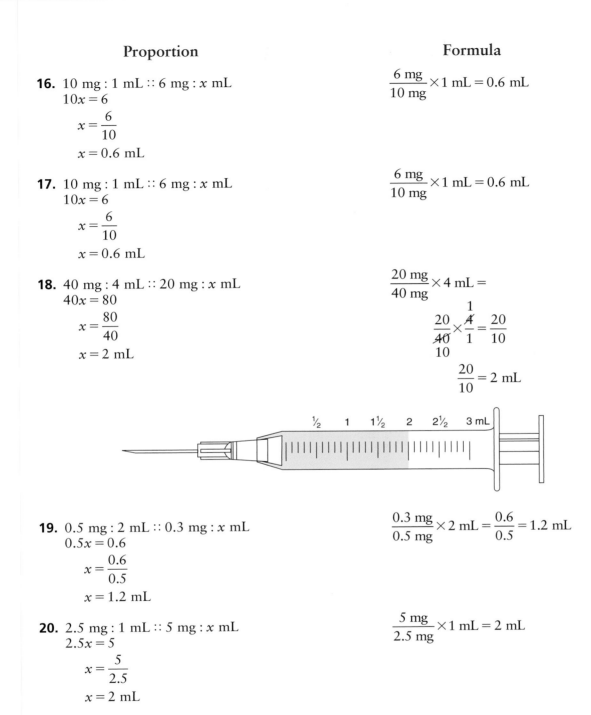

Proportion	**Formula**

16. $10 \text{ mg} : 1 \text{ mL} :: 6 \text{ mg} : x \text{ mL}$
$10x = 6$
$x = \dfrac{6}{10}$
$x = 0.6 \text{ mL}$

$\dfrac{6 \text{ mg}}{10 \text{ mg}} \times 1 \text{ mL} = 0.6 \text{ mL}$

17. $10 \text{ mg} : 1 \text{ mL} :: 6 \text{ mg} : x \text{ mL}$
$10x = 6$
$x = \dfrac{6}{10}$
$x = 0.6 \text{ mL}$

$\dfrac{6 \text{ mg}}{10 \text{ mg}} \times 1 \text{ mL} = 0.6 \text{ mL}$

18. $40 \text{ mg} : 4 \text{ mL} :: 20 \text{ mg} : x \text{ mL}$
$40x = 80$
$x = \dfrac{80}{40}$
$x = 2 \text{ mL}$

$\dfrac{20 \text{ mg}}{40 \text{ mg}} \times 4 \text{ mL} =$

$\dfrac{20}{\overset{}{\underset{10}{\cancel{40}}}} \times \dfrac{\overset{1}{\cancel{4}}}{1} = \dfrac{20}{10}$

$\dfrac{20}{10} = 2 \text{ mL}$

19. $0.5 \text{ mg} : 2 \text{ mL} :: 0.3 \text{ mg} : x \text{ mL}$
$0.5x = 0.6$
$x = \dfrac{0.6}{0.5}$
$x = 1.2 \text{ mL}$

$\dfrac{0.3 \text{ mg}}{0.5 \text{ mg}} \times 2 \text{ mL} = \dfrac{0.6}{0.5} = 1.2 \text{ mL}$

20. $2.5 \text{ mg} : 1 \text{ mL} :: 5 \text{ mg} : x \text{ mL}$
$2.5x = 5$
$x = \dfrac{5}{2.5}$
$x = 2 \text{ mL}$

$\dfrac{5 \text{ mg}}{2.5 \text{ mg}} \times 1 \text{ mL} = 2 \text{ mL}$

Chapter 14 Parenteral Dosages—Posttest 2, pp. 307–312

Proportion	Formula

1. 4 mg : 1 mL :: 2 mg : x mL
$4x = 2$

$x = \dfrac{2}{4}$

$x = 0.5$ mL

$\dfrac{2 \text{ mg}}{4 \text{ mg}} \times 1 \text{ mL} = 0.5 \text{ mL}$

2. 4 mg : 1 mL :: 2 mg : x mL
$4x = 2$

$x = \dfrac{2}{4}$

$x = 0.5$ mL

$\dfrac{2 \text{ mg}}{4 \text{ mg}} \times 1 \text{ mL} = 0.5 \text{ mL}$

3. 500 mg : 10 mL :: 400 mg : x mL
$500x = 4000$

$x = \dfrac{4000}{500}$

$x = 8$ mL

$\dfrac{\overset{4}{\cancel{400}} \text{ mg}}{\underset{5}{\cancel{500}} \text{ mg}} \times 10 \text{ mL} = \dfrac{40}{5} = 8 \text{ mL}$

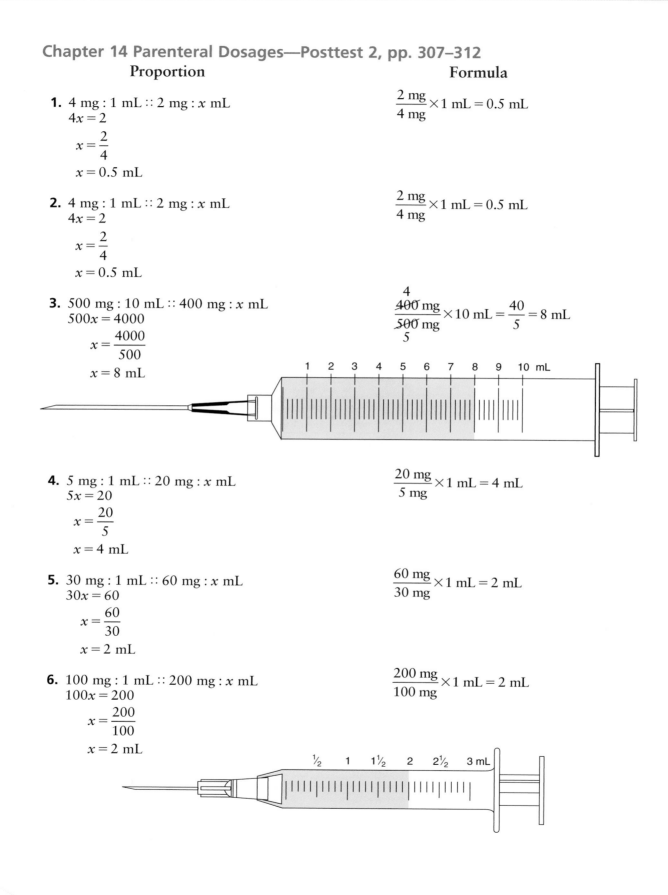

4. 5 mg : 1 mL :: 20 mg : x mL
$5x = 20$

$x = \dfrac{20}{5}$

$x = 4$ mL

$\dfrac{20 \text{ mg}}{5 \text{ mg}} \times 1 \text{ mL} = 4 \text{ mL}$

5. 30 mg : 1 mL :: 60 mg : x mL
$30x = 60$

$x = \dfrac{60}{30}$

$x = 2$ mL

$\dfrac{60 \text{ mg}}{30 \text{ mg}} \times 1 \text{ mL} = 2 \text{ mL}$

6. 100 mg : 1 mL :: 200 mg : x mL
$100x = 200$

$x = \dfrac{200}{100}$

$x = 2$ mL

$\dfrac{200 \text{ mg}}{100 \text{ mg}} \times 1 \text{ mL} = 2 \text{ mL}$

Proportion	Formula

7. $0.4 \text{ mg} : 1 \text{ mL} :: 0.3 \text{ mg} : x \text{ mL}$

$0.4x = 0.3$

$x = \dfrac{0.3}{0.4}$

$x = 0.75 \text{ mL}$

$\dfrac{0.3 \text{ mg}}{0.4 \text{ mg}} \times 1 \text{ mL} = 0.75 \text{ mL}$

8. $50 \text{ mg} : 1 \text{ mL} :: 25 \text{ mg} : x \text{ mL}$

$50x = 25$

$x = \dfrac{25}{50}$

$x = 0.5 \text{ mL}$

$\dfrac{25 \text{ mg}}{50 \text{ mg}} \times 1 \text{ mL} = 0.5 \text{ mL}$

9. $20 \text{ mg} : 1 \text{ mL} :: 100 \text{ mg} : x \text{ mL}$

$20x = 100$

$x = \dfrac{100}{20}$

$x = 5 \text{ mL}$

$\dfrac{100 \text{ mg}}{20 \text{ mg}} \times 1 \text{ mL} = 5 \text{ mL}$

10. $50 \text{ mg} : 1 \text{ mL} :: 75 \text{ mg} : x \text{ mL}$

$50x = 75$

$x = \dfrac{75}{50}$

$x = 1.5 \text{ mL}$

$\dfrac{75 \text{ mg}}{50 \text{ mg}} \times 1 \text{ mL} = 1.5 \text{ mL}$

11. $125 \text{ mg} : 1 \text{ mL} :: 200 \text{ mg} : x \text{ mL}$

$125x = 200$

$x = \dfrac{200}{125}$

$x = 1.6 \text{ mL}$

$\dfrac{200 \text{ mg}}{125 \text{ mg}} \times 1 \text{ mL} = 1.6 \text{ mL}$

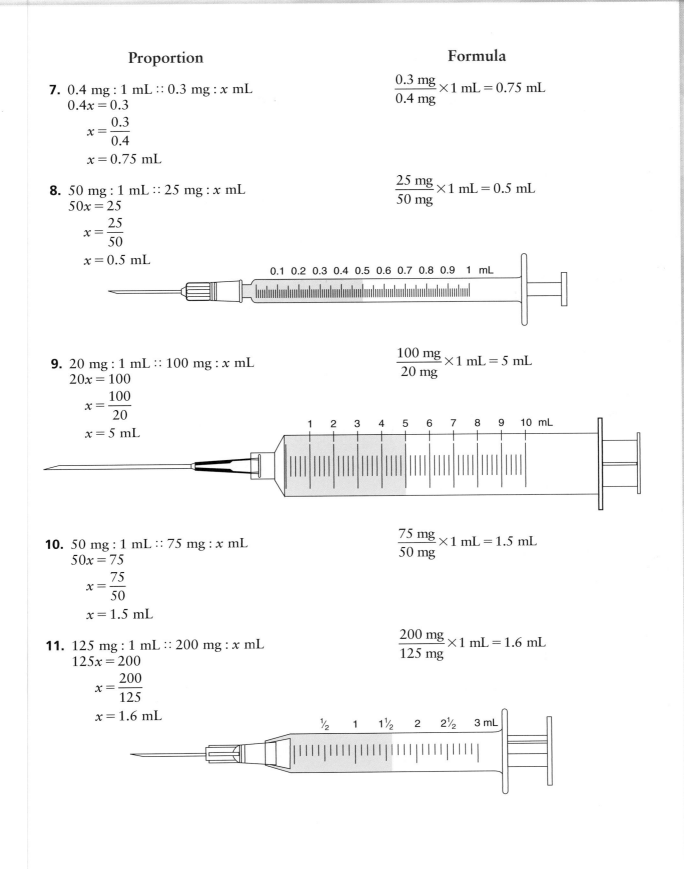

Proportion

Formula

12. $\frac{1}{200}$ gr : 1 mL :: $\frac{1}{150}$ gr : x mL

$$\frac{1}{200}x = \frac{1}{150}$$

$$x = \frac{200}{150}$$

$$x = 1.33 \text{ mL}$$

$$\frac{\frac{1}{150}\text{ gr}}{\frac{1}{200}\text{ gr}} \times 1 \text{ mL} =$$

$$\frac{1}{150} \times \frac{200}{1} = \frac{200}{150}$$

$$\frac{200}{150} = 1.33 \text{ mL}$$

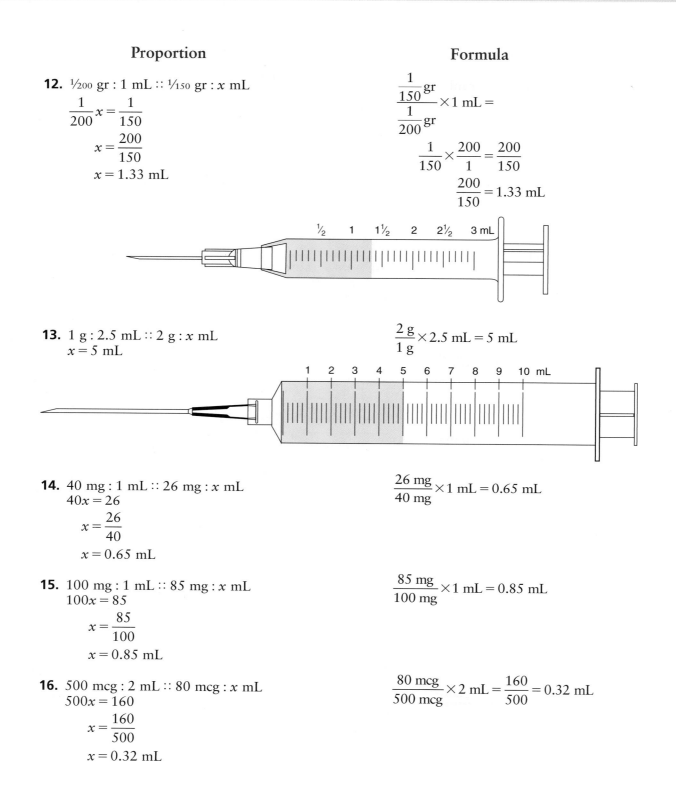

13. 1 g : 2.5 mL :: 2 g : x mL

$x = 5$ mL

$$\frac{2\text{ g}}{1\text{ g}} \times 2.5 \text{ mL} = 5 \text{ mL}$$

14. 40 mg : 1 mL :: 26 mg : x mL

$$40x = 26$$

$$x = \frac{26}{40}$$

$$x = 0.65 \text{ mL}$$

$$\frac{26\text{ mg}}{40\text{ mg}} \times 1 \text{ mL} = 0.65 \text{ mL}$$

15. 100 mg : 1 mL :: 85 mg : x mL

$$100x = 85$$

$$x = \frac{85}{100}$$

$$x = 0.85 \text{ mL}$$

$$\frac{85\text{ mg}}{100\text{ mg}} \times 1 \text{ mL} = 0.85 \text{ mL}$$

16. 500 mcg : 2 mL :: 80 mcg : x mL

$$500x = 160$$

$$x = \frac{160}{500}$$

$$x = 0.32 \text{ mL}$$

$$\frac{80\text{ mcg}}{500\text{ mcg}} \times 2 \text{ mL} = \frac{160}{500} = 0.32 \text{ mL}$$

Proportion	Formula

17. $8 \text{ mg} : 1 \text{ mL} :: 4 \text{ mg} : x \text{ mL}$

$$8x = 4$$

$$x = \frac{4}{8}$$

$$x = 0.5 \text{ mL}$$

$$\frac{4 \text{ mg}}{8 \text{ mg}} \times 1 \text{ mL} = 0.5 \text{ mL}$$

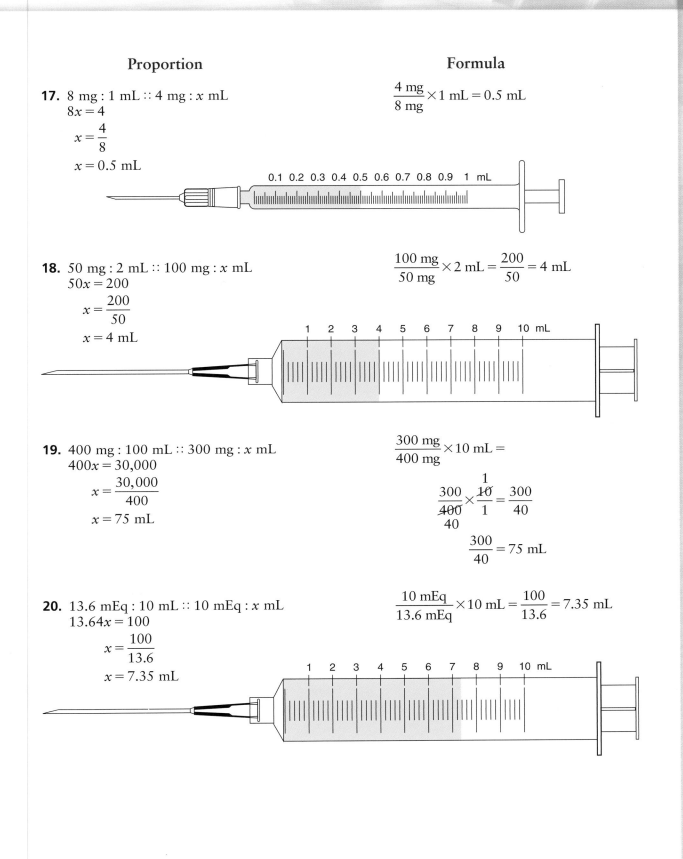

18. $50 \text{ mg} : 2 \text{ mL} :: 100 \text{ mg} : x \text{ mL}$

$$50x = 200$$

$$x = \frac{200}{50}$$

$$x = 4 \text{ mL}$$

$$\frac{100 \text{ mg}}{50 \text{ mg}} \times 2 \text{ mL} = \frac{200}{50} = 4 \text{ mL}$$

19. $400 \text{ mg} : 100 \text{ mL} :: 300 \text{ mg} : x \text{ mL}$

$$400x = 30,000$$

$$x = \frac{30,000}{400}$$

$$x = 75 \text{ mL}$$

$$\frac{300 \text{ mg}}{400 \text{ mg}} \times 10 \text{ mL} =$$

$$\frac{300}{\underset{40}{\cancel{400}}} \times \frac{\overset{1}{\cancel{10}}}{1} = \frac{300}{40}$$

$$\frac{300}{40} = 75 \text{ mL}$$

20. $13.6 \text{ mEq} : 10 \text{ mL} :: 10 \text{ mEq} : x \text{ mL}$

$$13.64x = 100$$

$$x = \frac{100}{13.6}$$

$$x = 7.35 \text{ mL}$$

$$\frac{10 \text{ mEq}}{13.6 \text{ mEq}} \times 10 \text{ mL} = \frac{100}{13.6} = 7.35 \text{ mL}$$

Proportion   Formula

1. 400,000 units : 5 mL :: 200,000 units : x mL

400,000x = 1,000,000

$x = \dfrac{1,000,000}{400,000}$

$x = 2.5$ mL

$\dfrac{200,000 \text{ units}}{\underset{80,000}{\cancel{400,000} \text{ units}}} \times \dfrac{\overset{1}{\cancel{5}} \text{ mL}}{1} =$

$\dfrac{200,000}{80,000} = 2.5$ mL

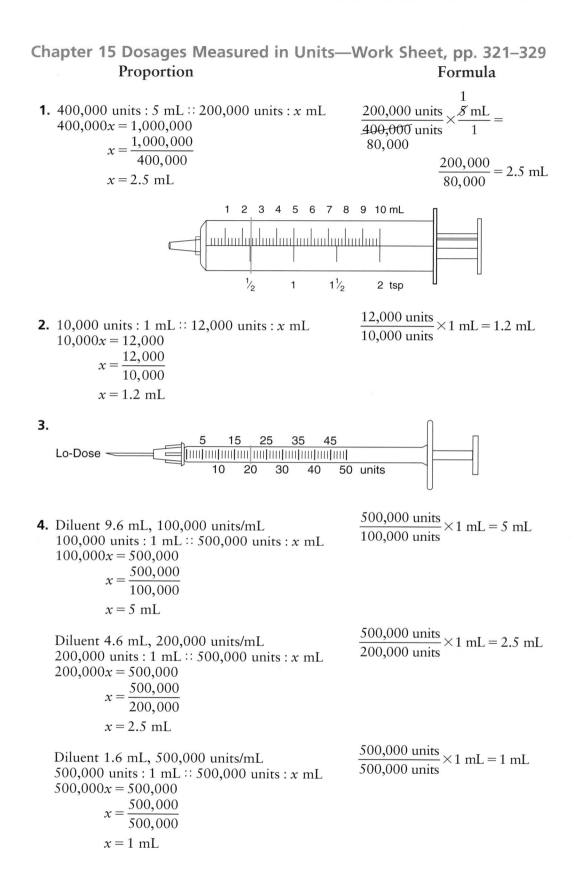

2. 10,000 units : 1 mL :: 12,000 units : x mL

10,000x = 12,000

$x = \dfrac{12,000}{10,000}$

$x = 1.2$ mL

$\dfrac{12,000 \text{ units}}{10,000 \text{ units}} \times 1 \text{ mL} = 1.2 \text{ mL}$

3.

4. Diluent 9.6 mL, 100,000 units/mL

100,000 units : 1 mL :: 500,000 units : x mL

100,000x = 500,000

$x = \dfrac{500,000}{100,000}$

$x = 5$ mL

$\dfrac{500,000 \text{ units}}{100,000 \text{ units}} \times 1 \text{ mL} = 5 \text{ mL}$

Diluent 4.6 mL, 200,000 units/mL

200,000 units : 1 mL :: 500,000 units : x mL

200,000x = 500,000

$x = \dfrac{500,000}{200,000}$

$x = 2.5$ mL

$\dfrac{500,000 \text{ units}}{200,000 \text{ units}} \times 1 \text{ mL} = 2.5 \text{ mL}$

Diluent 1.6 mL, 500,000 units/mL

500,000 units : 1 mL :: 500,000 units : x mL

500,000x = 500,000

$x = \dfrac{500,000}{500,000}$

$x = 1$ mL

$\dfrac{500,000 \text{ units}}{500,000 \text{ units}} \times 1 \text{ mL} = 1 \text{ mL}$

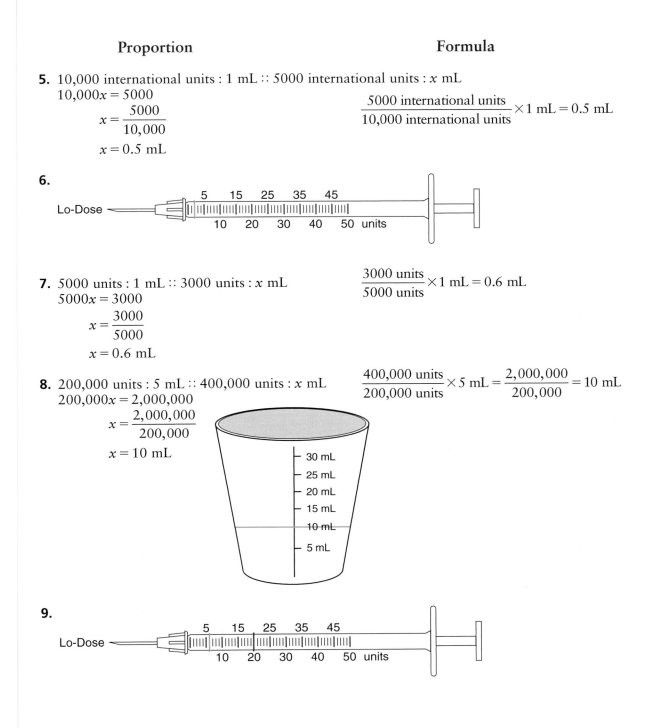

Proportion	Formula

5. 10,000 international units : 1 mL :: 5000 international units : x mL
$$10{,}000x = 5000$$
$$x = \frac{5000}{10{,}000}$$
$$x = 0.5 \text{ mL}$$

$$\frac{5000 \text{ international units}}{10{,}000 \text{ international units}} \times 1 \text{ mL} = 0.5 \text{ mL}$$

6.
Lo-Dose

5   15   25   35   45
10   20   30   40   50   units

7. 5000 units : 1 mL :: 3000 units : x mL
$$5000x = 3000$$
$$x = \frac{3000}{5000}$$
$$x = 0.6 \text{ mL}$$

$$\frac{3000 \text{ units}}{5000 \text{ units}} \times 1 \text{ mL} = 0.6 \text{ mL}$$

8. 200,000 units : 5 mL :: 400,000 units : x mL
$$200{,}000x = 2{,}000{,}000$$
$$x = \frac{2{,}000{,}000}{200{,}000}$$
$$x = 10 \text{ mL}$$

$$\frac{400{,}000 \text{ units}}{200{,}000 \text{ units}} \times 5 \text{ mL} = \frac{2{,}000{,}000}{200{,}000} = 10 \text{ mL}$$

30 mL
25 mL
20 mL
15 mL
10 mL
5 mL

9.
Lo-Dose

5   15   25   35   45
10   20   30   40   50   units

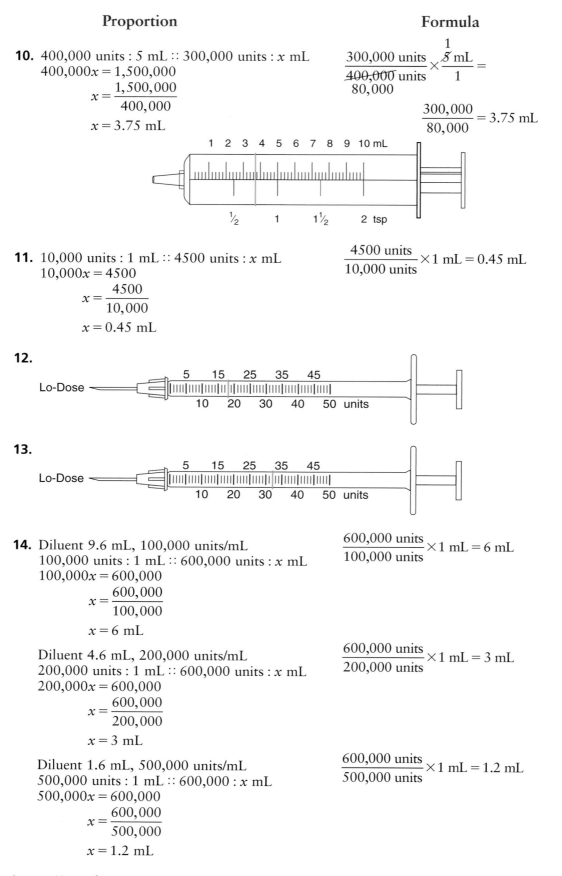

	Proportion	**Formula**

10. 400,000 units : 5 mL :: 300,000 units : x mL

400,000x = 1,500,000

$x = \dfrac{1,500,000}{400,000}$

$x = 3.75$ mL

$$\dfrac{300,000 \text{ units}}{\overline{400,000} \text{ units}} \times \dfrac{\overset{1}{\cancel{5}} \text{ mL}}{1} =$$

80,000

$$\dfrac{300,000}{80,000} = 3.75 \text{ mL}$$

11. 10,000 units : 1 mL :: 4500 units : x mL

10,000x = 4500

$x = \dfrac{4500}{10,000}$

$x = 0.45$ mL

$$\dfrac{4500 \text{ units}}{10,000 \text{ units}} \times 1 \text{ mL} = 0.45 \text{ mL}$$

12.

13.

14. Diluent 9.6 mL, 100,000 units/mL

100,000 units : 1 mL :: 600,000 units : x mL

100,000x = 600,000

$x = \dfrac{600,000}{100,000}$

$x = 6$ mL

$$\dfrac{600,000 \text{ units}}{100,000 \text{ units}} \times 1 \text{ mL} = 6 \text{ mL}$$

Diluent 4.6 mL, 200,000 units/mL

200,000 units : 1 mL :: 600,000 units : x mL

200,000x = 600,000

$x = \dfrac{600,000}{200,000}$

$x = 3$ mL

$$\dfrac{600,000 \text{ units}}{200,000 \text{ units}} \times 1 \text{ mL} = 3 \text{ mL}$$

Diluent 1.6 mL, 500,000 units/mL

500,000 units : 1 mL :: 600,000 : x mL

500,000x = 600,000

$x = \dfrac{600,000}{500,000}$

$x = 1.2$ mL

$$\dfrac{600,000 \text{ units}}{500,000 \text{ units}} \times 1 \text{ mL} = 1.2 \text{ mL}$$

Proportion	Formula

15. 8.2 mL of diluent
500,000 units : 1 mL :: 250,000 units : x mL
500,000x = 250,000
$$x = \frac{250,000}{500,000}$$
$x = 0.5$ mL

$$\frac{250,000 \text{ units}}{500,000 \text{ units}} \times 1 \text{ mL} = 0.5 \text{ mL}$$

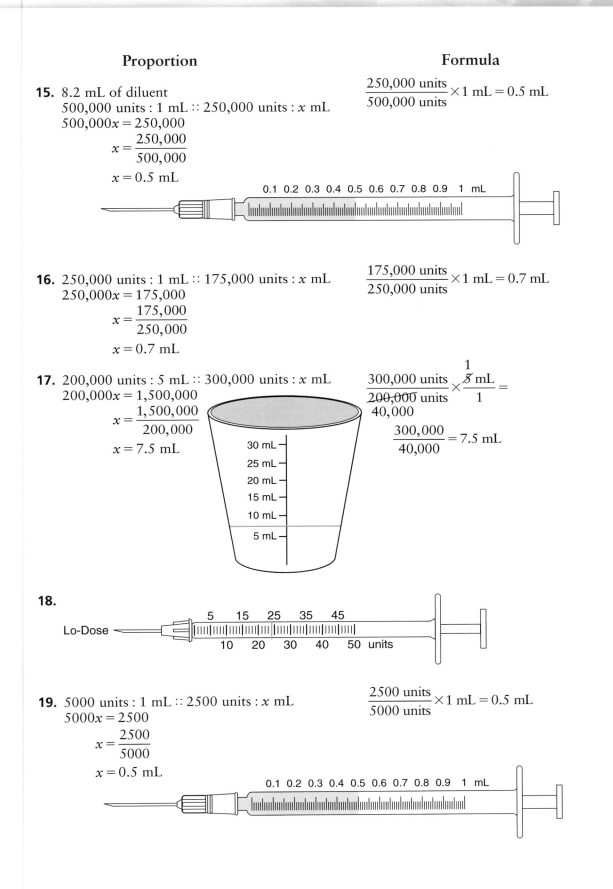

16. 250,000 units : 1 mL :: 175,000 units : x mL
250,000x = 175,000
$$x = \frac{175,000}{250,000}$$
$x = 0.7$ mL

$$\frac{175,000 \text{ units}}{250,000 \text{ units}} \times 1 \text{ mL} = 0.7 \text{ mL}$$

17. 200,000 units : 5 mL :: 300,000 units : x mL
200,000x = 1,500,000
$$x = \frac{1,500,000}{200,000}$$
$x = 7.5$ mL

$$\frac{300,000 \text{ units}}{200,000 \text{ units}} \times \frac{\overset{1}{\cancel{5}} \text{ mL}}{1} =$$
$$\frac{40,000}{300,000} $$
$$\frac{300,000}{40,000} = 7.5 \text{ mL}$$

30 mL
25 mL
20 mL
15 mL
10 mL
5 mL

18.

Lo-Dose

5 15 25 35 45
10 20 30 40 50 units

19. 5000 units : 1 mL :: 2500 units : x mL
5000x = 2500
$$x = \frac{2500}{5000}$$
$x = 0.5$ mL

$$\frac{2500 \text{ units}}{5000 \text{ units}} \times 1 \text{ mL} = 0.5 \text{ mL}$$

0.1 0.2 0.3 0.4 0.5 0.6 0.7 0.8 0.9 1 mL

Proportion   Formula

20. 250,000 units : 1 mL :: 200,000 units : x mL

$$250,000x = 200,000$$

$$x = \frac{200,000}{250,000}$$

$$x = 0.8 \text{ mL}$$

$$\frac{\overset{4}{\cancel{200,000}} \text{ units}}{\underset{5}{\cancel{250,000}} \text{ units}} \times 1 \text{ mL} = 0.8 \text{ mL}$$

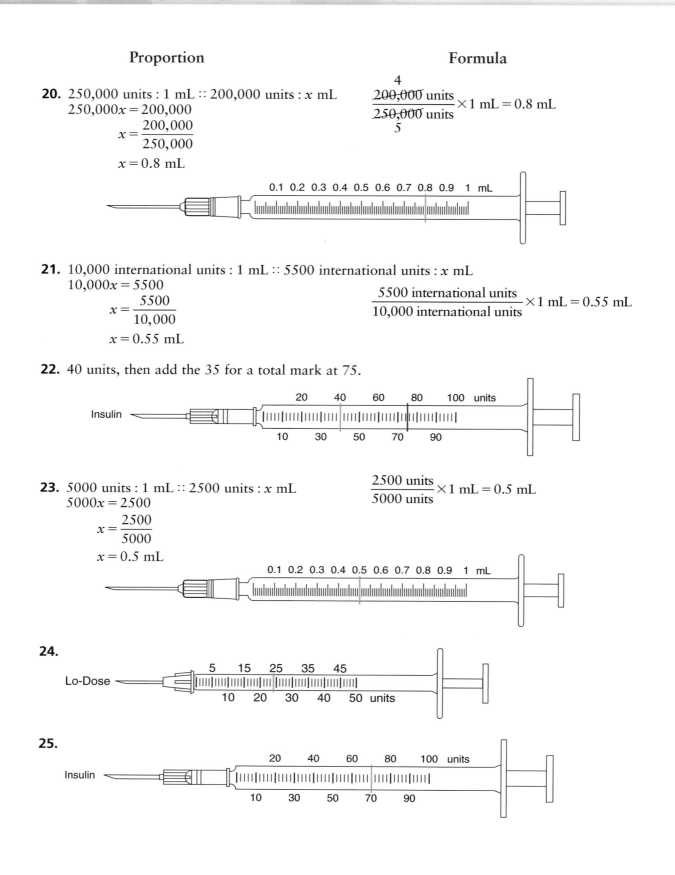

21. 10,000 international units : 1 mL :: 5500 international units : x mL

$$10,000x = 5500$$

$$x = \frac{5500}{10,000}$$

$$x = 0.55 \text{ mL}$$

$$\frac{5500 \text{ international units}}{10,000 \text{ international units}} \times 1 \text{ mL} = 0.55 \text{ mL}$$

22. 40 units, then add the 35 for a total mark at 75.

23. 5000 units : 1 mL :: 2500 units : x mL

$$5000x = 2500$$

$$x = \frac{2500}{5000}$$

$$x = 0.5 \text{ mL}$$

$$\frac{2500 \text{ units}}{5000 \text{ units}} \times 1 \text{ mL} = 0.5 \text{ mL}$$

24.

25.

Proportion	Formula

1. 400,000 units : 5 mL :: 500,000 units : x mL

400,000x = 2,500,000

$x = \dfrac{2,500,000}{400,000}$

x = 6.25 mL

$\dfrac{500,000 \text{ units}}{400,000 \text{ units}} \times 5 \text{ mL} =$

$\dfrac{25}{4} = 6.25$ mL

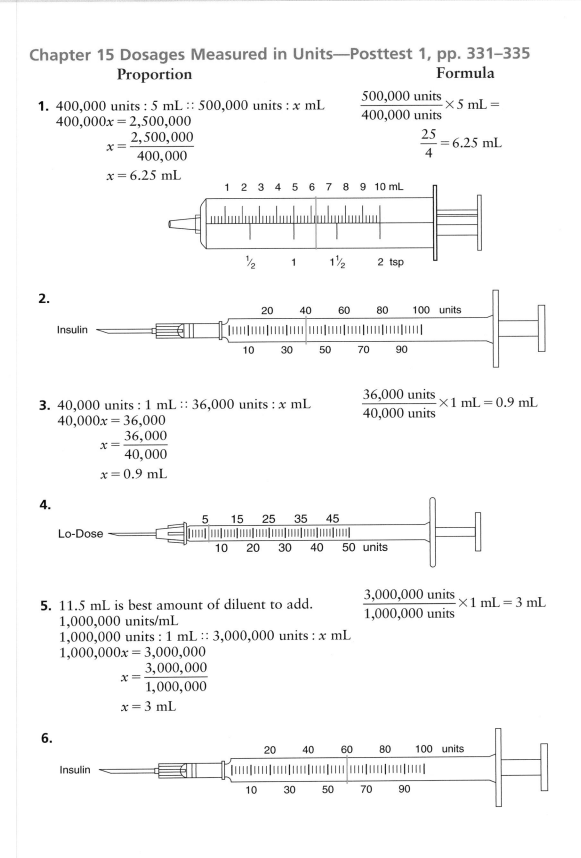

2.

3. 40,000 units : 1 mL :: 36,000 units : x mL

40,000x = 36,000

$x = \dfrac{36,000}{40,000}$

x = 0.9 mL

$\dfrac{36,000 \text{ units}}{40,000 \text{ units}} \times 1 \text{ mL} = 0.9 \text{ mL}$

4.

5. 11.5 mL is best amount of diluent to add.

1,000,000 units/mL

1,000,000 units : 1 mL :: 3,000,000 units : x mL

1,000,000x = 3,000,000

$x = \dfrac{3,000,000}{1,000,000}$

x = 3 mL

$\dfrac{3,000,000 \text{ units}}{1,000,000 \text{ units}} \times 1 \text{ mL} = 3 \text{ mL}$

6.

Proportion	Formula

7. Diluent added = 1.5 mL.
500,000 units : 1 mL :: 600,000 units : x mL
$500,000x = 600,000$
$x = \dfrac{600,000}{500,000}$
$x = 1.2$ mL

$\dfrac{600,000 \text{ units}}{500,000 \text{ units}} \times 1 \text{ mL} = 1.2 \text{ mL}$

8.

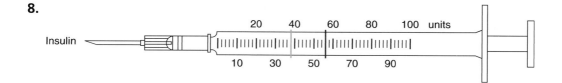

9. 200,000 units : 5 mL :: 300,000 units : x mL
$200,000x = 1,500,000$
$x = \dfrac{1,500,000}{200,000}$
$x = 7.5$ mL

$\dfrac{300,000 \text{ units}}{200,000 \text{ units}} \times 5 \text{ mL} =$

$\dfrac{15}{2} = 7.5 \text{ mL}$

10. Diluent added = 11.5 mL
Concentration is 1,000,000 units/mL
1,000,000 units : 1 mL :: 1,200,000 units : x
$1,000,000x = 1,200,000$
$x = \dfrac{1,200,000}{1,000,000}$
$x = 1.2$ mL

$\dfrac{1,200,000 \text{ units}}{1,000,000 \text{ units}} \times 1 \text{ mL} = 1.2 \text{ mL}$

11. 400,000 units : 5 mL :: 200,000 units : x mL
$400,000x = 1,000,000$
$x = \dfrac{1,000,000}{400,000}$
$x = 2.5$ mL

$\dfrac{200,000 \text{ units}}{400,000 \text{ units}} \times 5 \text{ mL} =$

$\dfrac{1,000,000}{400,000} = 2.5 \text{ mL}$

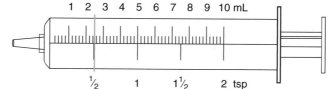

12. 2500 units : 1 mL :: 5000 units : x mL
$2500x = 5000$
$x = \dfrac{5000}{2500}$
$x = 2$ mL

$\dfrac{5000 \text{ units}}{2500 \text{ units}} \times 1 \text{ mL} = 2 \text{ mL}$

Proportion	Formula

13. 10,000 international units : 1 mL :: 8700 international units : x mL
10,000x = 8700

$$x = \frac{8700}{10,000}$$

$x = 0.87$ mL

$$\frac{8700 \text{ international units}}{10,000 \text{ international units}} \times 1 \text{ mL} = 0.87 \text{ mL}$$

14. 100,000 units : 1 mL :: 600,000 units : x mL
100,000x = 600,000

$$x = \frac{600,000}{100,000}$$

$x = 6$ mL

$$\frac{600,000 \text{ units}}{100,000 \text{ units}} \times 1 \text{ mL} = 6 \text{ mL}$$

15. 3000 units : 1 mL :: 2200 units : x mL
3000x = 2200

$$x = \frac{2200}{3000}$$

$x = 0.73$ mL

$$\frac{2200 \text{ units}}{3000 \text{ units}} \times 1 \text{ mL} = 0.73 \text{ mL}$$

Chapter 15 Dosages Measured in Units—Posttest 2, pp. 337–342

Proportion	Formula

1.

2. 10,000 units : 1 mL :: 14,000 units : x mL
10,000x = 14,000

$$x = \frac{14,000}{10,000}$$

$x = 1.4$ mL

$$\frac{14,000 \text{ units}}{10,000 \text{ units}} \times 1 \text{ mL} = 1.4 \text{ mL}$$

3. 200,000 units : 5 mL :: 500,000 units : x mL
200,000x = 2,500,000

$$x = \frac{2,500,000}{200,000}$$

$x = 12.5$ mL

$$\frac{500,000 \text{ units}}{\underset{40,000}{\cancel{200,000} \text{ units}}} \times \frac{\overset{1}{\cancel{5} \text{ mL}}}{1} = 12.5 \text{ mL}$$

4.

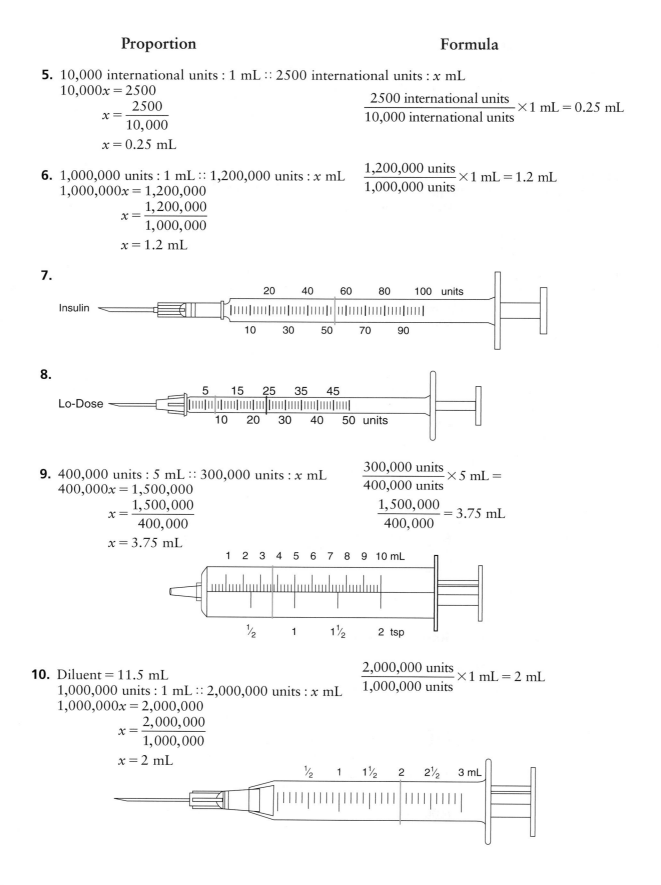

Proportion	Formula

5. 10,000 international units : 1 mL :: 2500 international units : x mL
10,000x = 2500

$$x = \frac{2500}{10,000}$$

$$\frac{2500 \text{ international units}}{10,000 \text{ international units}} \times 1 \text{ mL} = 0.25 \text{ mL}$$

$$x = 0.25 \text{ mL}$$

6. 1,000,000 units : 1 mL :: 1,200,000 units : x mL
1,000,000x = 1,200,000

$$\frac{1,200,000 \text{ units}}{1,000,000 \text{ units}} \times 1 \text{ mL} = 1.2 \text{ mL}$$

$$x = \frac{1,200,000}{1,000,000}$$

$$x = 1.2 \text{ mL}$$

7.

Insulin

8.

Lo-Dose

9. 400,000 units : 5 mL :: 300,000 units : x mL
400,000x = 1,500,000

$$\frac{300,000 \text{ units}}{400,000 \text{ units}} \times 5 \text{ mL} =$$

$$x = \frac{1,500,000}{400,000}$$

$$\frac{1,500,000}{400,000} = 3.75 \text{ mL}$$

$$x = 3.75 \text{ mL}$$

10. Diluent = 11.5 mL
1,000,000 units : 1 mL :: 2,000,000 units : x mL
1,000,000x = 2,000,000

$$\frac{2,000,000 \text{ units}}{1,000,000 \text{ units}} \times 1 \text{ mL} = 2 \text{ mL}$$

$$x = \frac{2,000,000}{1,000,000}$$

$$x = 2 \text{ mL}$$

Proportion
Formula

11. 9.6 mL diluent, 100,000 units/mL
100,000 units : 1 mL :: 600,000 units : x mL
100,000x = 600,000
$$x = \frac{600,000}{100,000}$$
$x = 6$ mL

$$\frac{600,000 \text{ units}}{100,000 \text{ units}} \times 1 \text{ mL} = 6 \text{ mL}$$

4.6 mL diluent, 200,000 units/mL
200,000 units : 1 mL :: 600,000 units : x mL
200,000x = 600,000
$$x = \frac{600,000}{200,000}$$
$x = 3$ mL

$$\frac{600,000 \text{ units}}{200,000 \text{ units}} \times 1 \text{ mL} = 3 \text{ mL}$$

1.6 mL diluent, 500,000 units/mL
500,000 units : 1 mL :: 600,000 units : x mL
500,000x = 600,000
$$x = \frac{600,000}{500,000}$$
$x = 1.2$ mL

$$\frac{600,000 \text{ units}}{500,000 \text{ units}} \times 1 \text{ mL} = 1.2 \text{ mL}$$

12. 250,000 units : 1 mL :: 400,000 units : x mL
250,000x = 400,000
$$x = \frac{400,000}{250,000}$$
$x = 1.6$ mL

$$\frac{400,000 \text{ units}}{250,000 \text{ units}} \times 1 \text{ mL} = 1.6 \text{ mL}$$

13.

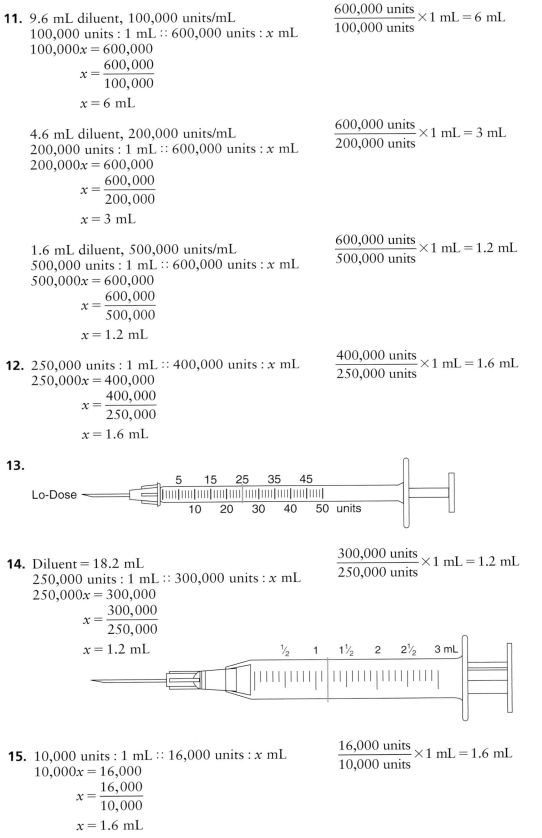

14. Diluent = 18.2 mL
250,000 units : 1 mL :: 300,000 units : x mL
250,000x = 300,000
$$x = \frac{300,000}{250,000}$$
$x = 1.2$ mL

$$\frac{300,000 \text{ units}}{250,000 \text{ units}} \times 1 \text{ mL} = 1.2 \text{ mL}$$

15. 10,000 units : 1 mL :: 16,000 units : x mL
10,000x = 16,000
$$x = \frac{16,000}{10,000}$$
$x = 1.6$ mL

$$\frac{16,000 \text{ units}}{10,000 \text{ units}} \times 1 \text{ mL} = 1.6 \text{ mL}$$

1. $\dfrac{500 \text{ mL}}{24 \text{ h}} = 20.8 \text{ or } 21 \text{ mL/h}$

2. $\dfrac{100 \text{ mL}}{1 \text{ h}} = 100 \text{ mL/h}$

3. $\dfrac{100 \text{ mL}}{\overset{}{\underset{2}{\cancel{30} \text{ min}}}} \times \overset{1}{\cancel{15}} \text{ gtt/mL} = \dfrac{100}{2} = 50 \text{ gtt/min}$

4. $\dfrac{3000 \text{ mL}}{12 \text{ h}} = 250 \text{ mL/h}$

5. $\dfrac{100 \text{ mL}}{\overset{}{\underset{3}{\cancel{30} \text{ min}}}} \times \overset{1}{\cancel{10}} \text{ gtt/mL} = \dfrac{100}{3} = 33.3 \text{ or } 33 \text{ gtt/min}$

6. $\dfrac{500 \text{ mL}}{6 \text{ h}} = 83.3 \text{ or } 83 \text{ mL/h}$

7. $\dfrac{100 \text{ mL}}{\overset{}{\underset{6}{\cancel{60} \text{ min}}}} \times \overset{1}{\cancel{10}} \text{ gtt/mL} = \dfrac{100}{6} = 16.6 \text{ or } 17 \text{ gtt/min}$

Proportion

8. $60 \text{ mEq} : 250 \text{ mL} :: 20 \text{ mEq} : x \text{ mL}$
$60x = 5000$
$x = \dfrac{5000}{60}$
$x = 83.3 \text{ or } 83 \text{ mL/h}$

9. $\dfrac{50 \text{ mL}}{\overset{}{\underset{1}{\cancel{30} \text{ min}}}} \times \overset{2}{\cancel{60}} \text{ gtt/mL} = \dfrac{100}{1} = 100 \text{ gtt/min}$

10. $\dfrac{1000 \text{ mL}}{10 \text{ h}} = 100 \text{ mL/h}$

11. $\dfrac{50 \text{ mL}}{\overset{}{\underset{1}{\cancel{15} \text{ min}}}} \times \overset{4}{\cancel{60}} \text{ gtt/mL} = 200 \text{ gtt/min}$

12. $400 \text{ mg} : 200 \text{ mL} :: 200 \text{ mg} : x \text{ mL}$
$400x = 40{,}000$
$x = \dfrac{40{,}000}{400}$
$x = 100 \text{ mL/h}$

Formula

$\dfrac{\overset{2}{20 \text{ mEq}}}{\underset{6}{\cancel{60} \text{ mEq}}} \times 250 \text{ mL} =$
$\dfrac{500}{6} = 83.3 \text{ mL or } 83 \text{ mL/h}$

$\dfrac{200 \text{ mg}}{\underset{2}{\cancel{400} \text{ mg}}} \times \overset{1}{\cancel{200}} \text{ mL} =$
$\dfrac{200}{2} = 100 \text{ mL/h}$

	Proportion	Formula

13. $\dfrac{1000 \text{ mL}}{\underset{6}{\cancel{60} \text{ min}}} \times \overset{1}{\cancel{10}} \text{ gtt/mL} = \dfrac{1000}{6} = 166.6 \text{ or } 167 \text{ gtt/min}$

14. $\dfrac{1000 \text{ mL}}{8 \text{ h}} = 125 \text{ mL/h}$

15. $\dfrac{25 \text{ mL}}{\underset{1}{\cancel{15} \text{ min}}} \times \overset{1}{\cancel{15}} \text{ gtt/mL} = 25 \text{ gtt/min}$

16. 20 mg : 100 mL :: 0.5 mg : x mL
$20x = 50$
$x = \dfrac{50}{20}$
$x = 2.5 \text{ mL/h}$

$\dfrac{0.5 \text{ mg}}{\underset{1}{\cancel{20} \text{ mg}}} \times \overset{5}{\cancel{100}} \text{ mL} =$

$\dfrac{0.5}{1} \times 5 = 2.5 \text{ mL/h}$

17. $\dfrac{25 \text{ mL}}{\underset{3}{\cancel{15} \text{ min}}} \times \overset{4}{\cancel{20}} \text{ gtt/mL} = \dfrac{100}{3} = 33.3 \text{ or } 33 \text{ gtt/min}$

18. 2 g : 100 mL :: 1 g : x mL
$2x = 100$
$x = \dfrac{100}{2}$
$x = 50 \text{ mL/h}$

$\dfrac{1 \text{ g}}{\underset{1}{\cancel{2} \text{ g}}} \times \overset{50}{\cancel{100}} \text{ mL} =$

$\dfrac{50}{1} = 50 \text{ mL/h}$

19. $\dfrac{250 \text{ mL}}{\underset{12}{\cancel{240} \text{ min}}} \times \overset{1}{\cancel{20}} \text{ gtt/mL} = \dfrac{250}{12} = 20.8 \text{ or } 21 \text{ gtt/min}$

20. $\dfrac{500 \text{ mL}}{\underset{24}{\cancel{240} \text{ min}}} \times \overset{1}{\cancel{10}} \text{ gtt/mL} = \dfrac{500}{24} = 20.8 \text{ or } 21 \text{ gtt/min}$

21. 40 mEq : 200 mL :: 10 mEq : x mL
$40x = 2000$
$x = \dfrac{2000}{40}$
$x = 50 \text{ mL/h}$

$\dfrac{10 \text{ mEq}}{\underset{1}{\cancel{40} \text{ mEq}}} \times \overset{5}{\cancel{200}} \text{ mL} =$

$\dfrac{10}{1} \times 5 = 50 \text{ mL/h}$

22. $\dfrac{1350 \text{ mL}}{10 \text{ h}} = 135 \text{ mL/h}$

23. 2 g : 50 mL :: 1 g : x mL
$2x = 50$
$x = \dfrac{50}{2}$
$x = 25 \text{ mL/h}$

$\dfrac{1 \text{ g}}{\underset{1}{\cancel{2} \text{ g}}} \times \overset{25}{\cancel{50}} \text{ mL} =$

$\dfrac{25}{1} = 25 \text{ mL/h}$

Proportion   Formula

24. $\dfrac{200 \text{ mL}}{1 \text{ h}} = 200$ mL/h

25. $\dfrac{50 \text{ mL}}{\cancel{30}^{\,3} \text{ min}} \times \cancel{20}^{\,2} \text{ gtt/mL} = \dfrac{100}{3} = 33.3$ or 33 gtt/min

26. $\dfrac{50 \text{ mL}}{0.5 \text{ h}} = 100$ mL/h

27. $\dfrac{200 \text{ mL}}{\cancel{60}^{\,3} \text{ min}} \times \cancel{20}^{\,1} \text{ gtt/mL} = \dfrac{200}{3} = 66.66$ or 67 gtt/min

28. $\dfrac{500 \text{ mL}}{8 \text{ h}} = 62.5$ or 63 mL/h

29. $200 \text{ mg} : 250 \text{ mL} :: 5 \text{ mg} : x \text{ mL}$
$200x = 150$
$x = \dfrac{1250}{200}$
$x = 6.25$ or 6.3 mL/h

$\dfrac{5 \text{ mg}}{200 \text{ mg}} \times 250 \text{ mL} = \dfrac{1250}{200} = 6.25$ or 6.3 mL/h

30. $\dfrac{50 \text{ mL}}{\cancel{30}^{\,1} \text{ min}} \times \cancel{60}^{\,2} \text{ gtt/mL} = 100$ gtt/min

31. $\dfrac{250 \text{ mL}}{2 \text{ h}} = 125$ mL/h

32. $\dfrac{1000 \text{ mL}}{10 \text{ h}} = 100$ mL/h

33. $\dfrac{9600 \text{ mL}}{8 \text{ h}} = 1200$ mL/h

34. $\dfrac{100 \text{ mL}}{3 \text{ h}} = 33.3$ or 33 mL/h

35. $100 \text{ mg} : 100 \text{ mL} :: 20 \text{ mg} : x \text{ mL}$
$100x = 2000$
$x = \dfrac{2000}{100}$
$x = 20$ mL/h

$\dfrac{20 \text{ mg}}{\cancel{100}^{\,1} \text{ mg}} \times \cancel{100}^{\,1} \text{ mL} = 20$ mL/h

36. $\dfrac{100 \text{ mL}}{0.25 \text{ h}} = 400$ mL/h

Proportion   Formula

1. $\dfrac{500 \text{ mL}}{2 \text{ h}} = 250 \text{ mL/h}$

2. $\dfrac{500 \text{ mL}}{4 \text{ h}} = 125 \text{ mL/h}$

3. $\dfrac{120 \text{ mL}}{\cancel{60}\ 5 \text{ min}} \times \cancel{12}^{\ 1} \text{ gtt/mL} = \dfrac{120}{5} = 24 \text{ gtt/min}$

4. $\dfrac{1500 \text{ mL}}{8 \text{ h}} = 187.5 \text{ or } 188 \text{ mL/h}$

5. $\dfrac{\cancel{500}^{\ 50} \text{ mL}}{\cancel{240}\ 24 \text{ min}} \times 15 \text{ gtt/mL} = \dfrac{750}{24} = 31.2 \text{ or } 31 \text{ gtt/min}$

6. $\dfrac{250 \text{ mL}}{\cancel{180}\ 15 \text{ min}} \times \cancel{12}^{\ 1} \text{ gtt/mL} = \dfrac{250}{15} = 16.6 \text{ or } 17 \text{ gtt/min}$

7. $\dfrac{500 \text{ mL}}{\cancel{360}\ 24 \text{ min}} \times \cancel{15}^{\ 1} \text{ gtt/mL} = \dfrac{500}{24} = 20.8 \text{ or } 21 \text{ gtt/min}$

8. $4 \text{ g} : 250 \text{ mL} :: 2 \text{ g} : x \text{ mL}$
$4x = 500$
$x = \dfrac{500}{4}$
$x = 125 \text{ mL/h}$

                                         $\dfrac{\cancel{2}^{\ 1} \text{ g}}{\cancel{4}\ 2 \text{ g}} \times 250 \text{ mL} =$
                                                  $\dfrac{250}{2} = 125 \text{ mL/h}$

9. $\dfrac{150 \text{ mL}}{\cancel{60}\ 1 \text{ min}} \times \cancel{60}^{\ 1} \text{ gtt/mL} = \dfrac{150}{1} = 150 \text{ gtt/min}$

10. $\dfrac{2500 \text{ mL}}{24 \text{ h}} = 104.1 \text{ or } 104 \text{ mL/h}$

11. $30 \text{ mOsm} : 200 \text{ mL} :: 10 \text{ mOsm} : x \text{ mL}$
$30x = 2000$
$x = \dfrac{2000}{30}$
$x = 66.6 \text{ or } 67 \text{ mL/h}$

                                         $\dfrac{\cancel{10}^{\ 1} \text{ mMos}}{\cancel{30}\ 3 \text{ mMos}} \times 200 \text{ mL} =$
                                                  $\dfrac{200}{3} = 66.6 \text{ or } 67 \text{ mL/h}$

12. $\dfrac{25 \text{ mL}}{\cancel{15}\ 1 \text{ min}} \times \cancel{60}^{\ 4} \text{ gtt/mL} = \dfrac{25}{1} \times 4 = 100 \text{ gtt/min}$

Proportion	**Formula**

13. $100 \text{ mg} : 200 \text{ mL} :: 15 \text{ mg} : x \text{ mL}$

$100x = 3000$

$x = \dfrac{3000}{100}$

$x = 30 \text{ mL/h}$

$\dfrac{15 \text{ mg}}{\overset{}{\underset{1}{\cancel{100}}} \text{ mg}} \times \overset{2}{\cancel{200}} \text{ mL} =$

$\dfrac{15}{1} \times 2 = 30 \text{ mL/h}$

14. $\dfrac{200 \text{ mL}}{4 \text{ h}} = 50 \text{ mL/h}$

15. $\dfrac{100 \text{ mL}}{\underset{1}{\cancel{60}} \text{ min}} \times \overset{1}{\cancel{60}} \text{ gtt/mL} = 100 \text{ gtt/min}$

Chapter 16 Intravenous Flow Rates—Posttest 2, pp. 371–373

Proportion	**Formula**

1. $\dfrac{200 \text{ mL}}{6 \text{ h}} = 33.3 \text{ or } 33 \text{ mL/h}$

2. $\dfrac{50 \text{ mL}}{\underset{3}{\cancel{30}} \text{ min}} \times \overset{1}{\cancel{10}} \text{ gtt/mL} = \dfrac{50}{3} = 16.6 \text{ or } 17 \text{ gtt/min}$

3. $\dfrac{200 \text{ mL}}{6 \text{ h}} = 33.3 \text{ or } 33 \text{ mL/h}$

4. $\dfrac{500 \text{ mL}}{\underset{18}{\cancel{180}} \text{ min}} \times \overset{1}{\cancel{10}} \text{ gtt/mL} = \dfrac{500}{18} = 27.7 \text{ or } 28 \text{ gtt/min}$

5. $\dfrac{500 \text{ mL}}{\underset{12}{\cancel{180}} \text{ min}} \times \overset{1}{\cancel{15}} \text{ gtt/mL} = \dfrac{500}{12} = 41.6 \text{ or } 42 \text{ gtt/min}$

6. $\dfrac{50 \text{ mL}}{0.5 \text{ h}} = 100 \text{ mL/h}$

7. $100 \text{ mg} : 100 \text{ mL} :: 8 \text{ mg} : x$

$100x = 800$

$x = \dfrac{800}{100}$

$x = 8 \text{ mL/h}$

$\dfrac{8 \text{ mg}}{\overset{}{\underset{1}{\cancel{100}}} \text{ mg}} \times \overset{1}{\cancel{100}} \text{ mL} =$

$\dfrac{8}{1} = 8 \text{ mL/h}$

8. $\dfrac{50 \text{ mL}}{\underset{1}{\cancel{15}} \text{ min}} \times \overset{4}{\cancel{60}} \text{ gtt/mL} = \dfrac{200}{1} = 200 \text{ gtt/min}$

9. $\dfrac{50 \text{ mL}}{\underset{1}{\cancel{15}} \text{ min}} \times \overset{1}{\cancel{15}} \text{ gtt/mL} = \dfrac{50}{1} = 50 \text{ gtt/min}$

Proportion   Formula

10. $\dfrac{1000 \text{ mL}}{6 \text{ h}} = 166.6$ or 167 mL/h

11. $8 \text{ mg} : 100 \text{ mL} :: 0.4 \text{ mg} : x \text{ mL}$
$8x = 40$
$x = \dfrac{40}{8}$
$x = 5 \text{ mL/h}$

$\dfrac{0.4 \text{ mg}}{\underset{2}{\cancel{8} \text{ mg}}} \times \overset{25}{\cancel{100}} \text{ mL} =$
$\dfrac{10}{2} = 5 \text{ mL/h}$

12. $\dfrac{1200 \text{ mL}}{8 \text{ h}} = 150 \text{ mL/h}$

13. $\dfrac{25 \text{ mL}}{0.25 \text{ h}} = 100 \text{ mL/h}$

14. $\dfrac{1000 \text{ mL}}{\underset{18}{\cancel{180} \text{ min}}} \times \overset{1}{\cancel{10}} \text{ gtt/mL} = \dfrac{1000}{18} = 55.5$ or 56 gtt/min

15. $\dfrac{1000 \text{ mL}}{12 \text{ h}} = 83.3$ or 83 mL/h

Chapter 17 Critical Care Intravenous Flow Rates—Work Sheet, pp. 383–390

Proportion   Formula

1. $25,000 \text{ units} : 250 \text{ mL} :: 1000 \text{ units} : x \text{ mL}$
$25,000x = 250,000$
$x = \dfrac{250,000}{25,000}$
$x = 10 \text{ mL/h}$

$\dfrac{1000 \text{ units}}{\underset{100}{\cancel{25,000} \text{ units}}} \times \overset{1}{\cancel{250}} \text{ mL} =$
$\dfrac{1000}{100} = 10 \text{ mL/h}$

2. $100 \text{ units} : 250 \text{ mL} :: 12 \text{ units} : x \text{ mL}$
$100x = 3000$
$x = \dfrac{3000}{100}$
$x = 30 \text{ mL/h}$

$\dfrac{12 \text{ units}}{\underset{2}{\cancel{100} \text{ units}}} \times \overset{5}{\cancel{250}} \text{ mL} =$
$\dfrac{60}{2} = 30 \text{ mL/h}$

3. $100 \text{ units} : 250 \text{ mL} :: 8 \text{ units} : x \text{ mL}$
$100x = 2000$
$x = \dfrac{2000}{100}$
$x = 20 \text{ mL/h}$

$\dfrac{8 \text{ units}}{\underset{2}{\cancel{100} \text{ units}}} \times \overset{5}{\cancel{250}} \text{ mL} =$
$\dfrac{40}{2} = 20 \text{ mL/h}$

4. $10,000 \text{ units} : 500 \text{ mL} :: 1000 \text{ units} : x \text{ mL}$
$10,000x = 500,000$
$x = \dfrac{500,000}{10,000}$
$x = 50 \text{ mL/h}$

$\dfrac{1000 \text{ units}}{\underset{20}{\cancel{10,000} \text{ units}}} \times \overset{1}{\cancel{500}} \text{ mL} =$
$\dfrac{1000}{20} = 50 \text{ mL/h}$

	Proportion	Formula

5. $\dfrac{12\text{ mcg}\times 75\text{ kg}\times 60\text{ min/h}}{4000\text{ mcg/mL}}=\dfrac{54{,}000}{4000}=13.5\text{ mL/h}$

6. $\dfrac{10\text{ mcg/min}\times 60\text{ min/h}}{200\text{ mcg/mL}}=\dfrac{600}{200}=3\text{ mL/h}$

7. $\dfrac{5\text{ mcg}\times 80\text{ kg}\times 60\text{ min/h}}{8000\text{ mcg/mL}}=\dfrac{24{,}000}{8000}=3\text{ mL/h}$

8. 250,000 international units : 45 mL :: 100,000 international units : x mL

$250{,}000x=4{,}500{,}000$

$x=\dfrac{4{,}500{,}000}{250{,}000}$

$x=18\text{ mL/h}$

$\dfrac{\overset{10}{\cancel{100{,}000}}\text{ international units}}{\underset{25}{\cancel{250{,}000}}\text{ international units}}\times 45\text{ mL}=$

$\dfrac{450}{25}=18\text{ mL/h}$

9. $\dfrac{0.5\text{ mg/min}\times 60\text{ min/h}}{1.8\text{ mg/mL}}=\dfrac{30}{1.8}=16.66\text{ mL/h or }16.7\text{ mL/h}$

10. $\dfrac{3\text{ mcg}\times 70\text{ kg}\times 60\text{ min/h}}{200\text{ mcg/mL}}=\dfrac{12{,}600}{200}=63\text{ mL/h}$

11. $\dfrac{10\text{ mcg}\times 100\text{ kg}\times 60\text{ min/h}}{4000\text{ mcg/mL}}=\dfrac{60{,}000}{4000}=15\text{ mL/h}$

12. $\dfrac{30\text{ mcg}\times 75\text{ kg}\times 60\text{ min/h}}{15{,}000\text{ mcg/mL}}=\dfrac{135{,}000}{15{,}000}=9\text{ mL/h}$

13. $\dfrac{4\text{ mg/min}\times 60\text{ min/h}}{8\text{ mg/mL}}=\dfrac{240}{8}=30\text{ mL/h}$

14. $\dfrac{10\text{ mcg/min}\times 60\text{ min/h}}{8\text{ mcg/mL}}=\dfrac{600}{8}=75\text{ mL/h}$

15. $\dfrac{0.75\text{ mg/min}\times 60\text{ min/h}}{1.8\text{ mg/mL}}=\dfrac{45}{1.8}=25\text{ mL/h}$

16. $\dfrac{15\text{ mcg/min}\times 60\text{ min/h}}{16\text{ mcg/mL}}=\dfrac{900}{16}=56.25\text{ or }56\text{ mL/h}$

17. $\dfrac{2\text{ mg/min}\times 60\text{ min/h}}{8\text{ mg/mL}}=\dfrac{120}{8}=15\text{ mL/h}$

18. 25,000 units : 500 mL :: 750 units : x mL

$25{,}000x=375{,}000$

$x=\dfrac{375{,}000}{25{,}000}$

$x=15\text{ mL/h}$

$\dfrac{750\text{ units}}{\underset{50}{\cancel{25{,}000}}\text{ units}}\times \overset{1}{\cancel{500}}\text{ mL}=$

$\dfrac{750}{50}=15\text{ mL/h}$

Proportion	Formula

19. 100 units : 100 mL :: 10 units : x mL

$100x = 1000$

$$x = \frac{1000}{100}$$

$x = 10$ mL/h

$$\frac{10 \text{ units}}{\cancel{100} \text{ units}} \times \overset{1}{\cancel{100}} \text{ mL} =$$

$$\frac{10}{1} = 10 \text{ mL/h}$$

20. $$\frac{10 \text{ mcg} \times 90 \text{ kg} \times 60 \text{ min/h}}{8000 \text{ mcg/mL}} = \frac{54{,}000}{8000} = 6.75 \text{ or } 7 \text{ mL/h}$$

21. $$\frac{4000 \text{ mcg/mL} \times 13.5 \text{ mL/h}}{60 \text{ min/h} \times 75 \text{ kg}} = \frac{54{,}000}{4500} = 12 \text{ mcg/kg/min}$$

22. $$\frac{200 \text{ mcg/mL} \times 3 \text{ mL/h}}{60 \text{ min/h}} = \frac{600}{60} = 10 \text{ mcg/min}$$

23. $$\frac{1.8 \text{ mg/mL} \times 17 \text{ mL/h}}{60 \text{ min/h}} = \frac{30.6}{60} = 0.51 \text{ or } 0.5 \text{ mg/min}$$

24. $$\frac{15{,}000 \text{ mcg/mL} \times 9 \text{ mL/h}}{60 \text{ min/h} \times 75 \text{ kg}} = \frac{135{,}000}{4500} = 30 \text{ mcg/kg/min}$$

25. $$\frac{200 \text{ mcg/mL} \times 5 \text{ mL/h}}{60 \text{ min/h}} = \frac{1000}{60} = 16.66 \text{ or } 16.7 \text{ mcg/min}$$

26. $$\frac{1.8 \text{ mg/mL} \times 20 \text{ mL/h}}{60 \text{ min/h}} = \frac{36}{60} = 0.6 \text{ mg/min}$$

27. $$\frac{4000 \text{ mcg/mL} \times 15 \text{ mL/h}}{60 \text{ min/h} \times 80 \text{ kg}} = \frac{60{,}000}{4800} = 12.5 \text{ mcg/kg/min}$$

28. $$\frac{400 \text{ mcg/mL} \times 10 \text{ mL/h}}{60 \text{ min/h}} = \frac{4000}{60} = 66.66 \text{ or } 66.7 \text{ mcg/min}$$

29. $$\frac{3.6 \text{ mg/mL} \times 15 \text{ mL/h}}{60 \text{ min/h}} = \frac{54}{60} = 0.9 \text{ mg/min}$$

30. $$\frac{2 \text{ mg/mL} \times 15 \text{ mL/h}}{60 \text{ min/h}} = \frac{30}{60} = 0.5 \text{ mg/min}$$

31. Bolus: 1 kg : 70 units :: 60 kg : x units

$x = 4200$ units IV bolus

Infusion: *Step 1*

1 kg : 17 units/h :: 60 kg : x units/h

$x = 17(60) = 1020$ units/h

Step 2

100 units : 1 mL :: 1020 units : x mL

$100x = 1020$

$$x = \frac{1020}{100}$$

$x = 10.2$ mL/h

$$\frac{1020 \text{ units}}{100 \text{ units}} \times 1 \text{ mL} = 10.2 \text{ mL/h}$$

	Proportion	Formula

32. Yes, the heparin drip needs to be reduced by 2 units/kg/h.

Bolus: No bolus is needed.

Infusion: *Step 1* (17 units/kg/h − 2 units/kg/h = 15 units/kg/h
1 kg : 15 units/h :: 60 kg : x units/h
$x = 900$ units/h

Step 2
100 units : 1 mL :: 900 units : x mL
$100x = 900$
$x = \dfrac{900}{100}$
$x = 9$ mL/h

$\dfrac{900 \text{ units}}{100 \text{ units}} \times 1 \text{ mL} = 9 \text{ mL/h}$

33. Bolus: 1 kg : 70 units :: 80 kg : x units
$x = 5600$ units IV bolus

Infusion: *Step 1*
1 kg : 17 units/h :: 80 kg : x units/h
$x = 1360$ units/h

Step 2
100 units : 1 mL :: 1360 units : x mL
$100x = 1360$
$x = \dfrac{1360}{100}$
$x = 13.6$ mL/h

$\dfrac{1360 \text{ units}}{100 \text{ units}} \times 1 \text{ mL} = 13.6 \text{ mL/h}$

34. Yes, provide a bolus of 35 units/kg and increase the heparin drip by 3 units/kg/h.

Bolus: 1 kg : 35 units :: 80 kg : x units
$x = 2800$ units IV bolus

Infusion: *Step 1*
1 kg : 20 units :: 80 kg : x units
$x = 20(80) = 1600$ units/h

Step 2
100 units : 1 mL :: 1600 units : x mL
$100x = 1600$
$x = \dfrac{1600}{100}$
$x = 16$ mL/h

35. $\dfrac{100 \text{ mcg} \times 80 \text{ kg} \times 60 \text{min/h}}{10,000 \text{ mcg/mL}} = \dfrac{480,000}{10,000} = 48$ mL/h

Chapter 17 Critical Care IV Flow Rates—Posttest 1, pp. 391–394

Proportion

1. 500 units : 500 mL :: 9 units : x mL

$500x = 4500$

$x = \dfrac{4500}{500}$

$x = 9$ mL/h

2. 50,000 units : 500 mL :: 800 units : x mL

$50,000x = 400,000$

$x = \dfrac{400,000}{50,000}$

$x = 8$ mL/h

3. $\dfrac{5 \text{ mcg} \times 62 \text{ kg} \times 60 \text{ min/h}}{400 \text{ mcg/mL}} = \dfrac{18,600}{400} = 46.5$ mL/h

4. $\dfrac{5 \text{ mcg} \times 50 \text{ kg} \times 60 \text{ min/h}}{4000 \text{ mcg/mL}} = \dfrac{15,000}{4000} = 3.75$ or 3.8 mL/h

5. $\dfrac{20 \text{ mcg} \times 60 \text{ min/h}}{200 \text{ mcg/mL}} = \dfrac{1200}{200} = 6$ mL/h

6. $\dfrac{3 \text{ mg} \times 60 \text{ min/h}}{4 \text{ mg/mL}} = \dfrac{180}{4} = 45$ mL/h

7. $\dfrac{5 \text{ mcg} \times 60 \text{ min/h}}{4 \text{ mcg/mL}} = \dfrac{300}{4} = 75$ mL/h

8. $\dfrac{25 \text{ mcg} \times 50 \text{ kg} \times 60 \text{ min/h}}{10,000 \text{ mcg/mL}} = \dfrac{75,000}{10,000} = 7.5$ mL/h

9. 25,000 units : 250 mL :: 1050 units : x mL

$25,000x = 262,500$

$x = \dfrac{262,500}{25,000}$

$x = 10.5$ mL/h

10. $\dfrac{0.5 \text{ mg} \times 60 \text{ min/h}}{3.6 \text{ mg/mL}} = \dfrac{30}{3.6} = 8.3$ or 8 mL/h

11. $\dfrac{200 \text{ mcg/mL} \times 63 \text{ mL/h}}{60 \text{ min/h} \times 70 \text{ kg}} = \dfrac{12,600}{4200} = 3$ mcg/kg/min

12. $\dfrac{4 \text{ mg/mL} \times 45 \text{ mL/h}}{60 \text{ min/h}} = \dfrac{180}{60} = 3$ mg/min

13. $\dfrac{16 \text{ mcg/mL} \times 15 \text{ mL/h}}{60 \text{ min/h}} = \dfrac{240}{60} = 4$ mcg/min

Formula

1. $\dfrac{9 \text{ units}}{\overset{1}{\cancel{500} \text{ units}}} \times \overset{1}{\cancel{500}} \text{ mL} =$

$\dfrac{9}{1} = 9$ mL/h

2. $\dfrac{800 \text{ units}}{\underset{100}{\cancel{50,000} \text{ units}}} \times \overset{1}{\cancel{500}} \text{ mL} =$

$\dfrac{800}{100} = 8$ mL/h

9. $\dfrac{1050 \text{ units}}{\underset{100}{\cancel{25,000} \text{ units}}} \times \overset{1}{\cancel{250}} \text{ mL} =$

$\dfrac{1050}{100} = 10.5$ mL/h

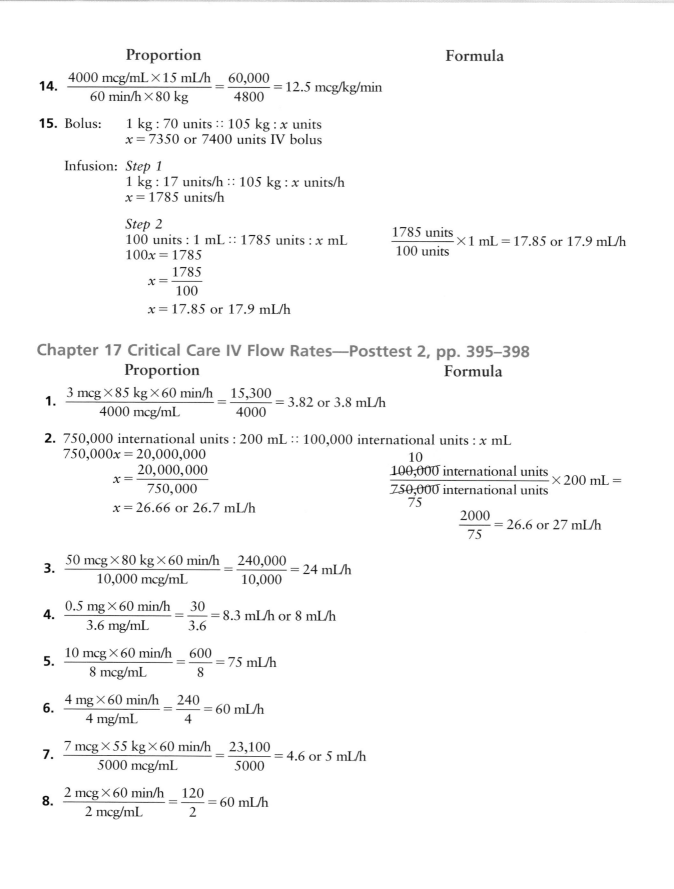

Proportion

Formula

14. $\dfrac{4000 \text{ mcg/mL} \times 15 \text{ mL/h}}{60 \text{ min/h} \times 80 \text{ kg}} = \dfrac{60{,}000}{4800} = 12.5 \text{ mcg/kg/min}$

15. Bolus: 1 kg : 70 units :: 105 kg : x units
           $x = 7350$ or 7400 units IV bolus

      Infusion: *Step 1*
           1 kg : 17 units/h :: 105 kg : x units/h
           $x = 1785$ units/h

           Step 2
           100 units : 1 mL :: 1785 units : x mL $\dfrac{1785 \text{ units}}{100 \text{ units}} \times 1 \text{ mL} = 17.85$ or 17.9 mL/h
           $100x = 1785$
              $x = \dfrac{1785}{100}$
              $x = 17.85$ or 17.9 mL/h

Chapter 17 Critical Care IV Flow Rates—Posttest 2, pp. 395–398
Proportion   Formula

1. $\dfrac{3 \text{ mcg} \times 85 \text{ kg} \times 60 \text{ min/h}}{4000 \text{ mcg/mL}} = \dfrac{15{,}300}{4000} = 3.82$ or 3.8 mL/h

2. 750,000 international units : 200 mL :: 100,000 international units : x mL
    $750{,}000x = 20{,}000{,}000$
        $x = \dfrac{20{,}000{,}000}{750{,}000}$ $\dfrac{\overset{10}{\cancel{100{,}000}} \text{ international units}}{\underset{75}{\cancel{750{,}000}} \text{ international units}} \times 200 \text{ mL} =$
        $x = 26.66$ or 26.7 mL/h $\dfrac{2000}{75} = 26.6$ or 27 mL/h

3. $\dfrac{50 \text{ mcg} \times 80 \text{ kg} \times 60 \text{ min/h}}{10{,}000 \text{ mcg/mL}} = \dfrac{240{,}000}{10{,}000} = 24 \text{ mL/h}$

4. $\dfrac{0.5 \text{ mg} \times 60 \text{ min/h}}{3.6 \text{ mg/mL}} = \dfrac{30}{3.6} = 8.3 \text{ mL/h}$ or 8 mL/h

5. $\dfrac{10 \text{ mcg} \times 60 \text{ min/h}}{8 \text{ mcg/mL}} = \dfrac{600}{8} = 75 \text{ mL/h}$

6. $\dfrac{4 \text{ mg} \times 60 \text{ min/h}}{4 \text{ mg/mL}} = \dfrac{240}{4} = 60 \text{ mL/h}$

7. $\dfrac{7 \text{ mcg} \times 55 \text{ kg} \times 60 \text{ min/h}}{5000 \text{ mcg/mL}} = \dfrac{23{,}100}{5000} = 4.6$ or 5 mL/h

8. $\dfrac{2 \text{ mcg} \times 60 \text{ min/h}}{2 \text{ mcg/mL}} = \dfrac{120}{2} = 60 \text{ mL/h}$

Proportion

9. 20,000 units : 200 mL :: 1500 units : x mL

$20{,}000x = 300{,}000$

$x = \dfrac{300{,}000}{20{,}000}$

$x = 15$ mL/h

10. 50 units : 100 mL :: 8 units : x mL

$50x = 800$

$x = \dfrac{800}{50}$

$x = 16$ mL/h

11. Bolus:　　1 kg : 70 units :: 75 kg : x units

$x = 5250$ or 5300 units IV bolus

Infusion: *Step 1*

1 kg : 17 units/h :: 75 kg : x units/h

$x = 1275$ units/h

Step 2

100 units : 1 mL :: 1275 units : x mL

$100x = 1275$

$x = \dfrac{1275}{100}$

$x = 12.75$ or 12.8 mL/h

12. $\dfrac{8 \text{ mcg/mL} \times 75 \text{ mL/h}}{60 \text{ min/h}} = \dfrac{600}{60} = 10$ mcg/min

13. $\dfrac{8 \text{ mg/mL} \times 30 \text{ mL/h}}{60 \text{ min/h}} = \dfrac{240}{60} = 4$ mg/min

14. $\dfrac{8000 \text{ mcg/mL} \times 3 \text{ mL/h}}{60 \text{ min/h} \times 80 \text{ kg}} = \dfrac{24{,}000}{4800} = 5$ mcg/kg/min

15. $\dfrac{200 \text{ mcg/mL} \times 50 \text{ mL/h}}{60 \text{ min/h} \times 60 \text{ kg}} = \dfrac{10{,}000}{3600} = 2.8$ mcg/kg/min

Formula

9. $\dfrac{1500 \text{ units}}{\cancel{20{,}000} \text{ units}} \times \overset{1}{\cancel{200}} \text{ mL} =$
${}_{100}$

$\dfrac{1500}{100} = 15$ mL/h

10. $\dfrac{8 \text{ units}}{\underset{1}{\cancel{50}} \text{ units}} \times \overset{2}{\cancel{100}} \text{ mL} =$

$\dfrac{16}{1} = 16$ mL/h

11. $\dfrac{1275 \text{ units}}{100 \text{ units}} \times 1 \text{ mL} = 12.75$ or 12.8 mL/h

Chapter 18 Pediatric Dosages—Work Sheet, pp. 415–420

Proportion

1. a.　2.2 lb : 1 kg :: 50 lb : x kg

$2.2x = 50$

$x = \dfrac{50}{2.2}$

$x = 22.7$ kg

Formula

1 kg = 2.2 lb

$\dfrac{50 \text{ lb}}{2.2 \text{ kg}} = 22.7$ kg

Proportion	Formula
b. 25 mg/24 h : 1 kg :: x mg/24 h : 22.7 kg	25 mg/kg/24 h $\times$ 22.7 kg = 567.5 mg/24 h
x = 567.5 mg/24 h	
50 mg/24 h : 1 kg :: x mg/24 h : 22.7 kg	50 mg/kg/24 h $\times$ 22.7 kg = 1135 mg/24 h
x = 1135 mg/24 h	
Safe dose range is 567.5 to 1135 mg/24 h.	
250 mg : 1 dose :: x mg : 4 doses	250 mg $\times$ 4 doses/24 h = 1000 mg/24 h
x = 1000 mg/24 h	

c. Yes, the order is safe to administer.

d. 250 mg : 1 cap :: 250 mg : x cap

$250x = 250$

$$x = \frac{250}{250}$$

$x = 1$ capsule

2. a. 2.2 lb : 1 kg :: 6.5 lb : x kg

$2.2x = 6.5$

$$x = \frac{6.5}{2.2}$$

$x = 2.95$ kg or 3 kg

b. 0.035 mg : 1 kg :: x mg : 3 kg

$x = 0.11$ mg/kg/day

0.06 mg : 1 kg :: x mg : 3 kg

$x = 0.18$ mg

The safe range is 0.11 to 0.18 mg/kg/day.

c. No, the order is not safe.

d. Question this order.

3. a. 2.2 lb : 1 kg :: 50 lb : x kg

$2.2x = 50$

$$x = \frac{50}{2.2}$$

$x = 22.7$ kg

b. 5 mg/24 h : 1 kg :: x mg/24 h : 22.7 kg

$x = 113.65$ mg/kg/24 h divided by four doses

c. $\dfrac{113.5 \text{ mg/kg/24 h}}{4 \text{ doses/24 h}} = 28.4$ mg/dose

Safe and therapeutic dose is 28.4 mg/dose, so the 25 mg ordered dose is safe.

d. 12.5 mg : 1 mL :: 25 mg : x mL

$12.5x = 25$

$$x = \frac{25}{12.5}$$

$x = 2$ mL

Proportion

4. a. 2.2 lb : 1 kg :: 28 lb : x kg

$2.2x = 28$

$$x = \frac{28}{2.2}$$

$x = 12.7$ kg

First 0–10 kg = 100 mL/kg/24 h
10 mL/24 h × 10 kg = 1000 mL/24 h
12.7 kg − 10 kg = 2.7 kg

Remaining 2.7 kg × 50 mL/kg = 135 mL/24 h
1000 + 135 = 1135 mL/24 h

b. $\dfrac{1135 \text{ mL/24 h}}{24 \text{ h}} = 47.3$ mL/h

5. a. 2.2 lb : 1 kg :: 22 lb : x kg

$2.2x = 22$

$$x = \frac{22}{2.2}$$

$x = 10$ kg

b. 70 mg : 1 dose :: x mg : 2 doses

$x = 140$ mg/24 h

$$\frac{140 \text{ mg/24 h}}{10 \text{ kg}} = 14 \text{ mg/kg/24 h}$$

Child is receiving the recommended dose.

c. 125 mg : 5 mL :: 70 mg : x mL

$125x = 350$

$$x = \frac{350}{125}$$

$x = 2.8$ mL

6. a. 30.3 kg

b. 20 mg/24 h : 1 kg :: x mg/24 h : 30.3 kg
$x = 606$ mg/24 h

30 mg/24 h : 1 kg :: x mg/24 h : 30.3 kg
$x = 909$ mg/24 h

c. $\dfrac{606 \text{ mg/24 h}}{2 \text{ doses/24 h}} = 303$ mg/dose

$\dfrac{909 \text{ mg/24 h}}{2 \text{ doses/24 h}} = 454.5$ mg/dose

303 to 454.5 mg/dose (single dose)
Yes, it is safe.

Proportion

d. 250 mg : 5 mL :: 300 mg : x mL
$$250x = 1500$$
$$x = \frac{1500}{250}$$
$$x = 6 \text{ mL}$$

7. a. 2.2 lb : 1 kg :: 94 lb : x kg
$$2.2x = 94$$
$$x = \frac{94}{2.2}$$
$$x = 42.7 \text{ kg}$$

b. 42.7 kg $\times$ 0.5 mg/kg/24 h = 21.4 mg/24 h
42.7 kg $\times$ 2 mg/kg/24 h = 85.4 mg/24 h
NOTE: 80 mg/24 h is the max dose.

c. No, the child would be receiving 90 mg/24 h.

d. No, call the physician who wrote the order.

8. a. 2.2 lb : 1 kg :: 40 lb : x kg
$$2.2x = 40$$
$$x = \frac{40}{2.2}$$
$$x = 18.2 \text{ kg}$$

b. 18.2 kg $\times$ 5 mg/kg/24 h = 91 mg/24 h
18.2 kg $\times$ 7 mg/kg/24 h = 127.4 mg/24 h

c. No, the order exceeds the recommended dose.

d. 30 mg : 1 tab :: 60 mg : x tab
$$30x = 60$$
$$x = \frac{60}{30}$$
$$x = 2 \text{ chewtabs}$$

9. a. 2.2 lb : 1 kg :: 68 lb : x kg
$$2.2x = 68$$
$$x = \frac{68}{2.2}$$
$$x = 30.9 \text{ kg}$$

b. $$\frac{750 \text{ mg} \times 4 \text{ doses/24 h}}{30.9 \text{ kg}} =$$
$$\frac{3000}{30.9} = 97.1 \text{ mg/kg/24 h}$$

c. No, it exceeds the recommended 40 to 60 mg/kg/24 h.

Proportion

10. a. 2.2 lb : 1 kg :: 42 lb : x kg

$2.2x = 42$

$x = \dfrac{42}{2.2}$

$x = 19.1$ kg

b. $\dfrac{19.1 \text{ kg} \times 25 \text{ mg/kg/24 h}}{2 \text{ doses/24 h}} = \dfrac{477.5}{2} = 238.8$ mg/dose

$\dfrac{19.1 \text{ kg} \times 50 \text{ mg/kg/24 h}}{2 \text{ doses/24 h}} = \dfrac{955}{2} = 477.5$ mg/dose

Single dose range is 238.8 to 477.5 mg/dose.

c. 125 mg : 5 mL :: 300 mg : x mL

$125x = 1500$

$x = \dfrac{1500}{125}$

$x = 12$ mL

11. a. $\dfrac{100 \text{ mL}}{30 \text{ min}} \times 60 \text{ gtt/mL} = 200$ gtt/min

12. a. 2.2 kg : 1 lb :: 58 lb : x kg

$2.2x = 58$

$x = \dfrac{58}{2.2}$

$x = 26.4$ kg

b. $\dfrac{26.4 \text{ kg} \times 10 \text{ mg/kg/24 h}}{3 \text{ doses/24 h}} = \dfrac{264}{3} = 88$ mg/dose

$\dfrac{26.4 \text{ kg} \times 20 \text{ mg/kg/24 h}}{3 \text{ doses/24 h}} = \dfrac{528}{3} = 176$ mg/dose

Single dose range is 88 to 176 mg/dose.

c. Yes, the dose is safe to administer.

d. 100 mg : 5 mL :: 150 mg : x mL

$100x = 750$

$x = \dfrac{750}{100}$

$x = 7.5$ mL

13. a. 2.2 lb : 1 kg :: 72 lb : x kg

$2.2x = 72$

$x = \dfrac{72}{2.2}$

$x = 32.7$ kg

Proportion

b. First 20 kg

Next $12.7 \text{ kg} \times 20 \text{ mL}$

$$
\begin{array}{r}
1500 \text{ mL/24 h} \\
+ 254 \text{ mL/24 h} \\
\hline
1754 \text{ mL/24 h}
\end{array}
$$

c. $\dfrac{1754 \text{ mL/24 h}}{24 \text{ h}} = 73.1 \text{ mL/h}$

14. a. $2.2 \text{ lb} : 1 \text{ kg} :: 52 \text{ lb} : x \text{ kg}$

$2.2x = 52$

$x = \dfrac{52}{2.2}$

$x = 23.6 \text{ kg}$

b. $23.6 \text{ kg} \times 5 \text{ mg/kg/dose} = 118 \text{ mg/dose}$

$23.6 \text{ kg} \times 10 \text{ mg/kg/dose} = 236 \text{ mg/dose}$

c. $100 \text{ mg} : 5 \text{ mL} :: 100 \text{ mg} : x \text{ mL}$

$100x = 500$

$x = \dfrac{500}{100}$

$x = 5 \text{ mL}$

15. a. $2.2 \text{ lb} : 1 \text{ kg} :: 81 \text{ lb} : x \text{ kg}$

$2.2x = 81$

$x = \dfrac{81}{2.2}$

$x = 36.8 \text{ kg}$

b. $\dfrac{36.8 \text{ kg} \times 25 \text{ mg/kg/24 h}}{4 \text{ doses/24 h}} = \dfrac{920}{4} = 230 \text{ mg/dose}$

$\dfrac{36.8 \text{ kg} \times 50 \text{ mg/kg/24 h}}{4 \text{ doses/24 h}} = \dfrac{1840}{4} = 460 \text{ mg/dose}$

Single dose range is 230 to 460 mg/dose.

c. Yes, 350 mg/dose is safe to administer.

d. $500 \text{ mg} : 5 \text{ mL} :: 350 \text{ mg} : x \text{ mL}$

$500x = 1750$

$x = \dfrac{1750}{500}$

$x = 3.5 \text{ mL}$

16. a. $2.2 \text{ lb} : 1 \text{ kg} :: 16 \text{ lb} : x \text{ kg}$

$2.2x = 16$

$x = \dfrac{16}{2.2}$

$x = 7.3 \text{ kg}$

Proportion

b. $\dfrac{7.3 \text{ kg} \times 15 \text{ mg/kg/24 h}}{3 \text{ doses/24 h}} = \dfrac{109.5}{3} = 36.5 \text{ mg/dose}$

$\dfrac{7.3 \text{ kg} \times 20 \text{ mg/kg/24 h}}{3 \text{ doses/24 h}} = \dfrac{146}{3} = 48.7 \text{ mg/dose}$

c. No, the order of 60 mg q8 h exceeds the safe range.

d. $\dfrac{60 \text{ mg} \times 3 \text{ doses/24 h}}{7.3 \text{ kg}} = 24.7 \text{ mg/kg/24 h}$

   Proof that the ordered dose exceeds the recommended 15 to 20 mg/kg/24 h

e. This is not safe, do not administer—call the physician or pharmacist to check.

17. a. $2.2 \text{ lb} : 1 \text{ kg} :: 19 \text{ lb} : x \text{ kg}$
   $2.2x = 19$
   $x = \dfrac{19}{2.2}$
   $x = 8.6 \text{ kg}$

b. $8.6 \text{ kg} \times 0.5 \text{ mg/kg/24 h} = 4.3 \text{ mg/24 h}$
   $8.6 \text{ kg} \times 2 \text{ mg/kg/24 h} = 17.2 \text{ mg/24 h}$

c. Yes, it is safe to administer.

d. $5 \text{ mg} : 5 \text{ mL} :: 8 \text{ mg} : x \text{ mL}$
   $5x = 40$
   $x = \dfrac{40}{5}$
   $x = 8 \text{ mL}$

18. a. $2.2 \text{ lb} : 1 \text{ kg} :: 32 \text{ lb} : x \text{ kg}$
   $2.2x = 32$
   $x = \dfrac{32}{2.2}$
   $x = 14.6 \text{ kg}$

b. $14.6 \text{ kg} \times 100 \text{ mg/kg/24 h} = 1460 \text{ mg/24 h}$
   The child may receive up to 1460 mg/24 h.

c. $400 \text{ mg} : 1 \text{ dose} :: x \text{ mg} : 3 \text{ doses}$
   $x = 1200 \text{ mg/24 h}$
   Yes, this order is safe.

d. $330 \text{ mg} : 1 \text{ mL} :: 400 \text{ mg} : x \text{ mL}$
   $330x = 400$
   $x = \dfrac{400}{330}$
   $x = 1.2 \text{ mL}$

19. $\dfrac{250 \text{ mL}}{3 \text{ h}} = 83.3 \text{ mL/h}$

Proportion

20. a. $10 \text{ mg} : 1 \text{ mL} :: 40 \text{ mg} : x \text{ mL}$

    $10x = 40$

    $x = \dfrac{40}{10}$

    $x = 4 \text{ mL}$

  b. $40 \text{ mL} \times \frac{1}{2} = 20 \text{ mL} \rightarrow 20 \text{ mL} - 4 \text{ mL} = 16 \text{ mL}$

  c. $\dfrac{20 \text{ mL}}{20 \text{ min}} \times 60 \text{ gtt/mL} = 60 \text{ gtt/min}$

Chapter 18, Pediatric Dosages—Posttest 1, pp. 421–424

1. a. $2.2 \text{ lb} : 1 \text{ kg} :: 55 \text{ lb} : x \text{ kg}$

    $2.2x = 55$

    $x = \dfrac{55}{2.2}$

    $x = 25 \text{ kg}$

  b. $\dfrac{25 \text{ kg} \times 4 \text{ mg/kg/24 h}}{2 \text{ doses/24 h}} = \dfrac{100}{2} = 50 \text{ mg/dose}$

    $\dfrac{25 \text{ kg} \times 6 \text{ mg/kg/24 h}}{2 \text{ doses/24 h}} = \dfrac{150}{2} = 75 \text{ mg/dose}$

    Single dose range is 50 to 75 mg/dose.

  c. Yes, 60 mg is ordered, and it falls within the 50 to 75 mg/dose range.

  d. $20 \text{ mg} : 5 \text{ mL} :: 60 \text{ mg} : x \text{ mL}$

    $20x = 300$

    $x = \dfrac{300}{20}$

    $x = 15 \text{ mL}$

2. a. $2.2 \text{ lb} : 1 \text{ kg} :: 44 \text{ lb} : x \text{ kg}$

    $2.2x = 44$

    $x = \dfrac{44}{2.2}$

    $x = 20 \text{ kg}$

  b. $\dfrac{20 \text{ kg} \times 25 \text{ mg/kg/24 h}}{4 \text{ doses/24 h}} = \dfrac{500}{4} = 125 \text{ mg/dose}$

    $\dfrac{20 \text{ kg} \times 50 \text{ mg/kg/24 h}}{4 \text{ doses/24 h}} = \dfrac{1000}{4} = 250 \text{ mg/dose}$

    Single dose range is 125 to 250 mg/dose.

  c. No, 500 mg q6 h exceeds the recommended dosage for weight.

  d. Question this order.

3. a. 2.2 lb : 1 kg :: 34 lb : x kg

$2.2x = 34$

$$x = \frac{34}{2.2}$$

$x = 15.5$

b. $\dfrac{300 \text{ mg} \times 3 \text{ doses/24 h}}{15.5 \text{ kg}} = \dfrac{900}{15.5} = 58.1 \text{ mg/kg/24 h}$

c. Dosage is safe and therapeutic; it falls in the recommended range.

125 mg : 5 mL :: 300 mg : x mL

$125x = 1500$

$$x = \frac{1500}{125}$$

$x = 12$ mL

4. a. 2.2 lb : 1 kg :: 78 lb : x kg

$2.2x = 78$

$$x = \frac{78}{2.2}$$

$x = 35.5$ kg

b. 35.5 kg $\times$ 0.1 mg/kg/dose = 3.55 mg/dose

35.5 kg $\times$ 0.2 mg/kg/dose = 7.1 mg/dose

c. Yes, it falls between 3.55 and 7.1 mg/dose.

d. 15 mg : 1 mL :: 4 mg : x mL

$15x = 4$

$$x = \frac{4}{15}$$

$x = 0.266$ or 0.27 mL

5. a. 2.2 lb : 1 kg :: 62 lb : x kg

$2.2x = 62$

$$x = \frac{62}{2.2}$$

$x = 28.2$ kg

b. 28.2 kg $\times$ 10 mg/kg/dose = 282 mg/dose

28.2 kg $\times$ 15 mg/kg/dose = 423 mg/dose

Single dose range is 282 to 423 mg/dose.

c. 160 mg : 5 mL :: 282 mg : x mL

$160x = 1410$

$$x = \frac{1410}{160}$$

$x = 8.8$ mL

160 mg : 5 mL :: 423 mg : x mL

$160x = 2115$

$$x = \frac{2115}{160}$$

$x = 13.2$ mL

6. $\dfrac{1000 \text{ mL}}{16 \text{ h}} = 62.5 \text{ mL/h}$

7. a. 2.2 lb : 1 kg :: 92 lb : x kg
$2.2x = 92$ lb
$x = \dfrac{92}{2.2}$
$x = 41.8$ kg

b. $\dfrac{41.8 \text{ kg} \times 15 \text{ mg/kg/24 h}}{2 \text{ doses/24 h}} = \dfrac{627}{2} = 313.5 \text{ mg/dose}$

c. Yes, 300 mg is a safe dose to administer.

d. 125 mg : 5 mL :: 300 mg : x mL
$125x = 1500$ mL
$x = \dfrac{1500}{125}$
$x = 12$ mL

8. a. 2.2 lb : 1 kg :: 25 lb : x kg
$2.2x = 25$
$x = \dfrac{25}{2.2}$
$x = 11.4$ kg

b. First 10 kg   1000 mL/24 h
Next 1.4 kg × 50 mL/kg =   + 70 mL/24 h
                              1070 mL/24 h

c. $\dfrac{1070 \text{ mL/24 h}}{24 \text{ h}} = 44.6 \text{ mL/h}$

9. a. 2.2 lb : 1 kg :: 96 lb : x kg
$2.2x = 96$
$x = \dfrac{96}{2.2}$
$x = 43.6$ kg

b. $\dfrac{650 \text{ mg} \times 4 \text{ doses/24 h}}{43.6 \text{ kg}} = \dfrac{2600}{43.6} = 59.6 \text{ mg/kg/24 h}$

c. Yes, it is safe; recommended is 40 to 60 mg/kg/24 h. Child is receiving 59.6 mg/kg/24 h.

10. a. 2.2 lb : 1 kg :: 95 lb : x kg
$2.2x = 95$
$x = \dfrac{95}{2.2}$
$x = 43.2$ kg

b. $\dfrac{300 \text{ mg} \times 3 \text{ doses/24 h}}{43.2 \text{ kg}} = \dfrac{900}{43.2} = 20.8 \text{ mg/kg/24 h}$

c. The child is receiving 20.8 mg/kg/24 h; recommended is 20 to 40 mg/kg/24 h. The ordered dose is both safe and therapeutic.

11. $\dfrac{100\ \text{mL}}{6\ \text{h}} = 16.7\ \text{mL/h}$

12. a. $250\ \text{mg} : 1\ \text{mL} :: 400\ \text{mg} : x\ \text{mL}$

$250x = 400$

$x = \dfrac{400}{250}$

$x = 1.6\ \text{mL}$

    b. $400\ \text{mg} \times \dfrac{1\ \text{mg}}{50\ \text{mL}} = 8\ \text{mL} \rightarrow 8\ \text{mL} - 1.6\ \text{mL} = 6.4\ \text{mL}$

    c. $\dfrac{8\ \text{mL}}{30\ \text{min}} \times 60\ \text{gtt/mL} = x\ \text{gtt/min}$

$x = \dfrac{480}{30}$

$x = 16\ \text{gtt/min}$

13. a. $\dfrac{60\ \text{mg} \times 2\ \text{doses/24 h}}{30\ \text{kg}} = \dfrac{120}{30} = 4\ \text{mg/kg/24 h}$

    b. No, the ordered dosage is more than the recommended of 0.5 to 2 mg/kg/24 h. Also, the maximum dose is 80 mg/24 h, and this is exceeded as well.

    c. No, check with the physician.

14. a. $2.2\ \text{lb} : 1\ \text{kg} :: 89\ \text{lb} : x\ \text{kg}$

$2.2x = 89$

$x = \dfrac{89}{2.2}$

$x = 40.5\ \text{kg}$

    b. $\dfrac{40.5\ \text{kg} \times 15\ \text{mg/kg/24 h}}{2\ \text{doses/24 h}} = \dfrac{607.5}{2} = 303.8\ \text{mg/dose}$

$\dfrac{40.5\ \text{kg} \times 20\ \text{mg/kg/24 h}}{2\ \text{doses/24 h}} = \dfrac{810}{2} = 405\ \text{mg/dose}$

Dosage range is 607.5 to 810 mg/24 h.
Single dose range is 303.8 to 405 mg/dose.

    c. Yes, 400 mg/dose is within the recommended single dose range.

    d. $375\ \text{mg} : 5\ \text{mL} :: 400\ \text{mg} : x\ \text{mL}$

$375x = 2000$

$x = \dfrac{2000}{375}$

$x = 5.3\ \text{mL}$

15. a. $2.2\ \text{lb} : 1\ \text{kg} :: 11\ \text{lb} : x\ \text{kg}$

$2.2x = 11$

$x = \dfrac{11}{2.2}$

$x = 5\ \text{kg}$

b. $\dfrac{90\ \text{mg} \times 4\ \text{doses/24 h}}{5\ \text{kg}} = \dfrac{360}{5} = 72\ \text{mg/kg/24 h}$

c. The order is both safe and therapeutic, between the recommended 50 and 100 mg/kg/24 h.

Chapter 18, Pediatric Dosages—Posttest 2, pp. 425–429

1. a. 2.2 lb : 1 kg :: 70 lb : x kg

$2.2x = 70$

$x = \dfrac{70}{2.2}$

$x = 31.8$ kg

b. $\dfrac{450\ \text{mg} \times 4\ \text{doses/24 h}}{31.8\ \text{kg}} = \dfrac{1800}{31.8} = 56.6\ \text{mg/kg/24 h}$

c. Yes, the child is receiving 56.6 mg/kg/24 h, which is between 40 and 60 mg/kg/24 h.

2. a. 2.2 lb : 1 kg :: 62 lb : x kg

$2.2x = 62$

$x = \dfrac{62}{2.2}$

$x = 28.2$ kg

b. 28.2 kg $\times$ 7 mg/kg/24 h = 197.4 mg/24 h
28.2 kg $\times$ 8 mg/kg/24 h = 225.6 mg/24 h
Dosage range is 197.4 to 225.6 mg/24 h.

c. $\dfrac{197.4\ \text{mg/24 h}}{2\ \text{doses/24 h}} = 98.7\ \text{mg/dose}$

$\dfrac{225.6\ \text{mg/24 h}}{2\ \text{doses/24 h}} = 112.8\ \text{mg/dose}$

Single dose range is 98.7 to 112.8 mg/dose.

d. Yes, the ordered dose is both safe and therapeutic because it falls within the recommended 24-hour dosage and single dose ranges.

e. 125 mg : 5 mL :: 100 mg : x mL

$125x = 500$

$x = \dfrac{500}{125}$

$x = 4$ mL

3. a. 2.2 lb : 1 kg :: 58 lb : x kg

$2.2x = 58$

$x = \dfrac{58}{2.2}$

$x = 26.4$ kg

b. 26.4 kg $\times$ 25 mg/kg/24 h = 660 mg/24 h
26.4 kg $\times$ 50 mg/kg/24 h = 1320 mg/24 h
Dosage range is 660 to 1320 mg/24 h.

c. $\dfrac{660 \text{ mg/24 h}}{2 \text{ doses/24 h}} = 330 \text{ mg/dose}$

$\dfrac{1320 \text{ mg/24 h}}{2 \text{ doses/24 h}} = 660 \text{ mg/dose}$

Single dose range is 330 to 660 mg/dose.

d. $\dfrac{400 \text{ mg} \times 2 \text{ doses/24 h}}{26.4 \text{ kg}} = \dfrac{800}{26.4} = 30.3 \text{ mg/kg/24 h}$

e. $250 \text{ mg} : 5 \text{ mL} :: 400 \text{ mg} : x \text{ mL}$
$250x = 2000$
$x = \dfrac{2000}{250}$
$x = 8 \text{ mL}$

4. a. $2.2 \text{ lb} : 1 \text{ kg} :: 99 \text{ lb} : x \text{ kg}$
$2.2x = 99$
$x = \dfrac{99}{2.2}$
$x = 45 \text{ kg}$

b. $\dfrac{500 \text{ mg} \times 4 \text{ doses/24 h}}{45 \text{ kg}} = \dfrac{2000}{45} = 44.4 \text{ mg/kg/24 h}$

c. Yes, the recommended is 50 to 100 mg/kg/24 h.

d. $250 \text{ mg} : 1 \text{ cap} :: 500 \text{ mg} : x \text{ cap}$
$250x = 500$
$x = \dfrac{500}{250}$
$x = 2 \text{ capsules}$

5. a. $2.2 \text{ lb} : 1 \text{ kg} :: 66 \text{ lb} : x \text{ kg}$
$2.2x = 66 \text{ lb}$
$x = \dfrac{66}{2.2}$
$x = 30 \text{ kg}$

b. $\dfrac{200 \text{ mg} \times 2 \text{ doses/24 h}}{30 \text{ kg}} = \dfrac{400}{30} = 13.3 \text{ mg/kg/24 h}$

c. Yes, the order is safe to administer.

d. $125 \text{ mg} : 5 \text{ mL} :: 200 \text{ mg} : x \text{ mL}$
$125x = 1000$
$x = \dfrac{1000}{125}$
$x = 8 \text{ mL}$

6. a. $1000 \text{ g} : 1 \text{ kg} :: 2012 \text{ g} : x \text{ kg}$
$1000x = 2012$
$x = \dfrac{2012}{1000}$
$x = 2.0$

b. $2 \text{ kg} \times 100 \text{ mg/kg/24 h} = 200 \text{ mg/24 h}$
$2 \text{ kg} \times 200 \text{ mg/kg/24 h} = 400 \text{ mg/24 h}$
Dosage range is 200 to 400 mg/24 h.

c. $\dfrac{200 \text{ mg/24 h}}{4 \text{ doses/24 h}} = 50 \text{ mg/dose}$

$\dfrac{400 \text{ mg/24 h}}{4 \text{ doses/24 h}} = 100 \text{ mg/dose}$

Single dose range is 50 to 100 mg/dose.

7. a. $2.2 \text{ lb} : 1 \text{ kg} :: 35 \text{ lb} : x \text{ kg}$
$2.2x = 35$
$x = \dfrac{35}{2.2}$
$x = 15.9 \text{ kg}$

b. $\dfrac{180 \text{ mg} \times 3 \text{ doses/24 h}}{15.9 \text{ kg}} = \dfrac{540}{15.9} = 33.96 \text{ mg/kg/24 h}$

c. Yes, the ordered dose is within the safe and therapeutic range.

d. $125 \text{ mg} : 5 \text{ mL} :: 180 \text{ mg} : x \text{ mL}$
$125x = 900$
$x = \dfrac{900}{125}$
$x = 7.2 \text{ mL}$

8. $\dfrac{150 \text{ mL}}{180 \text{ min}} \times 60 \text{ gtt/mL} = 50 \text{ gtt/min}$

9. a. $2.2 \text{ lb} : 1 \text{ kg} :: 74 \text{ lb} : x \text{ kg}$
$2.2x = 74$
$x = \dfrac{74}{2.2}$
$x = 33.6 \text{ kg}$

b. $\dfrac{330 \text{ mg} \times 4 \text{ doses/24 h}}{33.6 \text{ kg}} = \dfrac{1320}{33.6} = 39.29 \text{ mg/kg/24 h}$

c. Yes, the dose ordered is safe to administer.

d. $250 \text{ mg} : 5 \text{ mL} :: 330 \text{ mg} : x \text{ mL}$
$250x = 1650$
$x = \dfrac{1650}{250}$
$x = 6.6 \text{ mL}$

10. a. $2.2 \text{ lb} : 1 \text{ kg} :: 20 \text{ lb} : x \text{ kg}$
$2.2x = 20$
$x = \dfrac{20}{2.2}$
$x = 9.1 \text{ kg}$

b. 9.1 kg × 0.1 mg/kg/dose = 0.91 mg/dose
    9.1 kg × 0.2 mg/kg/dose = 1.82 mg/dose
    Safe dose range is 0.91 to 1.82 mg/dose (nearest hundredth with narcotics).

c. Yes, 0.9 mg is within the safe range to administer.

d. 0.5 mg : 1 mL :: 0.9 mg : x mL
    $0.5x = 0.9$
    $$x = \frac{0.9}{0.5}$$
    $x = 1.8$ mL

11. $\dfrac{200 \text{ mL}}{6 \text{ h}} = 66.7$ mL/h

12. a. 50 mg : 1 mL :: 500 mg : x mL
    $50x = 500$
    $$x = \frac{500}{50}$$
    $x = 10$ mL

b. 500 mg × $\dfrac{1 \text{ mg}}{5 \text{ mL}} = 100$ mL → 100 mL − 10 mL = 90 mL

c. Drop factor = 60 gtts/mL = microgtt

$$\frac{100 \text{ mL}}{60 \text{ min}} \times 60 \text{ mL/min} = x \text{ gtt/min}$$

$$\frac{6000}{60} = 100 \text{ gtt/min}$$

13. a. 1000 g : 1 kg :: 3036 g : x kg
    $1000x = 3036$
    $$x = \frac{3036}{1000}$$
    $x = 3.0$ kg or 3 kg

b. 3 kg × 6 mcg/kg/24 h = 18 mcg/24 h
    3 kg × 10 mcg/kg/24 h = 30 mcg/24 h
    Dosage range is 18 to 30 mcg/24 h.

c. $\dfrac{18 \text{ mcg/24 h}}{2 \text{ doses/24 h}} = 9$ mcg/dose

$$\frac{30 \text{ mcg/24 h}}{2 \text{ doses/24 h}} = 15 \text{ mcg/dose}$$

Single dose is 9 to 15 mcg/dose.
9 mcg = 0.009 mg
15 mcg = 0.015 mg

d. Yes, the ordered dose, 0.013 mg, is between 0.009 mg and 0.015 mg.

e. 50 mcg = 0.05 mg
   0.05 mg : 1 mL :: 0.013 mg : x mL
   $0.05x = 0.013$

   $$x = \frac{0.013}{0.05}$$

   $x = 0.26$ mL (a drug that is measured to the nearest hundredth)

14. a. 2.2 lb : 1 kg :: 9 lb : x kg
   $2.2x = 9$

   $$x = \frac{9}{2.2}$$

   $x = 4.1$ kg

   b. 4.1 kg × 10 mg/kg/dose = 41 mg/dose
   4.1 kg × 15 mg/kg/dose = 61.5 mg/dose
   Single dose range is 41 to 61.5 mg/dose.

   c. 80 mg : 0.8 mL :: 41 mg : x mL
   $80x = 32.8$

   $$x = \frac{32.8}{80}$$

   $x = 0.4$ mL
   80 mg : 0.8 mL :: 61.5 mg : x mL
   $80x = 49.2$

   $$x = \frac{49.2}{80}$$

   $x = 0.6$ mL
   Single dose range is 0.4 to 0.6 mL/dose.

15. a. 2.2 lb : 1 kg :: 37 lb : x kg
   $2.2x = 37$

   $$x = \frac{37}{2.2}$$

   $x = 16.8$ kg

   b. 16.8 kg × 4 mg/kg/24 h = 67.2 mg/24 h
   16.8 kg × 6 mg/kg/24 h = 100.8 mg/24 h
   Dosage range is 67.2 to 100.8 mg/24 h.

   c. Yes, 72 mg/24 h is within the recommended dosage range.

   d. 20 mg : 5 mL :: 72 mg : x mL
   $20x = 360$

   $$x = \frac{360}{20}$$

   $x = 18$ mL

Comprehensive Posttest, pp. 449–468

Case 1, pp. 449–452

1. 2 tablets
2. a. Digoxin 0.25 mg
  b. EC ASA gr v
  c. Cimetidine 300 mg
  d. Slow-K 10 mEq
3. 400 mL of $D_5\frac{1}{2}$ NS per shift
4.

2/3	Percocet								
	2 dose	p.o. route	q.4 h. interval	prn pain				
2/3	Tylenol								
	gr x dose	p.o. route	q.4 h. interval	prn pain or Temp >38° C				
2/3	MOM								
	30 mL dose	p.o. route	daily interval	prn constipation				
2/3	Mylanta								
	30 mL dose	p.o. route	q.4 h. interval	prn indigestion				
2/3	Restoril								
	15 mg dose	p.o. route	at bedtime interval	prn insomnia				

5.

2/3	Digoxin							
	0.25 mg dose	p.o. route	daily interval	09			
2/3	E.C. ASA							
	gr V dose	p.o. route	daily interval	09			
2/3	Cimetidine							
	300 mg dose	p.o. route	Three times daily interval	09	13	17	
2/3	Lasix							
	20 mg dose	I.V. route	q.8 h. interval	08		16	24
2/3	Slow-K							
	10 mEq dose	p.o. route	twice daily interval	09		17	

6. Restoril 15 mg po
7. 100 gtt/min
8. Milk of magnesia 30 mL
9. Lasix 20 mg

Case 2, pp. 453–455

1. Synthroid 0.15 mg
  Tagamet 300 mg
2. 1 mL
3. 600 mL/shift
  1800 mL/day
4. ½ tablet
5. a. Demerol
  b. Tylenol
6. 0.5 mL
7. 2 tablets

8.

2/3	Synthroid											
╱	0.15 mg dose	p.o. route	daily interval									
2/3	Tagamet											
╱	300 mg dose	p.o. route	daily interval									

Case 3, pp. 456–457

1. FeSO$_4$ 0.3 g
2. 300 mL
3. ½ tablet
4.

4/27	Perocet											
╱	600 mg dose	p.o. route	q.6 h. interval	prn pain								
4/27	Tucks											
╱	one dose	Peri route	interval	prn @ bedside								
4/27	Senokot											
╱	one dose	p.o. route	daily interval									
4/27	Tylenol											
╱	650 mg dose	p.o. route	q.4 h. interval	prn pain								

Case 4, pp. 458–460

1.

10/13	Allopurinol											
╱	50 mg dose	p.o. route	3 times daily interval									
10/13	Theophylline											
╱	16 mg dose	p.o. route	q.6 h. interval									
10/13	Prednisone											
╱	2 mg/kg dose	p.o. route	daily interval									
10/13	Vincristine											
╱	5.0 mg/m^2 dose	I.V. route	× 1 now interval									
10/13	MVI											
╱	1 dose	p.o. route	daily interval									

2.

10/13	Compazine							
╱	0.07 mg/kg dose	IM route	daily interval	prn nausea				
10/13	Tylenol							
╱	120 mg dose	p.o. route	3 times daily interval	prn pain				

3. 1.42 mL
4. 0.5 mL
5. 12.73 kg
   2.5 mL
6. 50 gtt/min
7. 0.9 mL

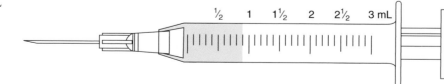

8. 200 mL
9. 0.66 mL

Case 5, pp. 461–463

1.

6/15	Heparin				
	5000 U (dose)	subcutaneous (route)	twice daily (interval)	09	21

6/15	Cefuroxime					
	1 g (dose)	IVPB (route)	q.8 h. (interval)	08	16	24

2.

6/15	Torecan			
	10 mg (dose)	IM (route)	q.4 h. (interval)	prn nausea

6/15	Mylanta			
	30 mL (dose)	p.o. (route)	(interval)	prn indigestion

6/15	Dulcolax Supp.			
	1 (dose)	pr (route)	q.shift (interval)	prn

6/15	Restoril			
	15 mg (dose)	p.o. (route)	at bedtime (interval)	prn insomnia

6/15	Tylenol #3			
	2 (dose)	p.o. (route)	q.4 h. (interval)	prn pain

6/15	Morphine			
	10 mg (dose)	IV (route)	q.10 min (interval)	250 mg/4 h. lockout

3. 1 mL

4. 1 mL/10 min

5. 1.0 mL

6. 400 mL/shift
1200 mL/day

7. 200 mL/h
3.33 mL/min
200 gtt/min

Case 6, pp. 464–466

1.

3/4	ASA			
	325 mg (dose)	oral (route)	daily (interval)	09

3/4	Plavix			
	75 mg (dose)	oral (route)	daily (interval)	09

3/4	Metoprolol				
	12.5 mg (dose)	oral (route)	2 times daily (interval)	09	21

2.

3/4	Tylenol			
	gr 10 (dose)	oral (route)	q.4 h. prn (interval)	

3/4	Ambien			
	5 mg (dose)	oral (route)	at bedtime prn sleep (interval)	

3. 3 mL/h

4. a. 5900 units
   b. 5.9 mL
   c. 14.3 mL/h
5. ½ tablet
6. 2 tablets

Case 7, pp. 467–468
1. 2.2 lb : 1 kg :: 7.5 lb : x kg
   $2.2x = 7.5$

   $x = \dfrac{7.5}{2.2}$

   $x = 3.4$ kg

   a. $\dfrac{160 \text{ mg} \times 3 \text{ doses/24 h}}{3.4 \text{ kg}} = 141.2$ mg/kg/24 h

   b. Yes, the neonate is receiving a dose that is within the recommended dosage range of 100 to 200 mg/kg/24 h.

   c. 250 mg : 1 mL :: 160 mg : x mL
   $250x = 160$

   $x = \dfrac{160}{250}$

   $x = 0.6$ mL

2. 80 mg : 0.8 mL :: 40 mg : x mL
   $80x = 32$

   $x = \dfrac{32}{80}$

   $x = 0.4$ mL

3. 12 mL/h $\times$ 6 h = 72 mL

Index

Page numbers followed by *f*, *b*, or *t* refer to
figures, boxes, or tables, respectively.